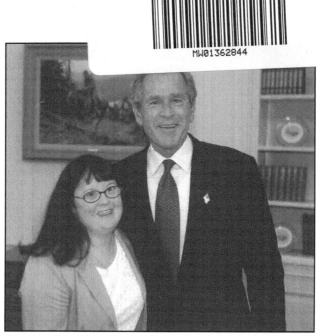

Windy with President Bush in Oval Office ~ 2006

* * *

This book contains many lessons for everyone—the abled and the disabled. Windy Smith, our heroine, was born with Down syndrome, but that did not keep her from the highest levels of national achievement. She learned that no matter her disability, God had also given her many abilities to be developed.

By reading this book, not only will the abled learn to value the disabled in our society, they will be amazed at their accomplishments. The lives of David and Vicki Smith, Windy's parents, are an example of showing love, exhibiting patience, creativity, and hard work to bring out Windy's abilities.

Read this book to be warmed with love and challenged with the possibilities that will enrich your life as you follow Windy through her first 40 years.

—Ronald G. Dolislager, author of *Following God's Call*
Brother, husband, and grandfather to people with disabilities.

BORN FOR THIS

From Disability to Destiny

Vicki Stansberry Smith

Copyright 2015 by Vicki Stansberry Smith

All official pictures are used with permission from the Office of George W. Bush, Dallas, Texas.

Born for This
From Disability to Destiny

Printed in the United States of America
Published by CreateSpace.com

ISBN-13: 978-1505351576
ISBN-10: 150535157X

All rights reserved. No part of this book may be reproduced or transmitted in any form or by any means without the prior written permission of the author.

Unless otherwise indicated, all Scripture quotations are taken from the *Holy Bible,* English Standard Version, copyright 2002. Used by permission of Crossway, Wheaton, Illinois 60187. All rights reserved.

To purchase additional copies of this book, visit **www.amazon.com**

Dedication

To my best friend, and the love of my life—
my husband, David L. Smith.

To the pieces of my heart living out there in the world:
Our children, Dave, Windy and Mikey.
Mom loves you very much!

To our wonderful grandsons:
Caleb, Jake, Lookens and Kensley.
The exact order we got you is a blessing to us all!
I love you, I love you, I love you, I love you!
May God bless you all on your own journey of life,
and may you give Him all the glory!

Thank you, God, for all of the family and friends
You have blessed me with,
and for allowing me to share the same time and space
in this world with them, *and in the one to come after!*

Acknowledgments

To write a book about our life with Windy
for her first forty years has been something
I felt God has called me to do.
Our family has been blessed in so many ways
because she was born to us.
I could not have brought this to fruition
without my wonderful husband, David,
our awesome sons, Dave and Mikey,
and all of our beloved family members and friends,
who have loved her (and me),
and who have prayed for us through all of these years.
Thank you. Thank you everyone!

I also want to thank two special people,
Phyllis and Ron Dolislager.
Without their diligent editing and 'fixing'
I would still be dreaming about finishing this book.

Finally, I want to thank our Lord and Savior,
Jesus Christ, for loving our daughter,
and for giving her miracles to live out
for ALL the world to see!

Introduction

I praise you for I am fearfully and wonderfully made.
                                              Psalm 139:14

When someone becomes aquatinted with Windy, inevitably they will ask us how she has gotten to do all the fabulous things in her lifetime: how she knows, on a first name basis, some former U.S. Presidents, former Cabinet members, former Governors, movie stars, sports figures, and so many, other people. David and I always smile before we answer. It's very hard to tell someone how it has all taken place: to sum up forty-plus years in a sentence or two is a weighty assignment. We try to be brief. We usually begin by explaining that God opened all the doors, through all the years, in amazing ways. Her story with Him is remarkable, and would be for any person, but especially for a person who was born with an intellectual disability called Down syndrome. And that's just the way she was born . . . with this medical diagnosis. We didn't let that fact limit or hinder her development or the growth of her faith in God, or her faith in her own abilities. In fact, we accepted the reality of raising a child with a disability *pretty* much in that first week of her birth, and we were determined to help her reach her *full* development, whatever that might be, or look like, down the road.

Her sweet disposition and strong determination enabled her to reach heights neither David nor I could have imagined. Not in a million, trillion years. Not *ever*!

The following is a story of Windy's remarkable life for the first forty years. This book has been years in the writing because it first had to be lived out, day by day, as her incredible story unfolded. Knowing her, the next forty years will probably fill another entertaining and engaging book.

Come along and experience with us the overwhelming joys we have felt. Feel as we did, the deep pain we went through at certain times in our lives, and laugh with us over some of Windy's hilarious antics. (Believe me there have been many antics!). Most of all, we pray you gain encouragement for your own life, as you read her story.

Preface / Previews

Sometimes I wonder what life would have been like for our entire family if at our daughter Windy's birth in 1973, we would have been allowed a glimpse into the future—like in a preview for a movie? Instead of feelings of grief and despair over the news at the birth of our baby, that she had a disability, we would surely have been jubilant and excited over the miraculous events that were to take place, and the honors that would someday be bestowed upon her.

What a surprise it would have been if we could have seen Windy as a saucy little seven year old being introduced to the Tennessee House of Representatives by our Representative Tom Wheeler, as the winner of the poster child for The Arc. (We had gone to school with Tom, and he and Windy would become friends at church.)

We would definitely have chuckled to see her seated in Tennessee Governor Lamar Alexander's desk chair in the State Capitol as he stood beside her two brothers, Dave and Mikey, looking on. She had pulled away from her family, present in the room with her, and had promptly run to sit in the Governor's big leather chair where she quickly picked up a pen with her right hand, leaned back with an authoritative air, as if to experience what it was like to be in charge, if only for a second, until the Governor himself gently picked her up, laughing with her over her actions! She would also make a televised public service announcement with the Governor's wife, Honey, that would be seen across our state.

As the movie of the future continued to play, we would have observed our daughter as a determined athletic preteen, as she received numerous gold, silver, and bronze medals for the Tennessee

State Special Olympics at Vanderbilt University in Nashville. Even more astonishing would be to watch her as she was awarded two bronze medals for her gymnastic routines at the International Special Olympics, hosted by the University of Notre Dame in South Bend, Indiana. (There would be seventy-four countries competing in the various events for ten days.) To see the medals swinging around her neck, as she walked with a sense of accomplishment, would have calmed our worst fears. (We were told that she might not ever learn to walk!)

If we could have seen just fourteen years down the road, would we not have thrilled at the sight of Windy, representing Special Olympics, running alongside a U.S. Olympic Gold Medalist runner, Florence Griffith Joyner (Flo Jo), in an opening ceremony, as Flo Jo lit the torch, along with Josh, a member of the AAU at the AAU Junior Olympic Games, on the University of Tennessee Campus in Neyland Stadium?

We would also have been impressed, no doubt about it, with her ease and friendliness as we saw her walking down the crowded halls of Farragut High in Knoxville, Tennessee. She would someday attend as a participant in the first LRE (Least Restrictive Environment Class) the high school had ever had, where she would also take regular classes and be treated as "normal" by her peers and teachers. We would surely have been flabbergasted to see our girl saying, Hi, to all she passed in the halls and being greeted and hugged by her *many* friends as she sashayed down the halls of her school. Some of her friends would have disabilities, but the surprising thing would be to find out that most of her close friends would be peers who had no disabilities. (This revelation of true friendship she was to experience would have been a real boost to our saddened countenance. We were doubtful that she would have many friends like we had had the privilege of having. In fact, she would someday have friends from all over the world!)

WOW! This part of our fast-forward movie would have been cause to pause the scenes and press repeat, I'm sure! (Windy would someday become so close to her siblings, and their wives, that she would be a bridesmaid in her brothers' weddings and in one of her best friend's wedding, Penel Roberson Croniser.) We would have loved to see our daughter holding onto her dad's arm standing on the football field, as a nominee for Homecoming Queen. (She got many votes from her classmates!) And, in 1996, we would have seen her addressing her graduation class of 500, and a crowd of over 4,000 at Thompson-Bowling Arena on the University of Tennessee Campus. Her speech would have left *us* speechless.

And, wonder upon wonder, would we have believed our eyes if we could have seen her, twenty-eight years from the time of her birth, speaking before a hushed crowd of thousands, plus a nationally televised audience of thirty-eight million more, at the 2000 Republican National Convention in Philadelphia, PA? We would have been shocked to see that she would be the *first* person with an intellectual disability to speak at such a key spot, just before the Vice President hopeful, Dick Cheney, spoke. (Wait, the doctor had just told us Windy might never speak words? Entire sentences? Really?)

What would we have done differently when Windy was born, if we had known that she would someday be appointed by a President of the United States, George W. Bush, to a federal level committee, which meets in Washington, D.C., four to six times a year? That she would become a self-advocate on such an elevated level? We would never have imagined any of this. In our small apartment in Memphis, Tennessee, we fearfully contemplated the future when we took our baby girl home for the first time. How could we have known that our daughter would be the catalyst for many flights to and from Washington, D.C., and beyond?

Would we have believed it if we had seen, in this "movie," how *she* would literally help change *history* because she would someday stand in the Oval Office of the White House with her fellow committee members, and watch as the President signed an Executive Order that changed the previous name of the Committee on which she served, to The President's Committee for People with Intellectual Disabilities? (This monumental event was to occur because she, her committee members, and another special committee member and self-advocate, Michael Rogers, had the courage and strong desire to propose a name change, ushering in a brighter future, for those who could not speak for themselves, and for *all* intellectually disabled Americans.)

If a peek into the future had been possible in 1973, we would have been overwhelmed with the gravity of knowing that she, in 2001, would be personally invited to sit at the coveted right-hand side of First Lady, Laura Bush, in the Upper Gallery of the Capitol, while President Bush gave his first speech to Congress. If we had seen her sitting and visiting with a former President and First Lady, George and Barbara Bush, could we have contained our excitement?

Our movie would have shown Windy meeting people with recognizable names; sitting with wrestler Darryl (The Rock) Johnston, visiting with actress Bo Derek, standing on stage with singer Chaka Khan, meeting boxer and heavyweight champion of the world, Evander Holyfield, as they stood backstage talking together, sitting at a table with actor Kirk Cameron (and Kirk telling Windy he had seen *her* on television!), meeting former TV host, Art Linkletter, Tennessee Senator Fred Thompson, meeting actor and self-advocate, Chris Burke, talking politics and make-up with the Secretary of Labor, Elaine Chao, talking to former Secretary of Commerce, Don Evans, and receiving personal letters from many other well-known people.

We would have been full of joy, to watch our grown daughter stand before thousands of undergrad and graduate students at Liberty University in Lynchburg, Virginia., in the spring of 2006, as she told several thousand students about her life, to encourage them in their lives.

And wouldn't we have jumped up and down with happiness at seeing Windy, at the age of thirty-two? This future movie would have shown her making a public service ad to encourage people to become Special Education teachers. It would be shown for several months on one of Knoxville's local television channels. She was with a friend, the Tennessee Commissioner of Education, Lana Seivers, and their mutual beloved friend, Bertie Bostic, one of Windy's first teachers, who would help *teach* her to read. (Wow. See. She was going to learn to *read*!) Windy would later email that commercial to First Lady, Laura Bush, explaining to us that "It would make Miss Laura happy because she was a teacher, and she wants people to become teachers."

Would we have ever thought this baby of ours would know heads of state on a first name basis, or fly to Washington, D.C. on a regular schedule as a paid special government employee? That she would be sworn into office on the grounds of the White House by the Secretary of Health and Human Services, Tommy Thompson? Uh, no . . . we wouldn't have imagined either one of us would ever know anyone in those positions, much less our tiny, little girl, who seemed to have so much going against her from the start. But most astonishing would have been her future friendships with a U.S. President, George W. Bush, and with his two Personal Aides, Blake Gottesman, and his predecessor, Jared Weinstein.

But let's face it, there was no way that we could have known *any* of 'what was to be' back in '73. It would have been wonderful and comforting to know, but instead, we had to live one minute at a time, in unfamiliar territory, filled with mind boggling "land mines". We found ourselves asking basic and simple questions about our perceived shaky future raising a child with a disability.

I suppose one of our most immediate, pressing concerns would have been focused on how she was going to look, not only as a child, but when she grew up. (After we realized she was strong enough to live, and was not going to die.) We would have been so happy just to see, if only for a moment, the beautiful young lady with dark hair and sparkling brown eyes she would grow up to be. Never would we have imagined the beautiful picture of her, standing next to her pretty blonde friend, Emily Garman, dressed in their high school graduation caps and gowns, on the Jumbo Screen in Times Square, for the Down Syndrome Buddy Walk, in 1997. What if we had been allowed to see *that* spectacle? We would have been assured that our baby girl would grow up to become a darling brunette, that's what!

To be sure, on a deeper level, we would have felt so blessed to have a daughter that would touch so many lives in such positive ways because she does not see race, or disability, or position in society, in any way other than with equality, true equality. I also know that we could not have resisted her beautiful, contagious smile that lights up a room, or her great big hugs handed out so freely to the loved, the unloved, and the unloving. We would have been so pleased to see the sweet spirit, strong faith, and admirable courage she possesses, even against all odds. We would have smiled at her cute personality and her quick sense of humor. Most of all, we would have been blown away with the positive effects she would have on us, her parents, on her two brothers, Dave and Mikey, on her sisters-in-law, Kari and Treva, and on her beloved nephews, and on all our extended families and friends.

The tears of sadness and fear we shed at first would certainly have become tears of joy. Our great expectations would have been so high if we could have known what was to be. (That David and I would be known in important circles, as "Windy's parents". They wouldn't know *our* names!)

At first there was no light at the end of the perceived dark tunnel, as we contemplated her future. Anyway, knowing her future would have taken no faith or obedience to follow God, and we might have missed out on all the joys we have experienced from the many great *and* small triumphs and blessings leading up to Windy's adult years. Even in our pain, probably *because* of our pain, we grew to be better people.

The birth of a child is usually a time of great joy and a celebration of life, but when the parents learn soon after the birth that the baby has a disability, they experience many different emotions. (One in ten families, an estimated thirty million people in the United States, is affected by a family member who has intellectual or developmental disabilities. It is believed that three percent of the general population, seven to eight million Americans, have an intellectual disability today.)

Parents struggle with the dreams they feel are lost forever—those dreams that we had for our child before we gave birth. However, new goals, hopes, and dreams do materialize. But just *getting* to that point can take quite some time. Dreams more achievable and attainable become top priority. Initially there are ***so*** many questions. Some can be answered right away, most cannot . . . only time can reveal the most pressing answers.

I don't mean to mislead anyone into thinking the day of Windy's birth was the happiest day of our lives, or that our life has been easy, or that it has been a breeze to raise a child born with a disability. Windy came into our family like a hard blowing wind . . . we were absolutely knocked down. It took some time to get our breath back. It took time to adjust, to mend our broken hearts, and to believe and trust that life would go on . . . just *not* exactly like we had planned.

This is the story and adventures of one *ordinary* family's journey through life with love and hope and prayers, and with a very *extraordinary* God. The story goes on in so many lives that Windy has touched and has yet to touch. We hope that by sharing our story, it gives *you*, the reader, real hope in your own life. God is always ready for any one of us to do great and mighty things to make this world a better place.

All these happenings were part of God's bigger plan for her life, although those Divine plans weren't always so clear to us, particularly at the time of her birth.

CONTENTS

	Dedication	v
	Acknowledgements	vi
	Introduction	vii
	Preface/Previews	ix
1	Memphis Daze	1
2	Birth and Meeting Big Brother	23
3	Finding Guidance	41
4	Family Background and Values	53
5	Learning about the World	79
6	Making Life-Long Friends	85
7	Facing Fears	95
8	Broader Horizons	99
9	WINDY'S LIFE LESSONS Begin	105
10	A Moving Experience	109
11	A Little Brother to Love	141
12	Daniel Arthur School Years	165
13	Change of Direction	175
14	Attending CAK with Brothers	183
15	Making Friends and Influencing People	205
16	Farragut High Living	219
17	Life after Graduation	281
18	Nine to Five: On the Job	289
19	The Remarkable Missive	299
20	Speech of a Lifetime	337
21	Box Seats Next to First Lady	371
22	Presidential Appointment	385
23	Proper Pleas, Persistence, and Possibilities	417
24	Windy Moments	467
25	Tidbits and Giggles	517

Afterword	545
Appendix	**551**
Times of Sadness	551
Call from President Bush	552
Family Update	553
Words of Wisdom	561
More Information on Down Syndrome	563
End Notes	564
About the Author	566

Chapter One
Memphis Daze

Memphis, Tennessee, was a great place to be in September, 1973. The beautiful early fall weather was great, and Elvis was alive and well and living in the city. The early seventies was certainly an interesting time: hippie dress, headbands, and wide bell-bottom jeans were all the rage, and rock music was rocking the country. To be sure, there were lots of fun times to be had in the now famous 70s era, and then there were very serious events taking place. The Vietnam War was still a major topic of concern. It had been fought for so long, so very far away, yet daily news reports about our country's involvement and the soldiers' and veterans' well-being kept the war close to home, and heart. To top all this off, an energy crisis threatened to disrupt our daily lives as we experienced long lines at the gas pumps.

It was also an exciting time to be born into the world. Windy Jeanne Smith arrived at a large, downtown hospital on the twenty-fourth day of September (on her great-great grandfather, Charlie Weaver's birthday) to me and my husband, David, with a little bit of dark hair and a cute little nose. She weighed 6 pounds, 8 ounces, and was 18 inches long. Our baby daughter looked so beautiful and so normal to us that, at first, we didn't realize she had a disability.

David and I were holding her for the first time, marveling at her particular beauty, and also, at the miracle of birth for the second time for us as a couple, when the doctor who had recently delivered her knocked three loud raps with his knuckles on the doorframe. He looked at us from his position across the room. He remained standing there in the doorway . . . evidently coming in and shutting the door for some privacy for us, protecting us from anyone passing by in the hall as he announced his news, was *not* an issue for *him*.

With a frown, no, more like a sneer on his face, he stated loudly and bluntly, "I guess you saw her face. She's a Mongoloid. She'll always be retarded. There's nothing you, or anyone can do. She will probably never walk or talk. She'll probably not live very long, either. Sorry, that's how it goes sometimes. I suggest you find a Home or Institution to put her in immediately before you get too attached. Don't even *think* about taking her home with you. I can give one of the nurses the go-ahead to find placement for her. Let me know. You all are young. You can have more babies. You need to put this behind you and, get on with your life."

With that, he turned on his heels and was gone. Vanished! He hadn't even taken the courtesy of stepping all the way into the room. It was obvious that he felt he had some disgusting facts to relate and he wanted to get it over with as soon as possible . . . for his own sake. To heck with his patient, and *especially* to heck with the child he had just delivered! We were shocked, stunned really! (We have since learned that this was *not* an uncommon way to inform the families of such news.)

We were so confused by our physician's reaction. What had he meant by "get on with your life?" Act like she hadn't been born today? Never look at her again? Pretend the last nine months hadn't happened? What *had* he meant?

David and I avoided looking into each other's eyes. We were very close to falling apart emotionally, and seeing pain and hurt in the eyes of each other would have been more than we could have taken. Instead we looked quickly, and inquiringly into Windy's pretty little face, as she lay sleeping so peacefully in my arms, so unaware of the 'bomb' that had just been dropped upon all three of us. We just *desperately* wanted our normal life back . . . the one we had been living, just a few seconds before . . . a happy couple filled with the joyful anticipation of raising a new baby, along with an adorable toddler at home waiting to meet his new sister. I began to pray silently. *Oh God, please turn back the clock. Make this all be just a bad dream! Make our baby whole and healthy! Right this second! Please God! Please!*

Because of our lack of knowledge, we called the nurses' station with a request for someone to come and quickly get the baby, so that they could monitor her vital signs and maybe save her life if she began to slip away from us as a result of the frailties we believed her to possess. We ascertained this diagnosis from the hastily spoken harsh words and the hasty departure of our physician. David and I thought she was going to die in our arms any second before we could get help for her! His prognosis had seemed such a 'death decree' that we, in our ignorance of Down syndrome, panicked. We wanted help for her before it was too late. Like NOW! STAT! (And like NOW we had already decided that we *wanted* help for her. She *belonged* to us.)

In just about sixty seconds, a middle aged nurse's aide answered our urgent call. She came hurriedly into the room, concerned over the panic she had heard in our voices over the intercom. (Couldn't they have sent a *real* nurse, or two, in for this dire need?) She asked about the problem in a very sweet Southern drawl. We repeated the doctor's words to her verbatim, and as she listened to us intently, she leaned over to peer into Windy's tiny face. She tenderly touched our baby's forehead with the palm of her hand. Then, after making a rather quick examination, (*Strangely* quick, we felt, for such a sick baby!), she stood facing us, placed her hands on her ample hips, and vowed confidently in a very loud voice that she had been on the OB/GYN floor for *years* and didn't think there was anything wrong with *this* baby girl. She said she had seen Windy in the nursery right after her birth, and that she had been the one who dressed and cuddled her. Her exclamations of "how cute, alert and healthy our baby looked to be" were strange words to hear after what we had been told, not two minutes earlier.

Obviously her sweet remarks were an effort to alleviate any fears she ascertained we possessed about new parenthood. Naturally she would think something was awry, derived from our panic, so obvious, as we hesitated to even hold our own child without a medical personal in attendance. We wanted her vital signs checked. We needed to be assured that she had received a thorough physical evaluation to determine if she was dangerously ill. The doctor had just "written her off". Her condition *must* be critical. Was this woman clueless? Despite her kindness, and because of her calmness, we were becoming even more confused. Was our baby sick? Was our baby "normal" or was she not? And just what was "normal" and just what was "not normal", we began to ponder in our confused minds. After a normal pregnancy (at least medically speaking) all this had come as a totally shocking surprise. We reiterated to her that the doctor *must* have been right.

"Well," she conceded, "if the doctor said it, I guess it's true. But if this baby *is* Down syndrome . . . she ain't *much*! You remember that, you hear?" We heard her, but we still didn't know what her words meant at the moment, or what they would mean to us in time.

There are times in life when an insignificant moment becomes very significant in one's memory, and you can instantly play back in your mind that event just as if you had hit the play button on an iPod. This was one of those times, and that phrase has given us much joy and laughter over the years. That dear lady set the tone and the way we would react to Windy's birth and her early years of development. We were to find out in the following years just how encouraging and prophetic a statement that nurse's aide had made. She was really just telling us to see the bright side of life. If our baby had a disability, it could have been worse, much worse, and we needed to search for what she *could* do, not what she could not do. It was as simple as that. She might not have been a registered nurse, but as it turned out, she was the perfect person to come into our room and answer our call for help that morning. We hadn't needed any medical help . . . we needed hope. We remember her as a woman on a mission of mercy, delivering her news in a happy tone, very unusual for such a somber moment for us. Our first response for help had been unfulfilling. Now we get it. When we called for help, God sent us who we needed in *His* perfect timing.

At the time, our future didn't look happy or simple to figure out. Truth be known, we feared we would never smile again. When your heart is truly breaking, you can't even muster a fake smile. We felt we were literally swept off our feet and had lost our footing on the earth, and on life as we had known it, and it would never be the same for David and me. Our lives would, from this moment on, always be different. Different, from our dreams that we had dreamed for our little family, different from our friends and family member's lives, and now even our prayers would be different than we had ever thought. Our life lesson was beginning for us as a couple. No one on this earth could give us a definite answer: no medical professional, no family member, no friend. We were going to have to trust the God we had heard about all our lives and thought we knew. We now had to believe, *really* believe, that He was holding us up in His mighty grip in the middle of this crisis. Or, we were going to have to decide . . . was He *really* there, and did He care?

God had been so wonderful in many events of our lives, but this was BIG. Could He really handle *this* one? Didn't He want us to be happy in life? Was it really so hard for Him to give us a healthy baby? He had given dozens of 'normal' babies to all the other women on the maternity ward that weekend, so why couldn't we celebrate with a lovely dinner like all the other couples on the OB/GYN floor were doing that night? It seemed as if we could only hear silence as we cried out in deep anguish. We were seeking specific directives, and there were *none* . . . at least there didn't seem to be any.

While in the hospital, not many hours after Windy was born, David and my mom, Flo, had made numerous long distance phone calls back home to our family members to tell of Windy's arrival and of the circumstances. They had to make the calls from the pay phones in the Father's Waiting Room. I'm sure they had to speak in low voices since the maternity ward was full that September day. I remained in the private room, hidden from the world. David had spoken with his mother and father, Juanita and Bill. His maternal grandmother, Jessie, along with my maternal grandmother, Emma were at our apartment keeping our toddler, Davey. They sent their love and prayers, and were going to call and tell his two older brothers, J.W. and Richard, and their wives. Mom had called my older sister, Dianne, her husband, Jack, and my younger brother, Chip, as well as some of their closest friends. Everyone was upset over the news, and all sent their love and prayers.

David and my mom were terribly weary by the evening of the first day because of their deep concern over me, and for the tiny, little girl (still nameless) that was resting peacefully in the nursery. I encouraged them to go home. It hurt me to see them looking so distraught.

Whenever I was going through a particularly difficult time when I was growing up, my mama, a "pull yourself up by your boot straps" kind of woman, would always try to encourage me by saying, "You can do this, girl!" On this day she would lean over and kiss my cheek and squeeze my hand hard. All her years of playing basketball and golf had given her hands strength, but her positive words were conspicuously absent. We both felt the burden and futility of her unsaid words. She now carried my pain with her. I guess she wasn't sure if any of us could overcome this happening, this challenge in our lives. No one had any answers. Really, we didn't even know what questions to ask!

David leaned down to kiss me, and hugged me tightly. They left knowing I was going to be in the good care of my father, Charles, who had just arrived by plane. He had abruptly left home in Clinton, Tennessee, where he was an Optometric Physician. He had hopped on the first plane to Memphis he could find. He knew all of us needed the support. He was a great comfort to me and a great companion that first dark, dark night.

I had never seen my dad cry. That night, at the hospital with me, he cried in big sobs, but only for a few seconds. Then he regained composure, pulled out his ever ready white, crisp, cotton handkerchief he always carried in his pocket, blew his nose, and then held my hand like I was a six year old again. He had scooted his chair up close to the bed, and we held hands through the raised bed rail. He held on like he was trying to prevent me from crossing a busy highway attempting to keep me safe from harm and pain. He couldn't stop this pain though. He was devastated about that, and so was I. Daddy had always made things right for me. He couldn't now. It was out of his hands.

Dad and Mom had led an interesting life. My father was the youngest of his family and the seventh child. His father, O.R. Stansberry, had owned drug stores (one later became Hoskins drugstore), and then he became an eye doctor. He had been an athlete in high school where his future father-in-law, R.B. Wallace, was the Principal. He learned to play golf in school and played until he was eighty-nine. As a youth he even met *the* Henry Ford, of the automobile industry, one night while walking down the main street of Clinton. (He enjoyed retelling that story so!) When he graduated from the University of Tennessee, and mom had graduated with a teaching certificate from Carson Newman College, they married in 1940. He became a Captain and a flight instructor during WWII, and one of the first Thunderbird squadron formation pilots, a member of the Air Corps, which became the Air Force. The Air Force always held a special place in their hearts.

He had even been in a movie made in 1941 entitled, *I Wanted Wings*, starring William Holden, Ray Milland, and Veronica Lake. The bulk of it had been filmed at Randolph Field near San Antonio, Texas. Dad got to fly his plane in formation with his flying buddies, in full view of the cameras rolling, with his plane number in the foreground. (A part he and Mama loved to see on the DVD of the movie we got for them years later, as a surprise for their sixty-ninth anniversary party.) This was the strong man who sat beside me that first night and wept.

My mind was reeling in a confused daze, but I kept asking things in my mind, circling uncontrollably in a sort of continual silent prayer: *If you hear me God, please don't let our lives and our baby's life be out of Your hands. Hold tightly to us. Don't let us fall into the deep, dark abyss we are standing right on the edge of. Don't let us fall in and lose our way now. Hold us!* I didn't really even know what I meant by those words. I just know I couldn't stop saying them, pleading with a God I hoped was close by and I hoped with all my heart that He was listening. Some football game was on television that night, the flashing bluish-green light seemed to invade the dark room, and Dad and I kept it on as background noise, and pretended to be interested in it. We didn't talk much.

I wrote in my journal from that time, "Our brains were sort of 'on stand-by', frozen and numb. Somehow the bright game in view on the wall above my bed in that semi-dark room, with players shouting, running, and tackling each other, helped my frame of mind in a strange sort of way. I felt like I was running with them, down that long, grassy green field, under those blearing bright lights, sometimes catching the ball and sometimes dropping it in front of a crowd with the world watching the accomplishments and the failures. And the tackles felt good to me, especially when they hit hard and fell down flat. At least I knew how to react to the pain as I saw someone suddenly, in mid-stride, hit the ground. That was it! *That's* the way we felt, David and I, we had been stopped in our tracks, and we felt like we had been blindsided."

We were now trying to get our breath back. Our eyes were open, but we were definitely still stunned. We didn't want to think at all about what lay ahead. Reality was *far* more complicated and too hard to face at that moment. We didn't care who won this complicated game of life we were playing, we just prayed we would have the stamina and endurance to finish. It felt like we had been thrust into the most difficult game in the world. And you know what? It was one of the most difficult things a parent will ever have to face. This was big league. We felt so little league! So unable to face the future.

Day two started out as a very difficult day. We felt like we were ill prepared for the rearing of a child with a disability. Dad went to our apartment to see Davey and check on Mom. David had come back after a fitful night's rest (Rest?) and sat on the side of my bed, tightly holding my hand in the quiet, stark hospital room. I couldn't let my mind think how tough a night it must have been for my guy. He must have gone back into our bedroom, empty without me, and had to face returning to that sad hospital room, with the even sadder brown-eyed girl he had married, waiting on him to come back to her.

I knew I couldn't ask even one question about his time away from me, or we both might start crying.

We could hear the muffled excitement and the happy voices of the friends and families of the other new moms as they passed by our closed door, on their way to visit them and their new babies in the nursery. The joy in their voices seemed to bounce onto the shiny terrazzo tiled floor by our door and then skip on past us, as if we could not take part in any of the joy. Their happiness seemed to make the pain and silence we felt that much more intensified. It was as if the baby we had so excitedly waited for during the past nine months seemed to have died, and in her place was this little stranger we didn't know how to take care of. We were grieving. Out of our deep love, we were silently hurting for each other, too.

David was so distressed for me, and he wondered how I was going to be able to take care of a toddler not yet two, *and* a baby with a disability, while our families lived over three-hundred and fifty miles away. I was so worried about David and all the heavy responsibilities he would face as a Daddy as he began a rigorous program in Optometry school. He was already missing his registration and first *full* day because he didn't want to leave me alone to face the unknown. I needed to tell him to go on to school, but I just couldn't let him go.

We had been in a Biology class in college together only two years earlier. (It was strange, but because of the tragedy we perceived ourselves going through, it seemed as if it had been twenty years ago. We seemed to have aged in a very short amount of time.) Oddly enough we recalled the *very* day our Biology professor, Mrs. West, had inscribed the words, **Down syndrome**, across the blackboard. Now even stranger, it felt as if those very words were written across our hearts.

We knew that Down syndrome, or DS, caused an irregular cell division and that there were different types, but we didn't recall much more, particularly any details of the chromosomal abnormality. We had both excelled at genetic equation solving. It had been a fun game for us to try to beat each other in speedily solving an equation on paper. (We even made the Dean's List as we competed in our classes.) Now we had a gigantic genetic equation that looked impossible to solve.

As we were contemplating our plight, we heard a knock on the hospital door and heard an unfamiliar male voice asking if he could come in. In strolled a very distinguished, older gentleman dressed in a suit that hung a bit loosely from his tall, slender frame. He introduced himself as Dr. Miller and explained to us that he was a pediatrician there in Memphis. He said he had received a call from his daughter-in-law, Ann Britt, telling him that her mother, Ann Watson Threefoot, had a special dear friend named Flo. They told him Flo had a brand new granddaughter in his hospital, and asked if he would stop by on his rounds to see the gorgeous baby. He said he loved babies, and so, of course, he couldn't refuse. He said he had heard about this 'Flo' for years, and what a fun personality she had, and so naturally he wanted to see her grandchild in person. He also said he had already been by to meet our daughter and thought she was beautiful, and as *healthy* as could be. He stood grinning brightly at us.

We were stunned by his medical opinion, *and* his smile, and asked if all this was true. Was our baby going to live, and if so, we eagerly asked him when could we take her home? He emphatically said that he was happy to report she had an unusually healthy heart. It is not unusual for DS babies to be born with a hole in their heart that requires surgery several months after birth, and so, theoretically, he said she could go home "today". I, as her mother however, should wait a day or two to recover from giving birth, he advised. Wow!

What good news! We simultaneously smiled. Our first smile since hearing the news of Windy's condition. *Maybe, just maybe, there was something in life to smile about again. Too soon to tell.*

Dr. Miller then promptly sat down in a chair by my bedside, as if he were there to talk awhile. (We had forgotten all our manners in our astonishment and had failed to ask him to sit down. But, in our defense, doctors had not stayed around very long in our room, and so we figured he would be dashing out the door any second!) He even propped his loafer-shod feet up on the lowest bed railing. A trick, we surmised, he had learned in residency to catch any little rest he could get in between patients. I leaned back on my pillows satisfied that he was going to remain with us for a while, and David quickly sat down on the bed next to me as the wise, senior doctor began to talk. He explained all he knew about mongolism, as he called the term the medical community used at the time to describe this particular chromosomal condition.

> Thank goodness that awful word was changed to Down syndrome soon after Windy's arrival, and we are grateful to all these who were responsible for the tremendously positive change. Wonder upon wonders . . . Windy herself would play a huge future role in changing the lives of individuals born with disabilities by helping to change the 'R' word to intellectual disabilities on a federal level which would filter on down into verbiage for laws and bills in government, in education, in medical dictionaries and in everyday language!

With all Dr. Miller's wisdom gained from his years of experience, he urged us to take her home and love her and to treat her no differently than our other children. He said to teach her, discipline her, and not to forget to love each other as a couple in the process. He gave us the greatest gift anyone could have given at the time, and that gift was *hope*. Hope deferred almost paralyzes a person, but true hope was something we could grasp and act upon. We had temporarily been downed by hopelessness and sorrow. We suddenly possessed a concrete feeling we could relate to—something to hold on to. Life had forever changed for us as a family. We needed to huddle together and to come back out of the huddle with action and intent. All the previous plans for our family were obsolete. Now, we needed a new game plan.

We bid Dr. Miller goodbye, and we thanked him from the bottom of our hearts for taking the time out of his busy schedule to come by and see us, to talk to strangers and encourage them at a very low time in their lives. David shook his hand. I motioned for Dr. Miller to lean over, and I hugged his neck. He teared up, and then turned to go. He stood at the doorway, almost as if to make a mental picture of the two of us, and then he walked out the door. We sat still, as if frozen, until the sound of his footsteps dissipated, as he walked down the hallway, and the ding of the elevator bell told us he had gone. Regrettably, we never saw him or spoke to him again. He was preparing for retirement, and we were busy raising a family.

We're sure he was a real man with flaws like anyone else, but we remember him as an angel that came to visit us, albeit, dressed in a normal suit and tie. God sent him right to our door of that big old hospital. By heeding his daughter-in-law's request to stop by and see us, he allowed God to help him make a stop in his routine rounds that *forever* changed one family's outlook on life, as we dealt with a disability. Nothing routine about it for us.

We were, from that day forward, going to live up to our own full potential, every one of us, *including* our new little daughter. We were young and this was only the first few minutes of the first quarter, I guess you could say. There was too much life out in front of us to stop us now. Sure we had been sidelined, but there was no time to lose. David and I had the desire to stand up, take a deep breath, and get back out there. Thank you Dr. Miller!

We started talking at the same time and we could see the light shining again in each other's eyes. We were breathing deeply again, and it didn't hurt as sharply anymore. Maybe I would get up and sit next to the window and feel the sunshine. (I wasn't numb anymore.) When they brought our baby back in, I wondered if she might like to feel the sun for the very first time. I kissed David on the cheek and said, "How's our Davey? Does he miss me? I sure miss him. Please kiss him and tell him his mama and baby sister will be home real soon!"

"That's my girl!" he said, as he beamed that smile at me that still, today, makes my heart beat faster. "I can't wait to take *my* girls home!" He was squeezing me so hard, I knew he was feeling like we could do this thing, whatever it took. We were going to live through it . . . and so was our tiny daughter!

Midmorning feeding brought the nurses and babies back to the waiting mothers and fathers, and our daughter was laid in my arms again. This time it felt different. It was as if God was saying somehow it was going to be all right. All we had to do was trust Him for the unknown future.

As David looked at us, he decided, then and there, that we should call our daughter Windy, spelled W-I-N-D-Y, not Wendy, the usual spelling. (None of the previous names we had picked out for a girl seemed to fit or suit her.) He said she was not going to be common but unique, like the spelling of her name, and she would be like the wind, sent by God to cleanse the air and bring in a new season. It was a new season in our lives, that's for sure.

There was a song popular from our high school years titled, *Windy,* by the musical group, The Association. It was about a girl who, "Smiling at everybody she sees . . . everyone knows it's *Windy*". The song continued to say "And Windy has stormy eyes that flash at the sound of lies and Windy has wings to fly above the clouds". (Many times in the months to come David would sing it softly to her, and I think she took it to heart because it describes her *perfectly*.) I liked the name. It seemed so fitting and right as we said the name out loud to the tiny person we held in our arms, and we agreed she would be Windy! I'll swear she smiled!

It was then that I insisted that David leave and get to class. I suddenly felt that we were not going to be taken down by this strange news in our lives. I assured him I was going to be fine. He had our future at stake, and he was going to have to go forward and 'hit the books' hard. He leaned down and kissed my cheek like a true 'school boy' stealing a kiss on the playground and bounded out of the room. I put on a brave face for his sake, but despite myself, I felt a buoyancy I didn't understand at the time. That true trust in God's plans for our lives felt so freeing, especially when we couldn't understand, and maybe would never fully understand, the reasons why things had happened the way they had happened. All I know for sure: When David left my room, I did not feel the panic I expected to feel. I felt the presence of our Lord and Savior in that room with Windy—and I knew in my heart that we were never going to feel alone again!

At the time, there were not many medical or parenting resources about her condition, and the ones that were available were atrocious. My sister flew down to be with us and went searching for the first load of books. She knew her way around Memphis. She and Jack had lived there for four years, almost ten years before us, when they had both attended Optometry school. She went to the Public Library and came home with everything available: a stack of outdated medical books that described someone born with DS (not the terminology used in those books, but I refuse to spell out here the very word Windy has helped to eradicate!) and the old "R" word was repeated with abandonment in very depressing and unkind ways. Cold and clinical, these books left little, if *any*, hope of a child's potentially positive development.

One particular book left an impressionable image. It had a black and white photograph of a grown woman who had been born with Down syndrome, dressed in a poorly fitted dress, sitting awkwardly on a swing set. She was holding onto the chains that held the swing up, and the toes of her feet were turning in toward each other. She looked into the camera with a haunting attempt at a slight smile. She appeared so lonely and unhappy and unhealthy. This was not the kind of future we envisioned, or hoped for, for our daughter. We wanted more for her in her adult years than playing on playground equipment like a little child. But, we also realized *if* that life was all she was going to be capable of, then we would love her and help her find a way to put a smile on her face, a true smile of joy and happiness. If it took all we had she was going to swing on a swing someday with *glee* because of her happy life at home that she shared with her brother and any other children we would be blessed with.

Surely God had intended her to lead a productive, meaningful life. Helping her reach her fullest potential would require our earnest endeavors, but wasn't that our job as caring parents? There *had* to be a reason for her life. We read all the information we could find, and then agreed to close the books (All those horrible books. Slam!) and open a new chapter together as a family.

After the initial state of shock and disbelief, David and I tried to be rational about our future. We took time to assimilate the facts and then to formulate ways to live with what positive facts we *had* found. David looked me in the eyes and grabbed both of my hands.

He went over the facts aloud; we had wanted another baby, a second child, and we had gotten one. Maybe not the one we thought we were getting, but a baby girl just the same. We decided on our own that we would take Windy home and love her and raise her like a normal child, along with her sixteen-month-old brother, John David (Davey), and any children who would come after. She was ours. We were hers. Facts are facts; we had read many facts, now we were listing our own.

We both remembered and spoke of a nice, large family back home, the Hamilton family, who had impressed everyone in town with their love and treatment of their daughter with special needs. All of her siblings were so unashamedly proud of that fragile young lady. They included her in all their activities. They never pushed the issue, but gently and quietly, they expected people to accept her as she was. They paved a way during a hard time when people judged anyone with a disability more harshly and stared at anyone that looked or behaved different from the expected. She was unable to participate in sports, but they took her to all of her siblings' ballgames and practices.

We wanted to be like that family, having that strong strength and faith, and yet lovingly asking others to accept our daughter as one of us. We were young, only twenty-one, but we knew something that our first doctor didn't know. Windy was already a big part of our lives. God had just made different plans, and we were going to be adaptable. (Years later, Windy said in a talk to the Rotary Club in our hometown, "My Mom and Dad never took me back to the doctor who said to give me away because I would never walk or talk. I have been on national TV twice this year, and I sure hope that doctor has been watching a lot of TV!" Windy's humor always wins out!)

As parents of a newborn child born with a disability, David and I had come to a major crossroads in our lives. There were two roads we felt were literally stretched out before us that led to our future as a couple and as a family. If I close my eyes and think back, I can still vividly see them as they looked on that night, beginning at our feet, much like the beginning of the yellow brick road in *The Wizard of Oz* as it was shown to Dorothy. The very beginning, where we would take our first steps, was clear, but it was as if a shroud of heavy fog veiled the direction and difficulty of both the paths. Both involved many unknowns, yet there were some known factors we had to take into consideration. We realized we had a choice on what our reactions would be to adversity and hardship in our lives together. One road was leading to a life without God: dark, lonely and full of obstacles, where we knew we could load up a lifetime of anger, bitterness, and broken hearts. We would have to travel down it alone, guiding ourselves, and no matter how we connived and willed things to be, we would fall short of a fulfilled life. That much we did know. (We'd seen people who had chosen this path, and it wasn't pretty.)

The other road was also dark, and we couldn't see where it would lead either, but we knew it was only initially dark because God would most certainly illuminate it as we followed Him, step by step. We knew this from previous experience and from a belief in the words we had read in the Bible. Granted, we had never had to trust to this great an extent and on such an elevated degree. We jointly came to the conclusion that we would trust and obey. We would rather wait and see what God had in store for us. (*Your word is a lamp to my feet and a light unto my path.* Psalm 119:105) We wanted to make Him the ruler of our lives. David and I clasped hands and chose the latter road, and we have never looked back.

If Windy could have talked at the time I think she would have said something like this….

> *I was born two weeks past my Mom's due date and on the first day of my Dad's professional education. I felt*

like he really needed to take his studies seriously, and so I reiterated it by the fact of my birth. Daddies know they have to take good care of their babies, and now my dad had two babies to feed and clothe. I was sorry about the added pressure, but hey, a little pressure spurs most on to great things. It was worth a try. I had been warned that there would be tears at first, but come on, enough was enough. There is a whole world out there waiting for all of us, and we have lots of living to do. And, that thing the nurse told them about me maybe not being able to suck on a nipple of a bottle very well . . . well, there sure is a lot to learn. But after that first night home, and poor Mommy up all night feeding me with a medicine dropper because she thought I would starve to death, I couldn't let her go through all that again. So I just put my little lips together and VOILA! I could drink from a bottle the very next day. Mommy let me sleep all night the second night and boy did I ever need the rest. Lord, don't let her panic again!

It is so good to be in my new home. My two wonderful great-grandmothers and an aunt were waiting with open arms to greet me, and I especially liked the hug and kiss I got from my big brother, Davey. I could tell we were going to be buddies someday. They brought me to this little apartment right in the heart of downtown Memphis, not too far from the mighty Mississippi River. It sure is cozy and warm and full of love. I fell asleep on that second night hearing the sweet voices of my parents whispering something about their love for each other and for us kids and for God. I tried to listen, but I was dog-tired; it's not easy being born. I was sure I'd find out later all the words they were murmuring in that dark, still night.

Back home, people were beginning to spread the word of Windy's birth. Both our families lived in the same town and had known each other for generations. News travels lighting fast by word of mouth, as it can only do in such a *unique* way in a small town. Some people were feeling so sorry for us, and some people (bless them!) were already praying for us. That's all we knew to do at the time: pray. *Lord help us all.* We couldn't come up with any more words to say than that at the time. It was enough for the time being. Numerous prayers were going up and up and up to heaven where they were heard. In His mercy, He sent help in so many ways, and through so many people, and over so many years, and He has never stopped. Praise be to God!

My parents mailed us a short, sweet note encouraging us to read a small paperback book they had found and mailed, entitled *Angel Unaware,* by Dale Evans, the wife of Roy Rogers. (David and I had watched their television show every Saturday morning when we were children. We had seen them on the big screen at the movie theatre. We had never known this part of their life.)

The book described the brief life of their daughter, Robin, who had been born with Down syndrome. It was a sad story, but so lovingly written about their special little girl and how her life had profoundly affected them, in Hollywood during the height of their careers. It was encouraging to read of their strong faith in Christ in the midst of tumult and difficulties. I started the book and would interrupt David's studying as I read passages aloud from where I sat up on our bed late at night while he studied at his big wooden desk in our bedroom. Then I would cry and sling the small paperback book to the floor, only to pick it up again a few minutes later to finish the chapter.

I cried for Dale and Roy. I cried for us. I read to the very end. From their compassion we took hope. From their faith we took strength. We desired to have that kind of faith, following their example, as we faced our future with Windy, and with Davey, and with any child that might be born to us in the future. As a young mother of a newborn I fervently pleaded with God to allow our little baby girl to live. *"Please God let her live and not die early like little Robin. With You, and for You, I'll be brave. I'll face the future boldly. Only please, please allow Windy to grow up to be a woman of faith."* I know now He heard my cry.

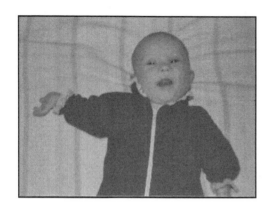

Windy at two months (1973) already showing off a cute personality

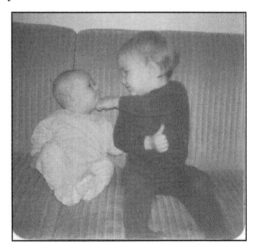

Seeing eye to eye with big brother Dave

Chapter Two
Windy's Birth and Meeting Big Brother

Do not be anxious about anything, but in everything . . . let your requests be made known to God. And the peace of God, which surpasses all understanding, will guard your hearts and your minds in Christ Jesus. Philippians 4: 6-7

Our names had been given by the hospital staff, with our permission, to a DS parent support group, that had just been formed with the help of the Child Development Center in Memphis, or CDC, as it was known as. A sweet young couple called us on the phone and asked if they could come to visit us and bring their two-year-old little girl, who had Down syndrome. The CDC paired parents of a newborn child with DS with a contact family for support and encouragement. In October, classes would begin at the center, what they called Early Intervention and Infant Stimulation classes for DS babies and toddlers. The first classes of the kind in the entire country, (make that the *entire* world!). This family, had been told the same news at their child's birth and wanted to come and meet us and invite us to enroll Windy. They were further down the road and willing to share their experiences with other new parents, they explained. We were quite anxious to meet the three of them. But, we had mixed emotions. Would we be glad to see this little one who shared the same diagnosis as our child? Would we be depressed after they left, because we were going to see what our reality was going to look like in the next year? We both wanted to face what was ahead sooner rather than later. And besides, something good *could* come from the visit. We were intrigued by their words "lightening the load". Yes, please!

We were home only a couple of days, when they stopped by to see us. Their love and concern for their daughter was impressive, and so was the time they spent with the many families they told us about who they had visited. David and I decided immediately that, in time, we wanted to pass along this same hope to others, (If we did find true hope to pass along!), to minister to people in this way. We have now lost count of the people whom God has sent our way, as we have spoken to them about raising a child with DS or other disabilities.

After we had talked for a few minutes, the young mom asked me if she could hold Windy. Only for a second was I hesitant, protective. She was passed around for them to cuddle as we waited for their comments. For the first time strangers were looking closely at her. We had to contain our joy as we heard . . . words of encouragement. They called our daughter *pretty*! (We knew she was pretty to us, but it was *so* nice to hear someone else say it and mean it, without staring or wondering what the correct words should be when they looked at a baby with a disability.) In addition, they found her to be very alert to voices and faces, as she already seemed to try to focus her attention on the person holding her. Stories of their own triumphs and struggles led us to realize that other people had gone through similar situations and had overcome the initial grief and pain. They had been where we were now. Stories of their child's antics as she developed gave us hope for the "normal" family life we wanted so much. Their visit was a God-send. Their daughter was precious, and like any toddler, she was getting into everything as she parallel played with our Davey.

It was so comforting to realize *our* baby would, someday soon, be running around our family room playing just like this with her big brother. We could see that we had a real little daughter to raise, who just happened to have DS. She was first, a person whose life had value. Having a child with a disability changed some things, of course, but we were learning it certainly didn't change everything.

Our very foundation as a family was shaken by her birth, much like an earthquake shakes up and breaks open the earth, and we had to ask the big questions in our early twenties. We needed answers, and fast. Did we believe what we had heard about God in the Sunday school classes of our youth? If so, were we going to live our faith out in a very difficult time of our lives? If not, were we going to try to find answers to LIFE out there without God's guidance and help? Were we going to run everything that happened to us through our own filters, or through God's filter? We decided together we would look to our Heavenly Father for the answers to our questions. Whether we ever understood it all was not as important to us as knowing in our hearts that He loved us through all of our hard, stormy times, as well as in our wonderful, joyful times.

We talked it over the next few nights and always came back to a shared belief that He would supernaturally take something we saw as not so good and make it into something good. We determined to live what we had read in the Bible in Romans 8:28, *And we know that for those who love God all things work together for good, for those who are called according to His purpose.* We knew with every fiber of our being that Windy had been born for a reason, and we desired to look to the Lord to show us why. We didn't think it would be a quick fix. We certainly wanted it to be quick, but we were rational enough to know it could, in reality, take years. We felt great peace in knowing *we* didn't have to find the answer . . . it would find us someday when the timing was right.

We figured the Bible would be a good starting point in our quest to discern a way of life for our family that would have substance and make sense in all the madness we were experiencing. Bottom line: we needed something real to ground us. Fast! Although it was an ancient book, we hoped there might be something in there, some mysterious something that helped people turn difficult situations and their lives around. We had seen it happen in other people's lives.

There had to be something in it we could discover. It was reputed to have been written for *everyone* in the world, and we hoped it could give advice that was just as significant for us as it had been for the people we were reading about who lived so long ago. We owned a Bible. Actually, we had two of them.

David had a tiny New Testament his grandmother, Jessie, had given to him, that he took with him to Alaska. Only a few days after graduation from high school, David flew away to find work with great pay. He went with a childhood friend of ours, Randall Sharp. They soon parted ways to find jobs to optimistically fulfill their dreams of making enough money for their upcoming college tuition.

David found work on the White Pass Yukon Railroad, between Skagway, Alaska, and Canada. He worked from dawn to dusk digging and laying train track. They fed them well and worked them hard. For several weeks he worked eighteen hour days, and yet he still took time to write me every day. His next job was on a commercial salmon fishing boat in Hoonah, Alaska. He was in charge of taking out the skiff to haul in the heavy nets. Reading that little book had a huge influence on his life while he was living away from home for the first time. Not to mention the real danger he was in from the tremendously dangerous jobs he was doing at the age of eighteen.

He traveled to Alaska to make his fortune. He came back flat-broke, but only financially. It hadn't broken his spirit; he was stronger than ever. He made great money, but the cost of living and travel was high. He spent most of his pay on extra clothing, camping gear, and chartered plane rides to and from job sites, and on phone calls to me from pay phones in Juneau and Skagway. Even though he hitchhiked down the Alcan Highway for free (Yes, he really did that!), he encountered heavy expenses. He told me he read at night as if his life depended on it . . . and it did. He left as a boy, and came back a man. He came home serious about his education, his future, his faith, and about me. He had had ample time to think about his future, and our future. He was but a "baby Christian," but he was certainly already on the right path.

That same summer I was working as a day camp counselor for underprivileged children, along with two of my first cousins, Bunnie Brown (Ison) and Ann Brown (Thomason), and some friends from high school. Each night I was reading Scripture from a Bible my parents had given to me years before. I was praying for David to come back safe and alive, and hopefully, back to me. Two and a half years later, after Windy was born, I would open that same Bible, and begin reading words that seemed to have the very thing we needed to hear . . . words with life-giving hope in them. As a young adult, I was never one of those people to know where a certain book in the Bible was located, so I began reading where the pages would fall open. It looked, and sounds, random, but I'll swear it was always pertinent to our day and circumstances. God was already guiding us and using something as simple as reading verses. We were beginning to gain the knowledge that would guide us through all the days of our future! And, we were learning something real, and good, and helpful that we could pass on to our children, whether they had a disability, or not.

The Child Development Center, later affiliated and consolidated with the University of Tennessee Medical Center, was conveniently located only four blocks away from our apartment. We didn't know about the CDC, or its location, its proximity to our little downtown, townhouse apartment. What was appealing to us about the apartments was the fact that the complex housed married students. It was brand new, and most importantly, contained a great playground and basketball court just outside our back door for our Davey. That playground was also for David as much as for the kids. He loved to play basketball, and it proved to be a great stress reliever when he took a break from his studies. We were not too far from his school. We were also neighbors to a couple from our hometown, Steve and Kathy Stewart, and their son, Stevie. They were there because Steve was in Pharmacy school. They had been a few years ahead of us in high school and married two years longer than us. Kathy taught a homesick, small town girl (me) how to drive in a big city, the shortest route to the grocery store, laundromat, and to my husband's school.

I was thrilled to be living near old friends. (Kathy and her sister, Dudley Bostic, would come to see me at our apartment a few times. Later on, Kathy and Steve would have two daughters, Carrie and Jessica. Carrie would be born with disabilities. Dudley's mother-in-law would be one of the teachers who would teach Windy to read someday.) Then when Windy was born, a "bigger plan" began to unfold, and we began to see Divine intervention. Here we were, living within walking distance of the most advanced classes ever offered for someone born with Down syndrome, classes one of our children would need.

We enrolled Windy in the CDC when she was three weeks old. Technically, she was in the second of the classes offered as there were children enrolled six months before. Both classes were closely monitored, and the results of their development were recorded for research. The cumulative information was regarded as the leading authority on the ground-breaking discoveries about the abilities of these kids. The data collected over a ten-year period was invaluable to health professionals and educators. It proved conclusively that the results of interacting with and teaching children born with intellectual disabilities were vital, beginning at a very early age. The studies changed the ways they would educate these children in the future.

(We would return to Memphis for the CDC ten year reunion. Windy was too busy with school obligations to attend the twentieth, and the thirtieth she missed because she was in Washington on federal business.)

Taking her to class was step one. Getting her there was challenging. David had to have the car to get to school early in the mornings, so we three walked to the Center most of the time. I would bundle our tiny girl, and our little Davey, until they resembled round-bodied snowmen, to keep out the cold and wind, on those fall and winter days. Rain or shine, we slowly made our way on foot and by stroller. We walked the few blocks twice a week, for ten week sessions, to meet experts in physical and speech therapy, and medical specialists, who flew in from around the country to give their input and follow the progress. It was a rather lonely walk past the apartments in our complex, then down the next few streets with empty office buildings and empty parking lots. I was more than a bit scared at times, but I was not going to let fear keep me from the help offered our child. Most of the time, we were the only ones out walking. I was acutely aware that I was obviously pretty helpless looking: a young mom with one baby on my hip, and one baby in a stroller.

I did some praying the whole walk to the CDC and the whole way back, *each* trip. There must have been a band of angels around us because we were never in harm's way. Our walk with the Lord was in spirit, *and* in reality. To us there was no doubt . . . God wanted us to go to the CDC. Go we did.

We met some very caring people whose main focus was educating and training the parents of the newborn children with DS with the purpose of facilitating physical and mental development by applying early intervention. Our group was spearheaded by two dedicated women, Faye Russell and Barbara Connolly. Under their guidance we all broke ground in this new frontier together. We were told the program originated with a female pediatrician, Dr. Margaret Giannini, in New York, where she had practiced for several years. She had been approached by parents of a DS child, in the 1960's, and from their desperation and determination to get quality health care for their child, a program emerged to help not only their child but thousands of children who participated in the courses. Dr. G. believed this group of people had so much untapped potential and set about proving their capabilities to the world.

It was here that we learned about genetic counseling. They suggested we have testing done, and David and I opted to have a blood test run on each of us to determine if either one of us had passed on to Windy anything in our gene pool to have caused her to be born with an extra chromosome. They were researching each parent who had a child in the new program.

It wasn't long before we were reacquainted with the facts: that people with DS, have an extra chromosome, on a critical portion of the number 21 chromosome (In 95% of the cases it is called Trisomy 21. Mosaicism is the name of the other 1% that occurs. Translocation is cause of the remaining 4%), present in all, or some of their cells. This alters development of the embryo and causes the characteristics associated with the syndrome. The most common traits are: muscle hypotonia, or low muscle tone, a somewhat flat facial profile, oblique palpebral fissures, or upward slant of the eyes, a single deep crease across the center of the palm, hyper-flexibility, an excessive ability to extend the joints, epicanthal folds, or small skin folds, on the inner corner of the eyes, and an enlargement of the tongue in relationship to the size of the mouth. Why this non-junction, or cell division, occurs at conception is still unknown. (DS affects people of all ages and all races and is the most frequent chromosomal abnormality, occurring once in approximately every 691 live births. About 6,000 babies are born with Down syndrome every year and over 400,000 people in the United States have Down syndrome today.) [1]

Whatever it was, or how it occurred, we wanted to know if we might pass on the syndrome to any future children. It is a frequently asked question (either aloud or silently), "Did I cause this to happen to my child?" Finally, after weeks of anxious waiting, all the genetic testing came back negative. Nothing we could have done would have made any difference in the way Windy was born into this world. At our age (of twenty-one), we learned there was a 1 out of 1,700 chance that we would have given birth to a child with Down syndrome. (The chances do increase with the advancing age of the mother, for by age thirty-five, the probability is 1 in 365; by age forty-four, it rises to 1 in 100 births.) Discovering the odds of her birth to us was all the more reason to believe she was born with a purpose; she was on a mission all her own.

We got busy learning about children who had disabilities, and it didn't leave a lot of free time. Between tending to Windy and Davey, and dealing with routine daily living—which by the way was a good thing because it didn't allowed us *any* time to sit back and reflect on our lives and to get down or depressed for very long. We had many reasons we could have been depressed because of some of the daunting information we were hearing, but we chose to take the good, the hopeful things out of all the info. We disregarded, or at least, did not dwell on, the negative. Neither did we look too far off into the future. We chose to take each day as it came. But we had our moments of sadness. They were rare, thank goodness, but I do remember one certain time.

One statement we heard during this time helped us so much. We hung onto it when almost everything else sounded bleak. We learned it from a young, female physical therapist, when she said to us, "It is important to know that people with Down syndrome *can,* and *do,* lead normal lives. I've seen DS people learn amazing things." There was that word "normal" again. What was normal and what was not? Wasn't this revolutionary thinking? Evaluation of the term was paramount for our family. How could we articulate our own thoughts on the subject until we got a grasp on all this? We began to make our own observations on Down syndrome and normal development, point by point, and we found our own inspiration in the things these children *could* learn. Watching them learn about the world around them eradicated the ambiguous concepts held by practically everyone else at the time.

As babies they generally develop like other babies, although the changes will, but not always, probably be delayed somewhat, i.e., the age they first learn to roll over, sit alone or pull up to stand and to walk will possibly be behind that of a child of the same age who is not born with Down syndrome. It was impressive to see the great desire these kids had to learn. They *did* learn to talk, but usually slower than their peers, and most required speech therapy to ensure better communication skills, and to help them develop understandable speech.

They *were* educable. Each child's individual mental and physical abilities and disabilities dictated a wide variety of learning levels and teaching modes. But they could all learn, regardless of their age or range of disability. We could already see this was true. As for the future, we felt that considering how quickly they were responding to this early therapy, students with Down syndrome were possibly capable of graduating from high school with some even going on to take college-level courses, obtaining a job, and even excelling in the job market. All this just hadn't been proven yet.

Why set a limit on the heights they could reach? There just were not many adults with DS living and working in society neither were they receiving much of an education, if at all. It was very rare in those days to see someone with DS.

We were excited over the possibilities. We came to the conclusion they could definitely obtain independence. The concept of independence was to be understood as a flexible term and only the future would tell just what could and would be achieved. Parents would need to be flexible on all future hopes and dreams for their child since independence would depend on several factors: on the person and the degree of disability they had, their family situation when they became an adult, and on the future desires of that individual. Lots of "If's and When's". It was all new.)[2]

Who knew that those classes would lead Windy to reach her full potential, and consequently do something to help *all* people with disabilities, someday in her future? It may have come as a surprise to us, but it was another plan of God's.

One of David's professors and his wife told me about the little booklets entitled *Sharing Our Caring*. They sent us the first year's subscription as a gift. It was a wonderful resource. Published six times a year, it was delivered to us by way of the small mail slot in our apartment front door, and it brought instant hope and encouragement in huge doses to our home. There were always photos of children from around the globe, with articles written by their parents, family members, friends or educators. There was always a section of specific questions and answers, purposefully left unanswered for parents to write in and tell something that had helped them in raising a child born with Down syndrome. There was another section that listed the many different answers the Editor received on previously asked questions. It really was all about "sharing our caring".

The format was excellent and more informative than anything we had ever seen on raising children with this particular disability. We kept them all, and reread them frequently as our daughter grew and changed and became the age of some of the children in the articles. It was as close to a great blog page as you could get at the time. The front inside page had a quote, "Written especially for parents of children with Down's Syndrome in order that they might help themselves and, thus, help their children." [3]

Even in the year 1974, parents were trying to work through the rude stares and comments of other people out in society. One mom's comment has always stuck in our memory. She had her six-year-old son in the grocery store with her when she had returned to her old hometown in Pennsylvania to visit her parents. A high school friend had recognized her in the check-out line and had come over to say, "Hello." She commented, "Oh, so this is the mongoloid child?" The mother said, "Before I could respond, the cute little fellow looked at the stranger, and quickly said, 'No. I'm Phillip.'" She went on to say she didn't have to say anything else. He had said it all! (I did not use real names here.) This one story gave David and me real hope for Windy. There were a lot of parents out there who loved their kids, and took pride in their accomplishments, and actions. In *all* countries! We weren't alone. Neither were our kids! Our Davey wasn't the only sibling with a special needs sister. That knowledge helped us tremendously. *Sharing Our Caring* was a wonderful parenting tool and a great gift. Thank heavens we found out about it when she was just a baby. It was a great companion-tutoring course to her infant stimulation.

Amazingly early intervention classes are now offered to each family of a child with a disability *by* law. So many babies are getting the necessary help to enable them to live up to their own potential. What a help this is to families. The first classes were only on a volunteer basis, and a very limited number of spaces were available, in only certain places in the nation. You could say David and I were lucky to have chosen an apartment so close to one of these rare classes, but our family knows luck had nothing to do with it. Even our move to Memphis was meant to be, and our paths were "being made straight". Somehow.

Many beneficial class sessions were offered to us. It was there that David and I learned about the 'football hold.' We began to carry our tiny one about on the plane of an extended arm—holding her on her stomach—to encourage her to strengthen her neck muscles. She learned to hold her own head up as she became curious about the sounds around her. Our parents were very leery over this different way to carry a baby around the house. Good thing they didn't get to (have to) witness it too often. (They sure were glad about that!) Her daddy and I became really good at it until she got too good at looking around, and too strong to continue the exercise. She was way too curious about life around her, and she gained fabulous control of her head way before anyone thought it was possible. She was off the charts.

I especially liked holding the other babies. Holding babies was a large part of our classes. We parents were encouraged to take turns with someone else's child as we put them through their exercise routines. Two or three physical therapists directed us. It allowed us to compare muscle tone and personalities of our children. It was really special to hold the different babies from Caucasian, African-American, Asian, and Jewish backgrounds. To be honest, it was also somewhat agonizing for me to see that the babies all seemed to look more like each other than they did their own siblings. (As they started growing into toddlers they began to look more like their families!) In a way that tugged at the hearts of the parents as they tried to identify family characteristics in their own babies that they wanted so desperately to fit into their own families, and so they could be as "normal" a family as possible.

We know this because we, David and I, were two of those in the group who were striving to have a regular family life despite our recent setbacks. We all had our own struggles to face. One of the mothers in our group could not get her husband to attend any of the meetings with her. You could hear the pain in her voice as she spoke about the man she loved. It was very hard for him to accept the fact that his first, and only son, had DS. (It would take a while for complete acceptance on his part, but it *did* happen over time.)

Another couple in Windy's class told us that they had had a difficult time getting pregnant, and after several miscarriages, over a wait of many painful years, had finally had a baby . . . a baby born with a disability. And, that was way beyond their ability to cope, for a while. There was another family that heeded their physician's advice and gave their baby girl up at birth. They left her at the hospital in the care of an agency. A social worker brought her to every one of our sessions, and we all took turns holding her and exercising her. I cannot express the joy we felt when, after hearing of their child's progress in just a few month's time, (I'm not sure who told them about her, the case worker or someone at CDC.) those parents walked into the room where we were all gathered and embraced their daughter for the first time. They sat in amazement as they watched her completing exercise routines, and they cried as they picked her up to take her home.

They had discovered she *was* a bright baby with a future all her own, despite the alarmingly heartbreaking diagnosis their own doctor had informed them at their baby's birth. Leaving them with what they felt was no hope, they had given her up to the "home" they thought would keep her comfortable for what they believed was a short life span. Every day they tried to forget her was "a day of hell on earth" for them, they told us later. Mornings they wondered if she was awake, and evenings they fretted over her feedings: was she lying in a baby bed hungry and wet because no caretaker had any extra time to give her the special attention she needed? When they could not stand another minute of speculation about her daily life, they asked permission to visit her, to set their minds at ease, so they could finally begin their lives afresh, without a baby girl who had Down syndrome.

Little known to them, they would walk out with more peace than they thought was possible. They walked in as a couple . . . but would go out as a family. Their daughter had surpassed their expectations, and they wanted to be there when she passed the next big milestone in her development. They were looking forward to witnessing her sitting up, crawling, and then walking, now that they understood all of those stages of development were possible for her. I can tell you even the toughest men present in that room on that day were moved to tears as we watched her parents clap their hands in joy, and to take turns holding their tiny daughter to their chests. Now that was a heartwarming scene if I ever saw one!

Davey, our friendly, cute, brown-eyed, blond-headed toddler had the privilege of playing with all the siblings of the children in the program. They all gathered in a large room filled with toys and books. They joined their brothers and sisters for some bonding time each session as they rolled on the tumbling mats with them and played with the beach balls that were used by the babies to stretch and bend their little bodies for their much-needed flexibility and coordination. Davey always looked forward to his playtime with all the children. We were still so concerned about him and his future with a sibling who had a disability. Would he get all the attention he needed to grow into a well-rounded individual, or would he resent the extra time Windy would probably require of us? Questions such as these kept interrupting our thoughts and prayers.

Thirty years later I came upon a journal I had kept, hidden away with the papers and baby books, in a box in our home's basement, and I read again our words as young inexperienced parents. The words written so many years before reflected our need of the assurance we wanted for Davey and for our other children, if we ever had any more: that they would always feel loved, and cared for. Both of our grown sons have told us *she* was the reason they were spurred on to achieve greater goals in their own lives. Bottom line: the guys say that Windy has always been their *inspiration.* They grew up watching her bravely attempt many hurdles in life, with strong faith and a strong will. She was an inspiration because she would not give up despite great odds against her. They witnessed *and* helped her to accomplish tasks, and many times surpass goals they set for her. And they were, in turn, inspired to reach out and try for goals they set for themselves.

They took courage in her courage, as they strove for things in life, even if it looked for all the world that it was a long shot: in grades, sports, businesses, the making of a musical CD, a law school degree, an environmental health and safety degree, or whatever the case happened to be. David and I cherish the words of our boys when they would tell of something they were facing, and then say, "If Windy can do what she has done, then I can do this!" They would take some of their sister's commitment, determination, and faith with them in their hearts and minds.

We really wish we could have known the wonderful effects Windy would have on her siblings in the future. The hours we spent speculating on this seemingly important aspect of our family dynamics could have been better spent on something really worthwhile! Now our Smith men are exceptionally tender and caring to those who have a disability. Each of our kids has different personalities, but they admire each other and have learned from each other. They do truly love each other. That's what matters to us.

I have one big regret, which youth and inexperience kept me from telling what was really in my heart of hearts . . . I kept silent in those early months at CDC and purposefully refrained from answering, at the opportune times, how deep and guiding my faith was to me. Specifically when some of the parents asked me how I could be so calm and assured at such a young age, with the burdensome future we were having to face so early in our lifetime. Most, if not all, of the parents present in those first early child development classes were older than us.

David and I had come to know in our hearts that Jesus was in control of our future, and we had an unexplainable peace. We now know it was "the peace that surpasses all understanding." Back then we didn't know that Bible verse to quote it. How could we verbalize and explain our beliefs when we didn't know exactly the how or why ourselves? We were not ready to testify that we trusted in God and held to the promises in His word, that we believed He would somehow work *all* things out for good. What exactly did that look like? We didn't know, but we just knew we had to trust and wait. But, when we look back at the many answers to prayer, and the many times we didn't get the answers we were seeking, we had the confidence, if not the proper patience, to hang on, to hold on to God's Word and His promises.

I wish I could have shared that truth with those strangers. With family and friends I could share more easily and openly talk about God, and our faith in Him, as He directed our lives. Whether everyone understood the depth of our faith when they heard our convictions, I can't say for sure. One thing I do know, I was shy and inarticulate with people I didn't know very well. I felt inadequate to share the things that I pondered in my heart. I didn't share openly then . . .but I promised God I would someday. Now, by the writing of this book, I am fulfilling that promise. The following verse sums it up for us. *In all your ways acknowledge Him and He will make straight your paths.* Proverbs 3:6.

Chapter Three
Finding Guidance

As Windy grew, we worked on fine and gross motor skills. We put her big brother through all the routines too. Raising a child like Windy would require a lot of special time and attention, and we were conscious of spending the same amount of attention on Davey as he grew. We didn't want him to develop any tendencies toward jealously because he felt left out or that we spent more time with her. Being so close in age made it fairly easy to work with them both on some of the same skills and academia. Besides, all the exercises only made him stronger and more coordinated.

Playtime with Daddy was always fun. David took study breaks and played "knee football and basketball." He literally walked around the living room carpet on his knees to be down on Davey's level. When they tired of these games, there was always wrestling and tickling sessions. The children lived for these treasured moments when they had Dad's undivided attention, and I treasured the times because it was basically the only free moments I had to myself. Either way, it was time well spent!

Our living room looked more like a nursery school than a living room. Standing next to one wall was a sizable, red wooden structure constructed with a ladder to climb onto a platform, with a small slide to come down on. We also had a balance beam and a bouncing board that their Uncle Jack and my dad showed David how to construct out of pieces of pliable wood. Our kids would jump on these, and they really learned to develop great balance.

We also had a gigantic beach ball to place Windy on her stomach, to learn to use her back and neck muscles. We rolled it gently from front to back, and side to side as we held her on the ball.

It was all great equipment for their motor skills, but it kept our apartment turned upside down. I learned to look past the mess. They wouldn't stay little kids for long. I told myself this too would pass.

Letters of encouragement and love came in the mail. How I loved getting those letters—they were a piece of home sent to brighten my days, sealed in small envelopes. My mom, David's mom, the grandmothers, my sister, and my Stansberry aunts: Bonnie, Kappie, Annette, and Lucille, all wrote me sweet words of encouragement and stuck in an occasional check for me to buy the kids a little something.

On rare days, (Most of the time I was upbeat and positive, always have been.) I contemplated our days ahead and the situations we might have to face, and the depressing thoughts would run freely. There were no Christian radio broadcasts that I knew about, no Internet to listen to a sermon to give me any hope. No Facebook to feel connected to anyone. I had friends, but they were all busy with school and their own plans for the future. Besides, long distance calls cost money then. There were no cell phones to give me the feeling that I could reach out and speak to someone at any given time. (The letters were great, but they didn't come every week.)

There was only me and God during the children's nap-times, and I learned more about Him as I opened up my Bible. I kept reading and praying for Him to illuminate my mind and heart as I tackled unfamiliar passages. I felt more familiar with Proverbs and Psalms, so I wore those pages out. It was a lonely time, but I know now it was necessary for me to grow stronger in my faith.

One particularly hard day I was feeling unusually sorry for myself. I lacked sleep because both of our babies hadn't slept through the night for a month. David was having a trying semester in school, and I felt as if he would *never* be done with his education or the endless amounts of study material. He was always sitting at his desk with an opened *Gray's Anatomy*, or some other tome just as thick and boring to me. To top it all off, I was homesick for family and friends. I was lonely and all of a sudden scared of the present *and* of the future.

My dear grandmother Emma, aged eighty-four at the time, and David's grandmother Jessie, aged seventy-eight at the time, had left us to go back home after staying with us for two whole months. It had been a great delight, and incredible help, to have the grandmothers in residence. Besides their wonderful wisdom in child-rearing they so graciously imparted to us, they gave us love like only grandmothers can. It didn't hurt one bit that they were both excellent cooks. I was still an inexperienced cook and had trouble making two things and having them ready to eat at the same meal!

Yes, our grandmothers' companionship and support was greatly missed. However, there had been a downside of them being with me . . . they were so impressed with Windy's strength and appetite that they kept telling me they thought the doctors had been wrong about her, that she was all right, that she would outgrow *this thing*. This belief made it even harder on me. I *knew (*or thought I did*)* what the diagnosis of Down syndrome meant. They even talked about her in this sweet, hopeful way when they didn't think I could hear them in another room as they quietly conversed. I could almost believe it could be true when they had been with me.

Windy's health *was* still a big unknown. Our pediatrician, Dr. Perry, was monitoring her heart at each check-up, to be sure her heart was still strong, and that she didn't require surgery. I was still fearful that she might get sick and die before I could get help for her.

I contemplated all these things on this particular day. I held Windy as she nursed her baby bottle. I was sitting in our old hand-me down, swivel-rocker from Juanita, and I began to cry, and then openly sob. I couldn't stop myself. I cried uncontrollably. Startled, Windy stopped sucking on the bottle and looked up at me. I will *never* forget the impact her look had on me.

I found this description of how she looked at me in my old journal from the year 1973:

> Her little brown eyes looked back into my eyes as if to draw out of my very being the reason for this sudden scary reaction in her usually happy, calm mother. Although she was only a few months old, her look was unexplainably like one of a woman *older* in age than me. Her steady gaze seemed to say to me that it was nonsense to shed tears over things I had no control over and that all would be well. I looked down at her and promised her aloud I would not allow myself to wallow in self pity too long. I was instantly reminded of the lines in a hymn David and I had sung in church as children, and that we had heard our grandmothers sing at home as they went about their daily tasks. Somehow the words came tumbling out of my memory, and I quietly sang to my baby:

Why should I feel discouraged, why should the shadows come,
Why should my heart be lonely, and long for heaven and home?
When Jesus is my portion, my constant friend is He:
His eye is on the sparrow, and I know He cares for me;
His eye is on the sparrow, and I know he watches me.

Refrain:
I sing because I'm happy,
I sing because I'm free,
For His eye is on the sparrow,
And I know He watches me (and you).

"Let not your heart be troubled," His tender word I hear,
And resting on His goodness, I lose my doubts and fear;
Though by the path He leads me, but one step I may see:
His eye is on the sparrow, and I know He watches me;
His eye is on the sparrow, and I know He watches me (and you).

Refrain

Whenever I am tempted, whenever clouds arise,
When songs give place to sighing, when hope within me dies,
I draw the closer to Him, from care He sets me free:
His eye is on the sparrow, and I know He watches me;
His eye is on the sparrow, and I know He watches me (and you). [4]

If God cared for the little birds of the air, then He surely cared for the details in our lives. Sure life was not so grand right at this moment. I had every right to be feeling sorry for myself. (It sounds pretty sad as I read my own written words about those early days of Windy's birth, but things had to get better, didn't they?) Depressing and trying times were always going to happen in life. We are not in control of these situations, but we have to learn that we do have control over how we react to the situations. It was not how we start, but how we finish, and we wanted to finish strong, and with God's help we had determined that we would do just that. I wanted to believe in the words "Fear Not." I had to lean on His strength because mine wasn't so strong after all. So this is what "taking a leap of faith" really meant, huh? I wasn't a "leaper" by nature . . . but I was now *willing* to learn how to become a "leaper".

Windy seemed satisfied with my song, and my smile at her, because she began to drink from her baby bottle again. I felt her take a deep breath, in and out, and she relaxed. I believe if she had been able to, she would have given me a big eye roll. No, now that I know her personality, I'm *sure* of it!

CDC held infant stimulation sessions two mornings a week. They began at nine and could last for three hours. That left five other mornings and seven afternoons and evenings to help Windy at home. We had some help for two days, but the bulk of her learning time was up to us. David and I made out a strict list of exercises and things to do with her. We were probably too hard on her and on ourselves. Our youth supplied the energy to stay on task, and we enjoyed the discipline of having a routine to follow, but it didn't leave a whole lot of down time for any of us. David finally had to learn to take a break from school, studying and parenting. He would go play some kind of ball: intramural football, join in a pick-up basketball game, or go ride his bike.

Unfortunately, I didn't learn that *much* needed attribute of taking some "me time," for many years. I don't know how I kept up the intensity of being a "teacher mom" to small children in their *every* waking hour. "You live . . . you learn."

We all became innovative when it came to teaching Windy. They say, "Necessity is the mother of invention," and I say, "A child's needs makes a mother invent ways to help them develop." I became *very* creative, and so did everyone around Windy. It became second nature.

As for making Windy more aware of her environment and surroundings, my sister, Dianne (nicknamed Dede), came up with an ingenious idea. She hand-sewed little elastic bands with small Christmas bells on them (we called them Win-De bells). We placed them around Windy's tiny ankles and wrists so she would be aware of her limb's movements. We'd lay her in the middle of a quilt we put down on the living room floor.

At first she was startled and surprised at the jiggling of the bells as she moved her hands and feet around. She would stop, and grow still, as if to listen for the source of the harsh sound. When all was quiet, she would move again, and the strange noise sounded again. She would shake a fist and look directly at the offending hand. Next, she would shake a foot, and then try to see her toes on the "loud ankle". It became an amusing game to occupy her time. We left them on for about thirty minutes at a time.

About three months passed with these ringing sessions until one day it was as if Windy had unlocked the "secret of the bells." The mystery was solved as far as she was concerned, and she soon grew bored with the whole game. She would pull to get the bracelets off, so she could move about unhindered. We took them off, and the 'Win-De' bell bands hit the recesses of our keepsake chest where they have remained to this day. They are a reminder to us of our simple strategies and hopeful endeavors to help our daughter grow and develop. Windy consequently learned to sit up, crawl, stand, and walk on a normal developmental rate. We kept meticulous notes. It was "so far so good" on the physical development issue. Her mental development was more obscure to us.

We didn't know how she would progress mentally, but we knew there were some important things we needed to teach her to help her reach her full potential. Full potential had become our goal for both our children. First, and foremost, we were *not* going to predetermine a limit to their achievements or to their potential—Windy's potential, as well as, Davey's potential. She *could* achieve, and *she* would be our best guide. We knew we had to encourage her, but not frustrate her to the point of defeating the whole purpose. Without sounding redundant, it called for a balance. We had to discover a balance in nudging her to try something new and knowing when to let it go and move on to something else.

In order to reach this potential we felt like there were some important hurdles we needed to cross. We wanted her to be disciplined just like our son and any other children we might have, so she would know how to behave and how to be safe in all situations. We wanted her to learn important social graces, so she would know how to act properly out in public and therefore not draw undue attention to herself. What she couldn't attain, we would learn to deal with. I wanted her dressed appropriately, cute and stylish, so people would be drawn to her positively. (Maybe I would have rethought the clothing thing if I could have known how conscious she would become about fashion and how much it would cost us. All you ladies who work at one of her favorite stores, Stein Mart, can attest to this, I know! She even has a letter from Jay Stein thanking her for wearing one of their outfits to the White House!)

We wanted her speech to be understandable to others, and we wanted her to be independent. (Another area we possibly over did, that independent part!) If we could teach her to read and write, it would be the icing on the cake . . . but that was *way* down the road. We'd love her . . . even if she never learned to do *any* of those things. She was ours, and we were hers.

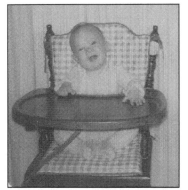

Hungry, but happy

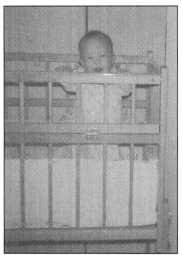

Joy in the morning

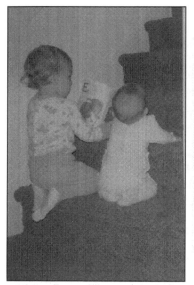

Big brother teaching reading and
stair climbing skills

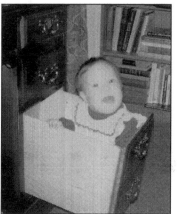

Getting into Daddy's desk drawer

Crawling on the floor with nothing but diapers on

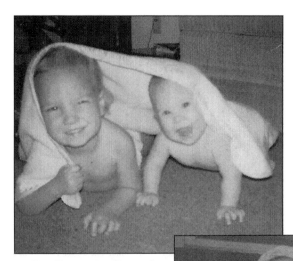

Anything for a laugh

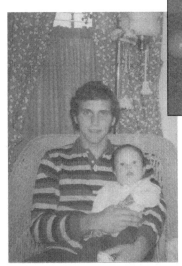

Daddy's girl

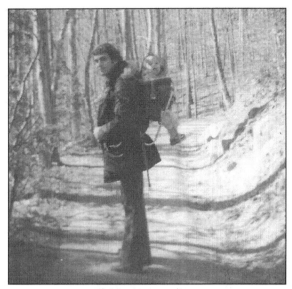

Hiking the Smokies

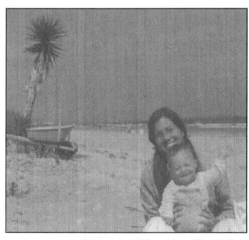

Mommy and Windy at Hilton Head in 1974

Chapter Four
Family Background and Values

We had read and heard from several sources by now, that a child with Down syndrome *did not* like change or large crowds. As far as we were concerned, that was nonsense! Call it ignorance, due to our youth, or just plain hard-headedness, but we were going to try our best to prevent Windy from developing those two traits. How was she going to have a normal life and not be able to adapt to change? Life's full of change. And, how in the world were we to keep her away from crowds? That was not gonna' happen! Someday, we wanted her to make her way down crowded hallways of schools, walk confidently on busy city sidewalks, be one of thousands at a firework display, a musical concert, or a member of a large church.

We figured the reading material and experts were outdated, and that it was time someone did the research to prove them wrong! David and I were up for the challenge! Our family's future happiness depended on the outcome of this. We wondered what chance children with disabilities really had experiencing real life, hidden away at home, or institutionalized from birth, or early childhood. How many people with special needs had been out in society up to this point, to test this "theory"?

Certainly we didn't disregard the brave and loving families who have shared their child who had a disability with the world, disregarded the stares, and at times, faced opposition others had about their child's inclusion. We had seen a few families choosing to raise their child in a loving home, and we had seen their older children with disabilities, who were loving, well groomed, with sweet dispositions. But, we only knew of a few families who made this decision.

We were going to find out if our daughter's environment could positively affect this natural aversion to change the experts said she would have. (If our Windy had an aversion.) We were a loud, fun group when our families all came together on holidays and vacations. She would have to be exposed early on to as many people and situations as we could muster up. That was easy enough when we went back home for a visit. All we had to do was walk in the front door of either of our family's homes. The testing grounds were ripe!

To better understand Windy's heritage and her personality, you have to know a little something about her family.

David and I grew up together in the Eastern part of Tennessee in the small town of Clinton, beside the beautiful Clinch River. (We Tennesseans make quite a to-do over the distinct three sections of the state: East, Middle, and West. They are all beautiful in their own right, but we love our Eastern Tennessee because it's been our homeland for many generations on both sides of our families.)

Our families had known each other for several generations. Our parents had even played together as kids. I guess one might think it was no big deal to meet and marry your childhood sweetheart in a situation such as this, but it *was*. It's a miracle anytime people find their soul mate. (David's mom, Juanita, told me she saw me for the first time when I was about a year old. She and David's dad had just moved back home after Bill had served as a medic's assistant in the Navy, and he had gone on to receive his degree in Accounting at Maryville College and had come back to work at one of the plants in Oak Ridge. She went home and asked David's dad who Flo was. He explained that she was one of his oldest sister, Margaret's, best childhood friends. Juanita told him all about meeting me. She had only boys, and remembers being delightfully entertained by my little girl antics as I pulled items within my reach into a shopping cart as my mom talked to everyone who came into the store. Mama knew simply everyone, and everyone knew Mama. She could be visiting for hours! Juanita told Bill she thought I was so cute. Now that little girl she liked back then is her daughter-in-law!)

Our shared history began when we were in church one Sunday morning. My family attended First Baptist Church, and David's family, all but his Mom's mother, attended United Memorial Methodist Church, located just down the main street from our church. On that fateful day David came to church with his grandmother, Jessie Webb, for some reason. It was his first visit to the Baptist Church. They sat on the ground level where Granny Jessie always sat. My friends and I were in the balcony talking before the service began. We had already moved once because Mrs. McGinley had asked us to move out of her aisle seat, her self-appointed seat.

She did me a huge favor that day because from my new vantage point I saw the cutest guy I had ever seen. He looked up at me from his seat in the second row all the way down front, and we locked eyes for a second. Really. A *second* was all it took. He had probably heard the ruckus we were creating by talking and giggling up there. I whispered and rudely pointed in his direction and asked if anybody knew who he was. Clinton had several elementary schools, and I knew he didn't go to mine. Some of my girlfriends attended the other schools and told me his name was David Smith. The church organ began to play, and the congregation grew quiet, but I had a difficult time keeping myself from looking at the boy with the curly brown hair, who was boldly turning around and looking up at the balcony.

I leaned over and whispered confidently to my girlfriends, "I'm going to marry that boy someday." With this comical confession, we all broke out in giggles and after a few stern stares from the people around us, not to mention my mom in the choir loft giving me one of 'those' looks, we quieted down to sing the worship hymn and to listen to the sermon. Well, I listened to *some* of the sermon. My heart would not be "quiet" but I'll bet I looked very attentive for a child. By staring straight at the minister, I could see every move the new boy named David made. I noticed he couldn't sit still for very long. (Still can't!)

On the following Monday afternoon I had some little girlfriends over to play, and we were in my home's unfinished basement playing dress-up, trying on my mom's old evening dresses that hung in a large, free-standing cedar closet. (Once a Beauty Queen always a Beauty Queen. Mom had been crowned Miss Anderson County and was a contestant in the Miss USA Pageant held in Florida when she was twenty years old. David's Aunt Margaret won the title of Miss USA that year. There were many lovely old dresses to choose from.)

I remember Mamaw Emma called down the open door, leading to the basement wooden stairway, to say that I had a visitor at the front door. Curious, I hiked up the long dress and raced up the steps, two at a time—no easy thing to do in high heels much too large for my feet. *That* cute boy, was standing at the door. The one I had seen at church the day before! I was startled to say the least. Somebody in my group of girlfriends must have "spilled the beans" and told him who I was and what I had said. I shyly, and politely, asked him to come in.

I was *so* embarrassed. He had caught me playing dress-up. We talked a little, neither one remembers about what, as my nephew, Jackie, and younger brother, Chip, ran around the room between us. They were so hyped up and excited because another boy had come to visit with all those girls in the house. He told me he was good with the younger kids because he had a nephew, Stevie Smith, who was the exact age of Jackie. I noticed his interactions with them. He was really kind.

David then told me he had a friend, Bob Miller, who had been too shy to come in with him, and he had promised him he wouldn't stay long. He stood up and told the little boys, "Bye" (I mentally gave him an 'A' for good manners.) and then turned and looked me in the eyes, and without a bit of shyness in his demeanor stated, "I'll come back and see you some other time." He didn't ask . . . he told me with assurance that he was coming back someday! It wasn't a goodbye . . . more like a promise, and with that he was out the door. Another boy, I correctly assumed was Bob, got up off the street curb where he had been waiting patiently. I watched them as they cut through the vacant lot across the street from my house and walked quickly out of sight.

He stayed just long enough to fall in love, he teased me later. I think he was just smitten with his first big crush. I know I had a big crush. Those gray-blue eyes had taken me in as he looked directly in my eyes. Funny thing, somehow I knew in my heart that this was not going to be the last time we saw each other.

We believe in love at first sight. Call it "first love" or "puppy love" but we both feel it was Providence. I tease him that it was that old black strapless formal dress and high heels I had been dressed in, but we both know it wasn't really. We were only *nine* years-old, and I had on a tee shirt and shorts under the dress. It *had* to be by Design.

We saw each other briefly over the next few years at ballgames, at Hoskins Drugstore, at Paul and Betty Smith's corner drugstore, at Saturday afternoon matinees at The Ritz, at local football, basketball and baseball games, and while riding bikes all around town with our friends. (We would pedal past each other as we rode to our respective grandparents' houses to visit.) We never really spoke to each other except for a brief "Hi" or "Bye." I even saw him walking down Main Street once with a cigar lit and hanging in the corner of his mouth, biting down on it to keep it from falling out. Real suave, huh? But it spoke volumes about his daring personality. He wasn't afraid of someone telling his mom, who worked at the city's utility's front office just over one block, about her juvenile-aged son walking on the streets smoking. And, it couldn't be just a cigarette. Oh, No, it had to be a cigar! I liked this guy's cavalier attitude. I liked it a lot. He made me laugh. (He still does!)

If it's true that opposites attract then we, as a couple, are another statistic for the record. I loved to read, took Ballet and Modern Dance for twelve years, played the flute in the band for seven years, was a Girl Scout, was a majorette with the marching band, won Freshman Beauty in our high school beauty pageant, was a Knoxville Teen Board Presentee, and was voted Most Feminine our senior year for the senior superlatives.

David played catcher for a baseball team (with a real gift for loudly mouthing off to the batters to throw them off their game and at many of these games I sat with his grandparents at their insistence), played varsity football in seventh and eighth grade, and in high school. He was *always* playing basketball every weekend, and he sang and played in a band. (Our good friend Steve Cochran played guitar with him and went on to be the Singer/Entertainer, Juice Newton's, lead guitarist for many years. He once wrote a song about our Windy. He and Steve also bought motorcycles and rode to Myrtle Beach a few times.)

David was dedicated to weight-lifting, and he also ran to stay fit. He was voted 'Most Masculine' our Senior year! He refused to be my escort at the Teen Board Presentation and Dance because he thought "it was ridiculous and pretentious". (I'm grateful to Tom McBryde for stepping in and acting like a big brother to me, and being my kind escort! Tom was *my* best friend, Martha's, brother and is a gifted musician. He grew up to become Dolly Parton's Music Director/Producer at Dollywood, and is a well-known pianist, composer, and music producer in Nashville.)

(All these great musicians, no wonder music has been so important to David and me all of our lives, and in special highlights in our lives, a tune will play in our heads that just fits the event taking place! Not to mention my parents *always* had beautiful music playing on their stereo system in our family room when we were growing up. Music is still an important part of our lives.)

David was a bit of a daredevil (okay, more than a bit), and he was never afraid to try something new. (He definitely got me out of my comfort zone in a hurry!) An example of his "daredevil behavior": Once when we were in high school, he (the youngest of three brothers) and a best friend, David Jones (the youngest of four brothers), came riding up to my front door one Saturday afternoon on horses, bareback . . . and wearing only blue jeans, no shirts and no shoes. Now if you don't think I envisioned my knight on horseback looking just like this, think again! The two of them were *so* cute, both a bit sunburned, both with curly medium brown hair and "killer smiles". All the girls in town were crazy about them, and they probably could have "lassoed-in" their pick. A fact not lost on the two of them, for sure! They had jumped on David J.'s horses on a whim, and ridden through the fields, up the hill, and down a neighborhood street or two, to come over to visit. They didn't ride up quietly, either. Nope. They sang the song *"Tennessee Stud"* at the top of their lungs in a serenade to me as they trotted into my front yard. (I'm not saying they had had a few beers before they had made the trip. But I'm not saying they *hadn't* either.)

I came out on the front porch to listen and laugh with them in their merriment. Then I shushed them up before my daddy came out to find them out! It was definitely official: I was hopelessly and helplessly in love with David Smith! Despite my parents' reluctance to me dating "that Smith boy" (I guess they had heard about some of his shenanigans too.), My parents grew to love him as a true son. (Even more miraculous.) I had always tried to obey my parents . . . note the word tried . . . but I could not eradicate him from my thoughts or heart. David says he loved my twinkling brown eyes and could see the light from within I seemed to have, and swears to this day he can't remember a time that he wasn't in love with me. For a rambunctious boy he sure grew up to be a romantic man, and he passed that know-how on to our sons. It's a gift for men to woo the woman in their life in a godly way—a rarity in today's world.

We spent hours and hours talking on the phone. We came to know each other's thoughts, hopes and dreams. (Still think God doesn't perform miracles today? David grew up to be an eye doctor who has tenderly cared for the vision of several of our school teachers as they grew older. I even went with him on several house calls to see them. That they knew him as a kid, and then would someday trust him with their vision, is a miracle to us!)

We both had friends of the opposite sex in school, friends that we talked to, and enjoyed going in large groups to ballgames and school functions with. We have always liked being around friends, but we basically dated only each other through high school. Our friends always considered us "a couple" We got mad and broke up a few times, to date other people—sometimes determined to be apart—to give ourselves a chance to maybe find someone else—only to find that these brief, miserable separations confirmed all the more that we didn't like to be away from each other. (The time away was made more profound by playing the big sixties hit song, *Walk On By*, written by Burt Bacharach, and sung by Dionne Warwick, really loud, and repeatedly, on my record player in my bedroom at home during those painful break-ups. Running around with friends helped ease that pain too. He would hang out with the Hedden boys or one of the Fox boys. I was always with Ann, Martha, Patti, Carolyn, Deane, Pat, Barbara, and others)

We both came to know about Christ in different ways. Sounds crazy I know, but I became a Christian in a mimosa tree when I was eleven years old. I had climbed up alone, but I climbed down with Jesus in control of my heart. I also knew I had somehow been forgiven for anything and everything I had ever done in my life so far because Jesus had died for me. I knew instantly that I was somehow of a different mindset. I had attended a Vacation Bible School at my church, and a special speaker's talk had made me ask questions of myself about my own existence, and made me wonder what this person named Jesus had to do with my life. (Our sweet housekeeper/substitute grandmother, Maude Webber, asked my brother and me this question all though our childhood.)

He was always there, I just had never known what to call Him or how to exactly please Him with my behavior and life. I wish I could say I came down out of that tree and instantly lived a God-led life. But I can't say that. I still acted like a self-centered child most of the time, but God was already teaching me about His great love for me, about His precepts, and how He wanted to guide me as I continued to attend church and began to read my Bible, little verse by little verse. It would be eight more years until I gave my whole life to Him: gave Him the seat of honor in my life, forever.

David took me to hear Billy Graham when he spoke at a large citywide crusade in Knoxville, at Neyland Stadium, in 1970, about a month before our high school graduation was to take place. When Evangelist Graham finished speaking in his simple, direct, powerful message, he stood and bowed his head, lifted his long arms up into the air, palms open and facing the thousands before him, and urged people to come forward, unashamed, to "Give your life to Jesus!" With our heads bowed, and eyes closed, I was feeling the strong urge to get up and make a public confession, and to make a movement toward the ministers placed down on the field when suddenly I was surprised to feel David patting me on the arm, "Let's go!" he said to me in a loving command. He got up from his seat, grabbed my hand, and we began the long walk to the stage down front. He asked Jesus to be the Lord of his life as he stood and prayed with one of the ministers. I rededicated my life to Christ as I bowed my head and prayed with them. I was impressed with how David was not ashamed to confess his sins and to openly vow to put Jesus first.

We didn't fully understand what we had just done . . . we just knew we had to do it, or we would have had no peace within our own hearts. In time we would learn how to live lives closer to how God wanted us to live. That He forgave us of our sins and would show us through his Word how to do that. It would take time—the rest of our lives. We would still make mistakes, still sin, but God would forgive us as we confessed and tried to do the right things. He would be with us, be in our hearts, to guide us every step of the way. It was a big night in our lives, we changed that night for the better. We would need that firm foundation for our future lives together. We also knew in our hearts that somehow, someday, we would be living our lives as husband and wife.

Our parents must have recognized the signs of love. My parents had gotten married at age twenty-two after paying attention to each other beginning at age twelve. They celebrated almost seventy years of marriage together. David's parents had gotten married when Juanita was only sixteen and Bill was eighteen. They were married almost sixty years when Papaw Bill passed away. The four of them *knew* what real love was.

We married during Christmas break of our Sophomore year in college, in the very same church we first saw each other. Married on my paternal grandparents' anniversary date (they were married for sixty-eight years). Our wedding was also in the same month, and in the same church my parents were married in thirty-one years before us. Already we were steeped in tradition even though we had just begun our lives together.

We were young and didn't have but a few hundred dollars between us (David sold his motorcycle to give us some spendable income), yet we were very much in love. We were excited and scared. Our schedules kept us busy. We had winter college classes to register for, and it was time to declare our majors. There were so many details to work out!

We learned early on to live each day to the fullest, and yet, to strategically plan for our future by writing out realistic goals. We were always inserting some dreams and hopes to work toward. We kept a running list of weekly goals, monthly goals, and on up to yearly goals. We liked to plan out each step in our education and future. We probably thought we were really pretty much in control of our own "destiny." So neat and orderly it all looked on the calendar for the year 1971. We were soon to learn that we were not in charge of anything, especially our future. Now, we can say we were blessed to learn early in our married lives that God was really in control of all things in our lives. But it didn't resemble anything close to a blessing to us, at first. No, not at first.

> David's tenacity and drive has helped make him a wonderful husband and father. God has tempered his take-charge attitude i.e., find a solution for a problem and

fix it immediately, with a tenderness and gentleness, which has complimented our different personalities. Over the years we have overlapped these traits, and at times even reversed them, emulating each other. A phenomenon we've found that happens when you're married for a while. (As Sylvester Stallone said in the movie *Rocky,* we "fill gaps.") It was helpful in raising children, especially a child with a disability. At different phases and times in their lives, we needed all those attributes as parents.

Our job was to be the best parents we could be. Mistakes would be made; we wouldn't be without imperfection, far from it, but we could strive for our personal best. It was a goal, and it kept us mindful and motivated.

We were ready to go back to East Tennessee for a visit. We had lots of family to introduce Windy to. We instinctively knew they would love her and treat her with dignity and respect, for she was one of us, after all. There was such comfort in that.

Windy grew into the cutest petite toddler. She was smaller in stature than her brother and looked younger than she really was. Everyone who saw her out and about always guessed her age quite a bit off the true answer. (The same thing still happens to her as an adult. Although we have tried to explain to her that people think it is really good to look younger than your actual age, she doesn't buy into all that. She wants to look older. Birthdays to her and to her friends are *very* big deals.)

Even while Windy was a tiny baby just catching on to the art of nursing, we would exercise her little legs and arms. This might be going overboard. Okay, it was going *way* overboard, and we did become conscious that we had to let the child rest some. But we were so intent upon helping her get stronger and developing her muscle strength, we felt like every second counted. We soon realized that downtime and rest is sometimes as important as the impending schedule, and we all needed to know when to implement both for balance in our lives. We learned as we went. One good thing about having children while you are young is ... you learn and grow up as they do. One bad thing about having children while you are young is . . . you learn and grow up as they do!

There are both advantages and disadvantages in being a younger parent. We tried our best with the knowledge we had to work with at the time. It doesn't mean we were the perfect parents, or the worst parents. We did try our best to be godly examples to our children, so they would hear and see us as we walked out our faith before them.

Day by day our daughter *did* grow stronger, and she learned to roll over, to sit up, and then to crawl. A milestone accomplished, she was mobile!

I fixed Windy's hair in little pigtails that bounced as she crawled. Boy, did she crawl! She crawled in a crab-like position with her fanny in the air, no knees on the ground, straight legged. Then Aunt Dede made more elastic bands, this time for her ankles only. She sewed them together, which kept her feet together, and she was forced to put her knees down and to crawl in the regular way, for the sake of full gross motor development. Bands weren't keeping her from being on the move. Then when she walked across our living room floor at thirteen months old, we screamed so loudly, she promptly plopped down to sit and grin at us. She thought about the whole process, and pondered our weird reaction for a few days until her next brave attempt.

Early on, Windy displayed a real cute sense of humor that she revealed in special ways, once she could move about unassisted. She discovered it was fun to hide from us, and she could get into the smallest of spaces. Once she hid in a large crock. It was a twenty-gallon size, and we had proudly displayed it in the corner of our living room. We never thought to look inside of it as the three us called out her name. We went all over our apartment in search of her. It took us awhile to discover her, crouched, still and silent, in her endeavor to fool us. She proved she could wait us out.

On another day, she proved she could also be a partner in crime with her brother. She had slipped quietly out of her stroller in Goldsmith's Department Store (Didn't know she could do that yet.), while I had my back turned preparing to pay for something. It was a wonderful department store, not too far from our home, and the kids always loved going there with me, especially at Christmas to see their spectacular Christmas Santa Land display in the tunnel leading from the parking area to a main entrance.

Sensing I was busy, they crawled under the rounder holding clothes on hangers, and she and Davey began to methodically pull off the price tags of as many items as they could. As it turned out, they were tremendously good at it, and very fast I might add. When I made my purchase and turned around, they came out with their hands full of tell-tale signs of their activities. Davey offered his pile to me remorsefully. Windy stood up and shrugged her shoulders with a large smile; she looked just like the little mouse in *Stewart Little*, only it was years before that movie would be released. You know the look I'm talking about here. I was *so* embarrassed, and we soon found out that the sales person waiting on me had a real humor deficiency. I confessed to their actions and apologized profusely. I had the kids apologize to help teach them a lesson in owning up to their actions, and we made a quick exit. Thank goodness it was before stores had cameras.

Like most moms, I always wanted my children to look clean and neat. I went beyond neat and clean with our daughter. (If strangers were bent on staring, then they were going to be pleasantly stunned by her cuteness!) So I would fix her hair everyday and tie gingham ribbons in it to match the color of her outfits. I wanted people to first see the pretty little girl before they saw that she had Down syndrome. I prayed they would think she was as beautiful as we thought she was.

We didn't have much income to spend on clothes, so it was a blessing when our moms would send us extra money for their grandchildren to have new outfits. Windy wore many of my niece, Kristi's, old clothes that she had outgrown. They were coordinated outfits with matching jackets, tights, and even matching hair bows. People always commented on how nicely we dressed her and how cute she looked.

One particular day Windy and Davey looked extremely cute playing on the playground at Edison Park where we lived. They wore new little shorts and shirts. They were a study in contrast: Davey was such a handsome little guy, tall for his age, with straight blonde hair trimmed in a Buster Brown haircut, and Windy was petite, short for her age, with long dark brown hair. Davey was holding onto a rung of a ladder while reaching out his free arm to Windy on a rung below him. He was always helping his little sis. (Davey watched her *so* carefully, even from the very first. I worried about him acting more like a grown-up and not a carefree little boy at times. He knew, almost innately, that he needed to look after her well-being. He felt she needed him, and he always wanted to help her.)

Playing in the sunshine, I thought they looked so beautiful. They caught the attention of a photographer for the *Memphis Press Scimitar,* who happened to be walking by on the way to an assignment. He had a large camera hanging on a strap around his neck. He stopped to smile at them, and then turned to ask me if he could take their picture for the paper! Not only did I think they were darling, but a stranger did too! It had been confirmed by an unbiased opinion!

My heart was brimming with pride as he stepped in to get a shot of them climbing on the huge wooden play structure with the tall downtown buildings in the background, and that's when I saw something different about her outfit. I suddenly noticed her discarded training pants not far from her feet, yet for the most part hidden behind a railroad tie at the backside of the ladder. I sure hoped the photographer hadn't noticed, and he didn't. He thanked the kids and went on his way. Thank heavens! Apparently she had quickly taken them off because she couldn't stand a wet diaper and had stepped back into her shorts while I was reading on the bench beside them. Detecting her movements in my peripheral vision as I read, lead me to think she was only playing in the sandbox. I had completely missed her "kid on a mission" motive. (She was real easy to potty train we can happily say, but not too easy on her mom's sense of propriety or modesty at times!)

We still have the newspaper clipping of the two of them, our precious little preschoolers, looking like they had just conquered the downtown Memphis skyline, from the angle it was snapped. Like Batman and Robin, or as the photographer described them: as "King Kong and Faye Wray". It was the first of many pictures Windy would have in a newspaper. We stuck it in a small photo album. If we had known then what we know now, we would have bought a really *big* album for *all* the pictures that she would have taken on future occasions by many more newspaper and television photographers!

Pictures by her, and of her, have hung in: the White House West Wing with First Lady, Laura Bush, and in New York's Time Square. Her artwork has hung in the Capitol Rotunda and in the Special Arts Office in D.C., in the Gymnastic Gym in Knoxville, and in the Office of the Knoxville Sports Association of the AAU Junior Olympics, Knoxville, Tennessee, in artist Robert Tino's studio in Highlands, North Carolina, in school classrooms around the country, and in Sam and Andy's Restaurant in Farragut on their "Wall of Fame", which is mainly comprised of the University of Tennessee's current and former athletes and coaches.

During those Memphis days, our daily routine was really no different than any other young family in their day-to-day lives. Davey was a busy little boy who loved to be outdoors, and Windy loved to be with Davey. They got to know all the kids in the apartment complex either at their backyard sandbox David made for them, or while riding Big Wheels on the empty basketball court. It was a challenge to get them to come in for a nap or for bath time.

David and I played music in abundance for them. They became familiar with the music of Gino Vannelli, Barefoot Jerry, The Beach Boys, Yes, Poco, Bert Bacharach, John Denver, Stevie Wonder and Kenny Loggins. (And yes, we do know our taste in music was, and still is, all over the place!) They loved to dance around our living room with us. They also memorized words to their favorite songs. (I wish I had a dollar for every time they sang the words "Rocky Mountain High...Colorado"!) They played with their good friends, Jason and Vanessa, Alisha, Heather and others.

They played with children from varied racial and ethnic backgrounds. This exposure to one another at a young age was healthy and beneficial. They were a diverse group of kids who liked to play together, and they learned to share and to get along.

Davey loved Windy from the minute we brought her home to him. He treated his sister like one of the gang, and the other children playing with them took their cue from him. This attitude proved greatly beneficial to Windy's overall social development. As he grew and matured, he became very sensitive to anyone with a disability and always took up for them in his school years.

He became a champion of someone weaker, just as their younger brother Mikey did while he was growing up. They educated others about the proper way to treat people who have disabilities, with respect by the words they used and by the example they set. A few times they even got into scuffles on the playground over defending their sister's, or someone else's, honor. If anyone ever made fun or said a derogatory word to someone with a disability, they wouldn't tolerate it. Now that they are grown men, both are still guardians of people with disabilities. It was a wonderful blessing for our young boys to develop this attribute, to protect those who need more protection, and it was a direct result of being raised with a sibling who has a disability. They loved her and wanted everyone to know that their sister, and all other children who had a disability, had the God-given right to be respected and to be treated with kindness.

David and I had been *exceedingly* concerned about the effects on our son, and any future children, when they became old enough to be conscious of the fact that they had a sibling who had a disability. What would it mean to their own development and relationships with us and with their friends? How would it negatively affect them? How could it positively affect them? This is a heavy-on-your-heart concern all families like ours face. We certainly were not intentionally going to spend more time with Windy and leave our other children to rear themselves. We wanted desperately to be fair to each child, with our love, and time and thoughts. Naturally some care for Windy would probably take more time, but if we remained conscious of it, we believed we could make up for the time to them in other ways, and at other times. One solid defining phrase of a great parent is "an accomplished juggler" of all the above mentioned attributes, and we did our best to achieve that.

Most importantly now, our sons say we did a wonderful job raising them and loving them. They have a confidence no one can take away because they know they are loved unconditionally for who they are as individuals. That's good enough for us; they are the authorities in this area after all, since they have lived it. We know that a lot of parents struggle with this issue as they seek to raise their family. It is a tough situation, but one that needs to be discussed openly between the parents, and also with their children. How super it would be to tell you that once that's decided, you won't have to think about it again, but that's not the case. This is something that is best reevaluated periodically. Kids need varying amounts of time and care at different stages of life. Families can easily get into "routine ruts" and have to take the time to stand back and see where each individual is at the time, and adjustments need to be made. But this would all still hold true, even without a special needs child in the mix!

> David and I have now seen many families that have a family member that has a disability, and our hearts have been touched by the grown siblings' compassion, and for the great strides they have made in society for this segment of the population they hold dear. In 2002 we were very impressed with a man we all met on the Presidential committee (PCPID) Windy would be appointed to, her fellow committee member, Jim Brett,

who had a brother born with a disability. Jim grew up to represent people like his brother in the political arena and sacrificed many an hour to make his home state of Massachusetts more acceptable for anyone with a disability. Like Jim, instead of hurting or hindering our boys by being a sibling of someone with a disability, it was the *making* of them. (This would have given us great hope. But at the time, we didn't know many families that fit into that category.)

Comprehendible speech had become one of our BIG goals. David and I brainstormed ways to conquer language skills. I wrote as fast as the ideas came to us. Here's where tenacity paid off. We weren't qualified speech therapists, but we didn't let that stop us from thinking up innovative strategies: ways to get Windy talking with *proper* diction. She had to learn the grammar and language skills while she was tiny. Once learned, we were afraid she would never relearn the right way. There was nothing out there to tell us anything about her speech. We just used good old common sense and applied the same teaching skills with her as we were using with her brother as we taught him proper speech.

By golly, it had to work! In college I was majoring in Early Education. I decided to stay home and teach my own children. There was no preschool for them to attend. There was certainly no preschool for a toddler who had a disability. This was groundbreaking education for all of us, and I took my job seriously. If I failed, they would ultimately be the losers. That just wasn't going to happen on my watch!

All the kids we've known that have Down syndrome, have always been wonderful communicators. It didn't matter too much that the words some of them spoke weren't readily understandable. They proved very adept at *nonverbal skills* to get what they wanted or needed. We watched some of the older kids in Windy's group sessions act out their wishes instead of using words. Windy was no exception. David and I agreed we weren't going to let her stubbornness in this area limit her communication. It obviously was going to be an ongoing battle. Thank goodness we had tutor Davey to help us with this!

We became *exceptionally* concerned about her speech being discernible. Verbal communication is a basic life skill that would assist her, not only in voicing her needs and wants as she began to interact with other people, but it would allow her to be more independent and accepted in society. When she did began speaking, she really didn't try to articulate any word clearly. We tried many times to say words to her, repeating them slowly and methodically, as we held up a toy or food or whatever it was that she wanted at the time, as she pointed to the item with a grunt or squeal. We were not above giving her bribes or enticing her to pronounce words correctly.

Windy loved the taste of peanut butter and became quite a mime at asking for a peanut butter cracker. She showed great thinking skills as she used many different approaches with us to get her way. It took planning and strategy on her part to "work us over" in this manner. Surely this was reason enough to believe she could learn to talk if she wanted to badly enough. We *knew* she was very smart.

Some parents during this time were beginning to teach their children with DS some sign language to be able to communicate with them better since their speech is generally delayed. They were starting a class for parents and children at the CDC. They called to invite us to join the class. We went to watch one day, and we declined. We felt in our particular situation that Windy might not try as hard if we went that route. Some children seemed to thrive on this new level of communication, and it made life a lot easier for their families, we were told later on. We were glad for them, but we wanted Windy to be able to interact with people everywhere we took her, and we knew not everyone would know sign language. We felt she would need to learn to speak, if it was possible. I know many children have learned sign language and use both modes, and that's terrific. This is our reasoning for choosing audible speech only. It's imperative to establish some form of communication, as early as possible, but each child, and each family situation is different. Of course, especially for those born with hearing impairments, sign language learned early is wonderful. We've seen entire extended families learn to sign together, and they grew in *all* their communication skills.

Since we had already had Windy's hearing tested, and she had no hearing problems, we opted out of sign language. It was the right decision for our family. We were going against the thinking of the popular medical professionals of the time. We were even dismissed as ignorant thinkers by one speech therapist we came into contact with at CDC, but we were determined "to stick to our guns". We probably looked foolish to her, but this was our kid in the real science lab of our lives, not some hypothetical situation. We felt we were on the right track, but with no backup, and we only had one chance to get it right. Pressure was high!

One afternoon, I became exasperated with Windy's nonverbal request for her favorite snack. I had reached my limit. She would swipe one hand over the palm of her open hand indicating she wanted a cracker with peanut butter spread on it, She had a way of ignoring what I said and pushing with her evident strong-willed determination to get what she wanted without having to say one little word. If minutes went by without her request being answered, she got more forceful with the gestures. She would slap her little hands and swipe harder to get my attention, sometimes accompanied by a vexed expression. Usually I gave in because I was in a hurry or busy doing something else. It was too easy to make a snack and hand it to her. She was a smart little cookie, a great mimic . . . she already had the system figured out, and to her advantage I might add!

On this certain day I was up for the "combat" I knew was bound to occur, and I decided I would not give in to her; I was going to try to *make* her talk. It was all for her sake, for her future, but I knew she wouldn't know or care about any of that. Instant gratification was her goal. Learning great communication skills was not a top priority for her at the moment. It was for her mom though! I knew she desperately needed to learn to speak clearly. If I had known she would speak to millions of people on a live, televised program someday, and have conversations with future Governors and Presidents, I would have been in a big hurry to teach her to speak, and I would have driven us both batty in the process.

That day in our little kitchen, I made a big production out of the object of her cravings. I showed her the jar of peanut butter and the box of crackers on the kitchen countertop, over her head and just out of her reach. I wanted her to get a good visual and to understand just what was at stake. She sat down on the floor to ponder this new situation, folded her legs and crossed them at the ankles, and then placed her elbows on her legs and set her chin on the two fists she had made of her hands. I promptly sat down beside her, purposely looking up at the food items, while repeating *over* and *over* the word "pea-nut-but-ter." I believed that if my enunciation was distinct and direct, hers would be also.

She grew frustrated with me, *very* frustrated, and laid down on the floor, on her back, glaring at me. (Thank goodness big brother was taking a nap. He could not have stood these intense moments as Windy was being denied food! I would have been in BIG trouble.) We remained on the floor for a *long* time. I lost track of time. Two stubborn Smith girls sat in that Memphis sunshine streaming in our small kitchen window, watching the shadows move across the floor, as time passed. Finally, in desperation, she yelled at the top of her lungs, "Pa-pun-nee." Now that may not sound like any word you have ever heard, but it was perfect diction to my ears. It was her first real word and her first verbal attempt to speak, albeit a stretch for the word peanut butter, but a real breakthrough nonetheless. Needless to say, she was so full of peanut butter crackers that night, after repeating her word and receiving crackers all afternoon, that she did not want any dinner. (We'd work on the words "Thank you" tomorrow.) That was fine with me!

That night big brother got to stay up alone to spend some special time with Mommy and Daddy because little sister hit the bed early, probably from sheer fatigue from talking too much! She had grinned so big at her daddy when I had related her breakthrough to him. She was really proud of herself, quite smug about it, really. She had discovered that the spoken word could bring her instant gratification, and she was really into *that*. It was a big turning point in her mental development, and she couldn't learn words fast enough in the days that followed. She repeated *everything* Davey said. It was as if he had a tiny parrot following him around all day. They both thought it was hilarious and would giggle like crazy over it. He was a natural teacher!

Windy was quickly developing her own personality. She learned to say, "Indy's turn" when she meant it was her turn at whatever the other kids were playing. She wasn't *about* to stand quietly back and be satisfied with watching everybody else have fun. She *wanted* in the games! We don't know if the other kids always understood what she said, but her brother interpreted for her when there was any doubt. He *always* knew what she was saying, even when *we* didn't. We were blown away about that. She would jibber something, because she loved to talk, and when we asked, or guessed, all the wrong things, Davey would chime in with the right choice of words, and she would nod her little head yes, as if to say, "OH, YES! Finally someone who understands me!"

If you have ever been to another country where they don't speak your native tongue and someone comes up who speaks your language and comprehends what you are trying to say, you know that feeling of relief and elation you have at finally being understood. Windy must have felt that on a daily basis—in her own country, surrounded by people who *supposedly* spoke her native tongue. In this language challenge, we witnessed her frustration with us and with other adults. We had to help her cross this language barrier somehow, or be prepared for her to be frustrated for a lifetime. We weren't going to accept this as a hurdle we couldn't cross. Better some frustration now, than a lot of frustration later.

Chapter Five
Learning about the World

Next hurdle, as far as David and I were concerned, came in under the appearance category. We had noticed that some of the people we had met, who had been born with DS, kept their tongue held slightly out of their lips. We learned there was a consensus of physicians who felt that many of the children were born with a smaller than normal palate, or roof of mouth, and some said they had a larger than normal tongue. Whatever caused this abnormality to happen, we wanted to know if there was anything *we* could do to help Windy keep her tongue *in* her mouth.

When we mentioned this to a nurse at the Child Development Center, she told us that we might try peanut butter placed on the roof of her mouth to make her aware of her tongue movements and hopefully to help her learn to control it better. I'm sure there is much newer research now on the subject but good old peanut butter sure came in handy, again. Wish we had bought stock in Jiffy or Peter Pan, or some other leading brand. (If you try this, please note: Just be sure there are no peanut allergies!) We used jars and jars of the stuff, and so did our friends with little kiddies. It was great for so many things: quick snacks, fold-over sandwiches, a great tool for teaching speech skills, and for taking bubble gum out of their hair. Don't ask. All I'm saying is Davey and Windy both needed this removal treatment on several occasions during a five-year period. I like to remember it as their 'bubble days'!

We were always applying a little scoop of peanut butter on our finger, out of an ever-ready jar that sat on the counter top and sticking it in Windy's mouth, while saying, "Tongue in, please!" Once again, it was big brother to the rescue! Davey became the self-appointed instructor in this. He tirelessly climbed up on a foot stool, swiped his little finger in the jar, and stepped back down to run and put his offering into his sister's mouth, *always* with the instructive words, "Tongue, please." She caught on quickly, and soon all we had to do was say the words.

    I had almost forgotten the work that had gone into helping her to be aware of her tongue-thrust when, *years* later, I looked over to see her put her tongue out before taking a basketball shot in our driveway at home. "Windy, tongue!" I admonished, out of old habit, as I walked by with bags of groceries in both hands, just returning from the store. "Mom, Michael Jordan does it this way, and I'm going to, too!" she said decidedly. "He does, Mom!" her younger brother, Mikey affirmed, while he shot a lay-up with his tongue mimicking his favorite pro athlete of the time. They were both right. We had all seen him do it on a televised game, and it sure hadn't hurt his game, or his tongue for that matter!

Our children loved to have us read to them, and they would always listen intently as we read aloud. They were learning about the great big world out there. At home we read to them from books before they could even understand the words. They would become so quiet and listened attentively to the melodious words of Robert Louis Stevenson's poems such as, *The Land of Counterpane,* sounding so strange and lyrical to their little ears. All I had to do was begin reading aloud, and they would stop whatever they were doing to walk over to look at the colorful pages, instantly drawn to the spoken words transporting them to another place and a different time.

    We read them story after story, night after night, before we said prayers and tucked them in bed. The routine was anticipated and expected. Whenever anyone asked what gifts they could give our kids, I always answered, "Books, please!" We built up quite a library of children's literature. We wore out *Good-night Moon,* by Margaret Wise Brown, and some other old favorites. Davey would follow along and Windy would try to turn the pages before we were ready to turn them. I would take her tiny hand and place it on my mouth and neck as I spoke, so she could feel the words as I formed them. I also took her finger, or Davey's, and would glide it over the words I was saying aloud.

It wasn't long before she began to "read" to her dolls in a "sing-song" way that made her laugh aloud at herself. Her little voice was a bit deep and raspy sounding, very common for someone with DS we learned. We all thought she sounded like an angel: she could talk in sentences! We had broken the language barrier. She began putting words together and experimenting with our reactions to them. She would still need speech therapy to perfect her diction, but we were relentless in making her repeat a string of words correctly: our attempt at preschool home-schooling.

I sometimes felt a bit like Anne Sullivan in Helen Keller's life story. I had read a book about her life when I was a teenager, and I had watched an old black and white movie with the role of Helen played by Patty Duke, when Patty was only a child herself. I figured if those teaching methods had worked for her—someone born completely blind and deaf, and yet successfully taught to speak—they would surely work for Windy, because she could *see* the formation of our mouths and facial expressions. She learned the word "No" and how to use it. At least it was a milestone, albeit not a pleasant one at times!

A bonus was her influence on Davey, and his influence on her. He became a great role model and instructed her on washing her hands, picking up toys, and he gave her verbal and physical instruction as he taught her in the many advantageous ways to move a chair around a room. Their favorite chair maneuver was to slide one from the dining room to the kitchen cabinet so they could climb up and get a cookie without having to bother Mommy or Daddy. Anything he told her to do, she never questioned. She was all in! His tutoring wasn't limited to the indoors. The great outdoors was a wonderful place to teach her about sports and gross motor skills. He taught her how to catch a ball and to run "like the wind". He was the perfect big brother, and she adored him . . . always has and always will!

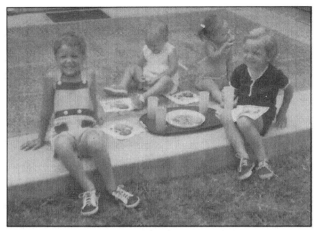
Picnicking on the patio with the Heady kids

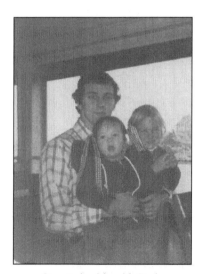
On a train ride with Dad

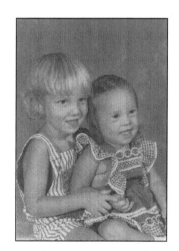
Sister (2 years-old) and
Brother (3 years-old)

Chapter Six
Making Life-Long Friends

Thankfully, some of life's pressure was lessening some. Our children were moving about on their own, starting to dress themselves some, and satisfied to play around the house for longer periods, without my intervention.

Family began to visit more frequently. God was so good! He didn't allow the loneliness period in our lives to last forever! My parents came numerous times. Bill and Juanita came several times and brought the grandmothers back to see us. My brother, Chip, and his friend, Gary Harbor, made the trip multiple times. They would watch the kids for me while I got things done around the house. (They were really good babysitters, especially since they were teenage boys, who had never babysat before!). Davey and Windy adored fun-loving Uncle Chip and Gary. Dede and her family piled in the car to come our way when they could. David's brother, Richard, came to see us, too. He had driven a rental truck to West Tennessee loaded with our furniture when we first moved in. He came back to see us, to see how we had arranged everything.

When family wasn't visiting, David and I felt it was a good time to start inviting people over, so our kids could get used to strangers and learn not to be shy. Sam Kincaid, a friend in medical school who lived nearby with his new bride, Janie, would stop in and stand on his head in the middle of our living room floor, just to make Davey and Windy laugh. His "off the wall antics" always made them laugh. (Come to think of it, he was also good at going into our kitchen and helping himself to something to eat without bothering 'Mommy and Daddy, too!' I think he always felt relaxed and at home, and since I cooked all the time, we always had leftovers in the fridge. Sam did *not* suffer from shyness!)

Linda and Ronnie Hendricks moved in just a few doors down from us with their daughter, Heather, and we visited numerous times with them. They were in Memphis while Ronnie attended dental school. We had gone to high school with them. Linda was kind enough to babysit our children some when I finally went back to school for a class. Martha McBryde (Borthen), my best friend from grade school days, came to see us from another state a few times and kept up with us via letters and phone calls. She later became a teacher of young children. My first cousin, Ann Brown (now Dr. Thomason), who grew up with us, enrolled in medical school in Memphis and came over to help with the kids' bath time on an occasion. She always enjoyed hearing of their recent escapades. Judy Brummitt (now Fuhrman), a friend from home, visited us a few times and always came to our parents' houses to see the kids when we went back to Clinton. Sam Brown, David's best friend from our high school days, more than once, drove over ten hours to see us. Sam was in Medical school at Duke and later became an orthopedic surgeon.

It was so good for us to have friends we could speak honestly with about our feelings and future dreams for our lives. It was, in turn, beneficial for them to learn from a parent's point of view what it was like to raise a child with a disability. To those in medical school, it would be enriching to their future medical practices, as it would give them a deeper appreciation of what their future patients with disabilities, and their families, were experiencing. We were all wading in waters we had never waded in before. The best way to learn to swim in those waters was to ask the hard questions and to give honest answers to those questions when they came up. We never minded answering anything asked us. This became part of David's and my mission in life—to educate and help others understand that people with an intellectual disability could learn and grow like all other children.

One vivid memory of Sam and the hard questions comes to the surface quiet poignantly. We doubt if he even remembers asking us this question back in '72, but we have never forgotten it because it was one of those hypothetical questions that we later had to ask ourselves in reality. David and I had gone over to his apartment and were sharing our excitement and amazement about our first baby on the way. The song *"Stairway to Heaven"* was playing in the background. David and Sam loved the musical run of the song by Led Zeppelin and to this day they still enjoy sharing good music with each other. We were all relaxing in beanbag chairs having a rare unhurried chat face to face with close friends with no pressing school assignment. In the middle of our conversation, Sam asked if we had ever considered what we would do if our baby were born with a disability, say for instance, a mongoloid child. (His choice of words before Down syndrome was the accepted medical term. He was in Pre-Med and had just studied the medical condition, so it was foremost on his mind that day.)

We answered by saying we honestly had not considered the possibility. Surely that couldn't happen to *us*. It was probably a hereditary trait that would cause a child to be born with any type of disability, right? We discussed what we would do . . . that we would accept the child as God sent him/her. It seemed so far reaching to us. We didn't need to think about that at all. And we were right, not with our first child.

Barely sixteen months later we would face that *very* question head-on. The great thing about that inquiry was a conclusion we arrived at together before the need arose to address it. We felt if God would send us a child, we would take the one He created, hidden away from human eyes, until the child's birth. (Just think, we were already educating one of those young future 'Docs' about the great potential of a child with special needs! Sam has had the privilege and honor of knowing Windy from her birth and witnessing her growth and grace as she grew up.)

Phil and Brenda Wenk and their daughter Andrea were more friends who came to our apartment, and we shared in the celebrations of our children's birthday parties. We had gone to school with Phil, another "hometown" boy. When his mom and dad, Phil Sr. and Pat, came to visit them, they always invited us out to go to dinner at a nice restaurant, and they insisted on paying for our meal. (Our parents reciprocated when they came to town.) What a treat it was to ditch the blue jeans, our everyday attire, and dress up to go out—a blessing for poor students, who had to watch every penny! Phil was a real help to Windy in those early years. He was in Dental school at the time, and when her teeth began to come in, he was concerned, as were we, that they were becoming discolored and much softer than normal. He set up an appointment for us to go to a dentist he knew, a professor of his. After assessing her dental health, they decided to put silver caps on her baby teeth to protect them and hopefully enable them to stay in until her permanent teeth appeared.

We took her to UT Dental School when she was two-years old to have the procedure done. They had to put her to sleep for the intensive process. She came out smiling with a really shiny smile, all her little front teeth were covered in tiny silver caps. It bothered me that she had a different looking smile. (One more thing to make her look different from everyone else. I was grateful, but sad, too. I have to be honest here.) I conceded to this beneficial alternative. When her permanent teeth came in later, they grew in white and beautiful! (She did have to wear braces to correct some crooked teeth later on, and so did her brothers, but not until years later when she became a 'Tween-Ager'. Thanks to the expertise of a compassionate friend and an excellent orthodontist, Dr. John Pryse, and thanks to another dentist, Dr. Mark Caldwell, her smile became even better. Then at age fourteen the braces came off, and her smile was finally perfect!)

We formed some very special bonds with friends in David's class at Southern College of Optometry during those years in Memphis. Dub and Lynn Moore, Ralph and Shirley Mullins, Tom and Carol Roberson, and Dan and Diane Schimmel came over to play Chinese Checkers or a board game of some type many nights. We went to the Memphis Zoo and picnicked at Overton Park on beautiful Saturday afternoons. It was cheap entertainment; we were all on student budgets, and there was no cable television or movie rentals invented yet! We shared many nights of food and fellowship. (Our Windy and Mikey ended up attending the same high school as the Schimmel boys. And the Moore kids, Joseph, Beka, and Margaret are very close friends to our three kids. The Roberson kids are friends of our kids, too. Even in adulthood they all keep up with each other!)

David met Dub, Tom, and Ralph in a unique way. It was their very first day of school, the day Windy was born. They were all standing in line to register for classes and they began to talk. David had been up all night, and he'd received the disturbing news of his tiny daughter's birth. He still had to go to his new school to register for classes and get all his books on that fateful September twenty-fourth. The guys directly in front, and behind him, began to talk as they waited. They introduced themselves to David, giving their names as Tom, Dub and Ralph. They asked if he was married, and if he had any children. At the time the three new guys were all married but hadn't started a family yet. David told them he had a daughter born that morning, in fact. Dub exclaimed that it was the *best* date to be born on, because it was his birthday! What a coincidence! Or, was it? (Tom and David are great friends and fondly say that they are "brothers from another mother". Dub and David became best buddies, and prayer warriors for each other ever since that day, too. And are now fly-fishing buddies along with their sons. Even on your worst days, you can find a tiny miracle. This conversation with these men turned out to be one.) David told them about his son, Davey, who would be two on May 8, and Ralph, standing directly behind David said, "No way, that's *my* birthday!"

(I know it sounds made up, but it's true. What are the chances? We had hit several of those long chances that day. But then again, it was all orchestrated from above, and not really left to chance.) The guys all became fast friends for the next four years in school, and so did we, their wives. I discovered that Lynn, Dub's wife, was a teacher at Madonna Day School, a private Catholic school that had started classes for children with intellectual disabilities. This was *really* ahead of its time, this educational program for special needs children. As an educator, Lynn was continuously encouraging to us in regards to what these kids *could learn*. With each new story she related about the smart children with Down syndrome in her classroom, I became happier. It gave us more hope for our little girl as she grew up to know that there *were* good schools and good teachers, who cared for the education of students with special needs. They were just few and far between. When the time came for Windy to attend school, we at least knew those good teachers were out there somewhere. We would just have to pray we would find them somehow.

We became close to the Roberson's, too. They now live on a farm not too far from Nashville. Their three kids, Penelope (Penel), Dustin and Jason became close to our kids as we visited back and forth. They would someday attend Special Olympics with us at Vanderbilt and cheer Windy over the finish line many times. Carol and Tom have fed us, hosted us for long weekends, and we've been there for each other through the years. Windy was even asked by Penel Roberson to be in her wedding as a bridesmaid. They were the same age and had always had a special bond. Later, Penel moved to Nashville, Tennessee and was a member of the Junior Chamber of Commerce. Windy visited many times with her and her good friends, Rachael, and Tracy. She ran around the "Country Music City" attending many special functions with the girls as their guest, and even worked at several of the functions as a volunteer-helper.

She was included in the wedding party with Penel's other best friends and looked beautiful in her pewter-gray, silky strapless bridesmaid dress, beaming a radiant smile as she watched her dear friend say her vows to Justin Croniser. Windy approved of him highly, I might add. At least by the time of the wedding! She had not remained silent when she offered advice about him, you can bank on that!

One weekend Penel had come to spend the night with us as business had brought her to East Tennessee. She worked for Cracker Barrel for several years. She and Windy would always stay up talking, and this night was no exception. Windy was stretched out on a chair, her legs on an ottoman where Penel was seated. I was lying down on the sofa, across from them. I was attempting to stay awake to talk and visit but I was just about to drift off to sleep with my head resting on the sofa arm when I heard Penel say, "Well, Win, Justin (her longtime boyfriend, who had been once been a policeman in Nashville) has graduated from Law school as you know, and he is going for an interview out of state, in Ohio, and he may be moving there. I would really miss him if he moves." Windy was silent for a second and then she said with all the wisdom of the world, "Justin needs to ask you to marry him before he leaves if he gets the job. I like him a lot, but if he doesn't do it, then you need to tell him goodbye!" Penel laughed so hard she nearly fell off the ottoman. "You know, Windy, I think you're right. This is it!" I woke up enough to giggle with them.

Some friends may have hesitated to say what was on their minds so openly. Not our girl. She is sensitive and never wants to hurt someone's feelings, but she always thinks it's important to tell the truth. She has so much good ol' common horse sense. (We're talking common sense here.) Penel called the following week on Windy's cell phone and told her Justin had gotten the job in Ohio, and she said that he *had* asked her to marry him. Windy was ecstatic and exclaimed, "I knew it! He loves you!" Penel immediately asked her to be one of her bridesmaids! Soon the wedding plan phone calls became more frequent between them, and we were all touched by Penelope (and Tom and Carol's) and Justin's true love and concern for Windy. Penel texts her all the time now about her two little boys. Windy never fails to say, "Oh how sweet! I have a text from Penel!" BFF is Windy's mantra.

Now after all these years, all of our grown children are friends, and so a whole new generation of Moores, Smiths, and Robersons have formed lifelong friendships. We families have vacationed together, laughed together, and mourned the loss of loved ones together, celebrated our children's weddings, and rejoiced in the births of our grandchildren.

We have Dub to thank for strongly encouraging us to go to church. He and Lynn were members at Bellevue Baptist Church.

David and Dub were beginning their freshman year, and Bellevue was located near Southern College of Optometry in downtown Memphis. Adrian Rogers was the new pastor there. We visited and felt so welcomed that we began attending regularly. Windy and Davey attended the nursery and played with all the other kids. There was no class for special needs children then. Windy started in the nursery and then joined regular classes and seemed to enjoy going.

David was baptized by Dr. Rogers after we had attended for a year or so. David teased the pastor that he had to have one of the 'big guys in God's lineup" because he required a heavy-hitter to dunk *him* and be sure it took. Nearing graduation in 1977, David will never forget shaking Pastor Roger's hand as we told him goodbye and hearing his wise words of godly wisdom as he looked him directly in his eyes and said, "Be sure and find your little family a Bible preaching church, and you take them to church and worship as a family together. It will be one of the most important leadership roles you have in life." David listened intently and took the advice to heart.

We sure are grateful David was standing just where he was in line with those men on the day Windy was born!

Chapter Seven
Facing Fears

Only one major time did the state of Windy's health really concern us in her toddler years, and it *greatly* concerned us. At the age of about eighteen months she began to tire easily, and she started bruising when she fell. After having fabulous muscle strength and coordination, she began to fall more frequently. She would play in the living room floor, stand up, and have a hard time walking across the floor from one side of the room to the other without stumbling. David and I thought she might be getting another ear infection, so I called her doctor's office. They asked me if she had a fever; I said, "No." They then recommended we give her baby aspirin for a day to see if we could stop a possible ear infection from happening.

After another day passed, we began noticing tiny dots appear as a rash all over her body. We rushed her to Dr. Perry, and he took a blood test. Her blood count was alarmingly abnormal, and he wanted her admitted to the hospital immediately to run more tests. As we questioned him, he told us one cause could be something not too serious, called petechiae, or the condition (rash-like appearance) of her skin, and the low blood count could possibly be a sign of leukemia. Having admitted he had only seen this less serious condition once before, he wanted to rule out the more serious condition.

Our hearts fell; we had accepted her as she came to us and had fought so hard to help her overcome insurmountable odds. Now were we going to lose her so soon? "*No, God, please! Help us find out what is invading her little body and don't let it be fatal,*" we prayed as we drove her to LeBonheur Children's Hospital, not far from our apartment. It felt like we had gone a hundred miles before we pulled up to the front door of the hospital.

They assigned us a room and had us dress her in the tiniest little hospital gown we had ever seen. It would have been so cute if the circumstances hadn't been so grave. They came to take blood samples, so many, from such a tiny baby's arm. Our hearts were torn apart as we kept her still and entertained her to distract her from the painful procedures. Dedicated doctors and nurses came and went as night turned to day and day to night. David tried to study for a test in the corner of the room, but he kept putting the book down to hold her when she held out her little hands and motioned her fingers for him to pick her up. In between enticing Windy to eat and reading to her, I kept calling to check on our Davey, who was at a friend's house for the time being.

Never will we forget the day the doctor came in to say we could take her home. Dr. P.'s hunch had been right. She had something called idiopathic thrombocytopenia purpura (ITP), a big word for a big scare. It was an atypical response her body had relating to a severe earache and possibly the baby aspirin prescribed for her treatment to keep her pain to a minimum. They felt it would possibly never happen again if we avoided giving her aspirin. They wanted to continue to check her blood level every month for the next six months, but it looked like Windy was going to be all right.

Life went on as to be expected in any active young family's life. Windy's health was surprisingly good. What a real praise! She and Davey had all the normal childhood illnesses: colds, sore throats and earaches, but nothing out of the ordinary. The ear infections were the only reoccurring health problems, and they had so many earaches that the pediatrician suggested they have tubes put in their ears. He suggested an Ear, Nose and Throat Specialist, a Dr. Morse, that was well known in the Memphis area. We made an appointment with him, and he felt it was best to insert tubes in both of their ears. They went into the children's hospital for an overnight stay, and the tubes remained in for two or three years, and the pain and infections subsided.

It was traumatic to have her blood tests run at Danny Thomas' inspirational hospital, St. Jude Children's Research Hospital, where they suggested we go for each testing. There they were set up for tiny patients and little veins. It was just about four or five streets over from our apartment complex. Windy was frightened, and so were we. She, of the needles, and we, of the possible results, each time we took her back. Her blood count returned to normal and remained there, thank heavens.

We met other parents and children who did not receive the same comforting news. We cried and prayed for the ones we met and for those we didn't know but had seen in that little waiting room area. We can't say enough good things about both hospitals and their tender care of their little patients. Six months later they gave Windy a clean bill of health and told us she would not have to come back unless symptoms reappeared, which they doubted would *ever* happen, they said to our tremendous relief. What a glorious day that was when we received the news that she was healthy again. After going through all that, nothing could be too hard for us as far as we were concerned. She wouldn't be just like the other children she played with on the playground, or in the church nursery. But the good news was that she *was* going to *live,* and by the grace of God, live for a *purpose.*

Chapter Eight
Broader Horizons

During this time, David was going to school and working part-time. He had found a construction job working on the building of Saint Joseph's Hospital in East Memphis. He was hammering away, up in the air, on the frame of the high new building. His pay check helped us buy gas to drive the long distance home. It was important for us to go back home as often as we could. Windy learned to interact with people at home and out in the world. We took her *everywhere*, and we made friends everywhere we went.

We became friends with Irene, the cashier at the grocery where we shopped. She always had a cookie from the bakery for the kids, or a piece of gum, or a little toy, and always a sweet word for all three of us. The children always looked forward to seeing her. (When it was time to move from Memphis, we went to the grocery for the last time and left with all of us crying, especially Irene.)

Broader horizons were found on our visits home. We took the kids to see and touch animals on our friends' farms, hiking in the Smoky Mountains, fishing on the Clinch River, and we traveled on vacations with family to the beach in South Carolina and Florida. We went swimming in Norris Lake, and rode horses on trails in the mountains—anything to have them experience life and new adventures, and to enable them to learn to adjust to change(s). If Windy was ever apprehensive, she got over it quickly. She seemed to reach for things to challenge and stretch herself. She never shrank back, but would *volunteer* to try something. She was always ready to embrace something she had never tried before, be it a taste of a new food, a ride at an amusement park, or any new lesson to be attempted.

David and I had tried our best to teach her to accept change. She learned to like change all right. She was *all about* change: change of scenery, change of climate, change of action. It had been worth all the effort to keep her from being the child described in those books about children with Down syndrome—those kids who they said didn't like change.

I got to relate all of this in a unique way. I was taking a correspondence class from Mississippi State during this time. I would study after our babies were asleep, something I personally didn't get to do much of . . . sleep that is. At the completion of the course, I wrote a paper about Down syndrome and told all about our daughter. I made an "A" in the class, and the professor, a basketball coach there at the time, wrote me a wonderful letter stating what an inspiration Windy was, and how the way we were raising her had been an inspiration to him personally, and to others that he had told about her. He had spoken of us to his boys on the team to give them encouragement to do their best on the court!

We realized then that we were on the cutting edge of a new concept: One that proved that children with special needs *could* learn, and that parents, siblings, family and friends could help them become more accepted in mainstream society. A bonus was that it could benefit and encourage everybody! We fully understood we had a story to tell to encourage others. The magnitude of that story was still hidden, but it was to be revealed in time.

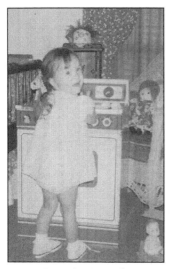
Learning to cook

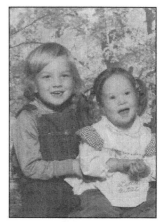
Happy kids

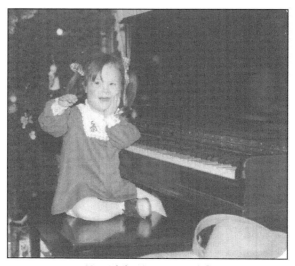
How'd that tune go again?

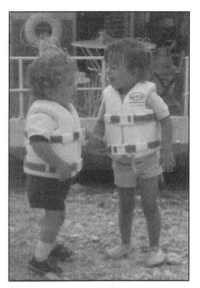

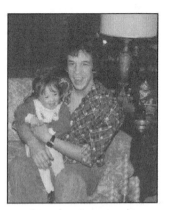

With beloved Uncle Chip

Taking younger cousin, Danny, in hand

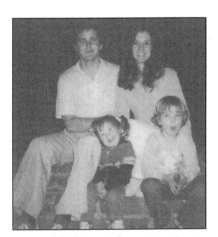

Finding out they were going to
have a new baby brother or sister

With cousins, Steve Smith and Keisha Smith

With oldest cousin, Jackie Pemberton

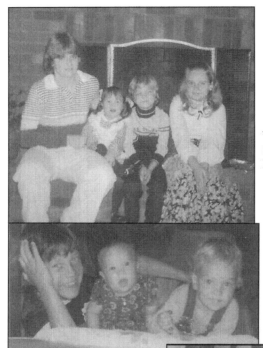

With cousin Kristi

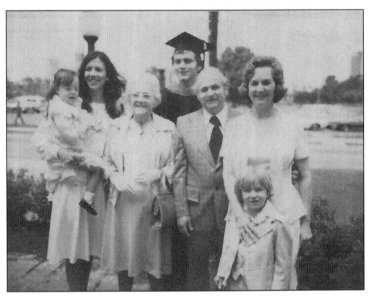
Daddy's graduation with Granny Jessie and the Smiths

Chapter Nine
WINDY'S LIFE LESSONS Begin

Inspiration came from a TV show. During this time a boy, several years older than Windy, began to appear with all the other little children on one of our children's favorite shows, *Sesame Street*. It was a surprise to all of the viewers I'm sure, especially to us. The first day I saw him singing and talking with the children, I sank down to sit on the floor right in front of the television with my children. I didn't want to miss a word he said, or an action he made. His name was Jason, and he had Down syndrome! It was so great for our Davey to see another child who favored his sister in some characteristics. He walked up close to the screen and pointed and said, "Look, Mommy, he looks like *my* Windy!"

Be still my heart! David and I were also thrilled to see a child with DS on TV! Our intention had been to expose Windy to the world and to expose the world to Windy . . . we didn't want to hide her away at home. We wanted society to accept her as a person whose life had value. Having this Jason in the public's sight helped encourage us, as parents, and it also helped the general public to see children born with DS as real people with 'normal' behavior and desires and dreams. He proved to all of us that children born with a disability could learn things like differentiating between colors, and numbers and letters! Thank you, thank you, thank you to Jason's mom, one of the producers of the program we later discovered, who chose to put him on the program and help lay the ground work for all of us who came after them.

We *all* stand on the shoulders of those who went before us. We are grateful for those who were courageous enough to do the right things, even if they were the *first* to do so. Having Jason on public television paved the way for kids like him to be more readily accepted in society. We knew his appearance would make it easier on our Windy's life, as we went out into the world to help her find her place in it.

Memphis was a wonderful place to bring up a child, especially one born with a disability. A bustling, growing southern city, filled with compassionate, kind people. People were friendly and sweet to our girl and her big brother. We will always love Memphis for the people we met in our children's first years of life. Some we still keep in contact with, and some we spoke with for only a moment—but moments that have lasted a lifetime in our memories.

After living in the big city for almost five years, it was time for David's graduation, and we were looking forward to getting back to the mountains where we had grown up. We bid farewell to friends with the promise to keep in touch, and we set off in a new direction that would include a huge step for our kids—preschool. An extensive search for a place to live helped us discover a small town for David to begin his practice. We had heard that their schools were good. It was located in a quaint college town, only forty-five minutes from our old hometown and family. Packing up everything we owned didn't take too long. We were a bit remorseful about leaving Memphis, but full of anticipation and hope for the future.

We felt our daughter had so much to learn, and as it turns out, so much to teach *us*. There have been so many things she has taught us that everyone in our immediate family now calls these moments, **WINDY LIFE LESSONS**—lessons that have caused us to be better, kinder, and more compassionate people.

As we packed, a group of painters, sent by our apartment manager, came in and walked among the boxes, to put a fresh coat of paint on the walls. They quickly covered up five year's worth of tiny handprints on the walls, and pencil marks on a bedroom doorframe from a homemade growth chart—hallmarks of how much our children had grown since we had lived there, only one street off of the city's well known Madison Avenue. Just as soon as we moved out, they had new renters ready to move in. It was sorta sad, but we could not look back at the past for long, we had an exciting future before us. We took a last walk-through . . . then we shut the bright-blue-painted front door for the last time, and headed back to East Tennessee.

Chapter Ten
A Moving Decision

Jefferson City, Tennessee, lies nestled near the beautiful Cherokee Lake, with every rise of the land revealing breath-taking views of the Smoky Mountains on one side and the Cumberland Mountains on the other side. Rolling fields and acres and acres of farmland span in between the two ranges. After living with pavement and concrete surroundings for five years, we found this environment refreshing. And it was quiet! The quiet took some getting used to: the hum of honey bees feeding on clover, the melodious call of the mockingbirds, the songs of the frogs in the nearby ponds.

Not one night did we miss the ambulance sirens or horns of the street traffic, but our ears had to readjust our sensory perceptions from city to country. I think it took about a week, and you would have thought we had been raised on a farm. Davey and Windy would hear a sound and say, "Don't worry, that was a cow, or a horse or a katydid," or whatever the source had been. They adjusted faster than David and I did.

Home was now a three-bedroom brick rancher, sitting amidst several hundred rural acres. The house and ten acres was ours for at least a year; we had signed a lease to rent. The day David graduated, we had loaded the U-Haul trailer and driven nearly the length of the state to settle in as soon as possible. He had found a place to begin a practice, and we were looking forward to registering the kids for school.

We had looked at many places. We had even considered New Mexico. David had gotten special permission to obtain credit hours for working on an externship in Fort Defiance, Arizona, with a friend, Dr. John Garber. He lived on the reservation for several weeks his senior year. In fact, his research and persistence in setting up the credit hours toward his degree was probably the first externship ever offered at SCO. He enjoyed the Native American people he met and felt blessed by being able to help them in a small way. They offered him a full-time position at the newly built Zuni hospital, on the reservation in New Mexico. It would have been a wonderful experience for all of us. All except Windy. She needed speech therapy and a preschool that could ensure her future mental growth. At the time there was nothing offered for special education there. Therefore, we had to turn down the offer. That's when we began looking at our other options and decided on Jefferson City.

On our move-in day help came by way of Lonas Tarr and his family. He had a Chevrolet dealership in the town, and he immediately took us under his wing. (There was a family connection. His mother had a brother named Everette Lewallen. Everette was married to my dad's sister. The Tarrs and I had memories of being together at large family gatherings in years past. Lonas and my dad had been pretty close growing up, and both became pilots in the Air Force.)

Lonas also sent us a tremendous gift; he sent his son Bill over to our house to help us move in. We not only gained immediate assistance, but we also gained dear lifelong friends in Bill and his wife, Deirdre. She stopped by with a pan of warm chocolate brownies, and we immediately loved her open heart and sweet spirit, not to mention her delicious brownies! (They have three grown sons now, two of them, Blake and Blane, have followed in David's footsteps. They are Optometric Physicians by profession. The youngest son, Brady, was a pastor of a church in Washington, D.C., and now in Alabama. (Brady's story is mentioned later on in another chapter). Our kids feel very close to the Tarr boys. It's been so good for Windy to run around with the five boys as she was growing up.

She learned to keep up with the guys, yet maintain her femininity. We have many, many special memories of hiking, camping, vacationing, heart-to-heart talks, and playing games before the "home fire" after consuming some scrumptious meals Miss Deirdre prepared. The Bill Tarr family's faith has always been a strong influence in our lives, and we hope we have been in theirs.)

Deirdre and Bill invited us to church, and we soon joined their Sunday school class. (Twenty-five years later, Windy's pastor at First Baptist Concord, Doug Sager, would be asked to be a guest speaker at their church, and during his sermon he would tell the congregation of Windy's story and faith and used her as an example of how one person *can* be used by God to make a difference in the world. He did not know the Tarr family, nor of the story of how she lived there long ago. Deirdre would call me to tell me about it, so touched and excited over hearing him speak about "their Windy." How interestingly and surprisingly wonderfully God weaves all of our life-stories together!)

In our new town we felt at home instantly with the kind, gentle people we met. We made friends with the people we met at church: Perry and Susan Brown, Earl and Claudia Ogburn, Carey and Shirley Herring, and many others. Our spiritual needs were met in the Bible studies we attended and in the sweet fellowship we experienced as we worshiped together and prayed for each other. That summer, Windy was accepted everywhere we went in our new town: the story hour at the library with her brother, the public swimming pool for swimming lessons, the church's Sunday school and children's choir. Everyone got to know her. She and her big brother quickly made new friends. Fall was approaching and we knew we must begin the task of finding a preschool for her to attend.

You may ask, why is this so unusual? Why would she not be accepted openly at all these places? Well, it was the 1970's. People who had disabilities were not widely integrated into normal society at the time. This was probably a result of the limited educational laws available for the public education of a child with a disability. It was an accepted, and almost expected thought in society to put a special needs child in an institutional, state-run home, so their varied and myriad needs could be meet in one place. Many people with intellectual disabilities still lived in institutions at the time of Windy's birth.

There were few legal rights or laws protecting people with intellectual and developmental disabilities. We were breaking new ground by taking our daughter with us wherever we went. We expected others to accept her, not on our terms, but on God's terms. Looking back, it was pretty daring behavior on our part. But we were proud of our children. *All* of our children. We got some stares when she was just a toddler. We got used to the stares. Some people even got brave enough to speak to us. Some asked us if she was a "mongoloid child." We hated that word ourselves and began the arduous process of educating people by introducing them to the *new* term, Down syndrome, to explain her condition.

Parents were talking up this new term all over the country, we just didn't know that at the time. Word spread across the nation rapidly. Every family member and friend was dedicated to making people aware of the term change. Most people were just curious, and when educated on just what DS was, they became friendly. Encouraged by our easy and natural attitude towards her, they became nice to Windy after they met her and saw that she was really just a kid like their kid. Just about everyone fell for her, *big* time, when they got to know her charming little disposition. She didn't push her way in . . . she lovingly and confidently walked into their lives!

The fall of 1977 would bring big changes in all our lives. Davey was entering kindergarten (the big "K"! How did he grow up so fast?), and we hoped his sister would be starting school as well. Windy needed to be with other children to play and grow. She needed to learn how to function on her own, without a family member about. There were several preschools in the area. Naively we thought it was going to be a cinch to enroll her in one. I had been told by several moms that we still had plenty of time to register.

I began making phone calls to the schools from a list I had been given by our new friends, a list of all the places where their children were attending. The preschools were all privately operated at the time and were not part of the city or county school system. We were willing to pay the fees required for a wonderful start to Windy's education.

I made myself comfortable as I perched upon a tall, metal kitchen stool near the wall phone, with the list balanced on my knees. I was far enough away to have a conversation, yet close enough to keep a watchful eye out on the kids. Davey and Windy were busy water painting on big sheets of white paper. I smiled at their concentrated efforts as I looked at their small hands creating their masterpieces. I couldn't wait until they began their education and took real art classes—just look how talented they are! I turned back to my task and I began to dial the first phone number.

I spoke to several teachers in a row and was flatly turned down by *all* of them, or rather, Windy was turned down from admission by all of them, "sight unseen," the moment I explained that she was a special needs child. Most curtly cut me off when I tried to explain that she would need no special treatment or care. In fact, I explained, we hoped they would treat her as a normal student. Most of the teachers, or directors, I spoke with were quite firm with their denials, and not one of them had any suggestions or a place to refer me to. They all ended our conversations hurriedly and with finality. Some told me they had been asked this countless times before and did not want to take on this extra "burden"!

At first I was stunned. I sat there listening to the faint dial tone as I held the phone loosely down at my side in defeat. The sun looked warm and bright outside beyond the large kitchen window, but things weren't as wonderful as they looked. I suddenly had a cold chill. I felt frustration and anger. I was flabbergasted. I wasn't trying to pass off a little monster that would disrupt their preschool classes. This was our well-behaved daughter we were talking about. She was a person with an intellectual disability—not a communicable disease! Surely there were other children with intellectual disabilities in this county! Where did they go for their early education?

Tearfully, I stopped my phoning to take out time to pray silently, *"God, our precious daughter needs a good education. Please direct us to the right people. Give us support and open a door, the right door. We need Your help, Lord. You sent her to us just like she is . . . so please show us the way. We're in the dark on this. We don't need to see every step, but we do need to see the next one!"* I guess you think the next call brought ready acceptance after such an earnest prayer. No, it didn't, and neither did the next one. I am not by nature a pushy person. It goes against my grain to do or say anything that could be considered pushy, but the *last* number on my list was our only hope.

Maybe on this last phone call I made that day, the woman on the other end of the line heard the tremor in my young mother's voice, or the hint of true desperation I must have had, as I pleaded with her to give our Windy a chance in her school. I remember I talked fast, before she could turn me down like her predecessors had done. She was initially silent on the other end of the phone line as I volunteered my presence on the first two or three weeks of school to help assist her, so any extra time would not be sacrificed from the teachers occupied with the other new students. (That idea had come to me in a flash. Maybe the teachers would be more receptive to the idea of her being in their class if they had some back-up.)

I said I would take her out if the director and the other teachers felt it was in the best interest of the other children, or if they thought it was best for Windy. I could deal with that. I presented her with a grace period. What could she say? Well . . . she could have said, no, like everyone else had before her. But she didn't. Instead she kindly said they looked forward to meeting us *both* on Monday. *Hooray! Thank you Lord!*

(That school number had been at the bottom of my list, but the list was in no real order. I had hurriedly jotted down phone numbers while talking with a group of moms at the public pool one day. I believe God had the list in perfect order . . . I needed to learn He was in charge of it all: her education, her future teachers, her placement. But I had to use the personality He gave me to help find a place for her. Inactivity would have gotten us nowhere. Plus, if the first school had accepted her immediately, I would not have been as grateful as I was for the great teachers and school she did attend! I know this now.)

I was so excited I nearly hit the floor in a faint. Thinking better of it, I swooped the children up and we took a surprise trip to get an ice cream cone at the local drive-in before we went by David's new office to tell him that our children, BOTH of them, were starting school in September! Life was looking up for the Smith family. We went to buy book bags, new tennis shoes and the works. Our kids were going to school! (Fourteen years later we related this story to a friend, Bill Stough, a missionary in Africa, who had also grown up in Africa as a Missionary Kid. He had come to stay at our house while he was on furlough. He couldn't believe it had been so hard to find a school for her. "This is America, isn't it?" he asked incredulously. That's exactly how we had felt—until we faced the very problem head on, time after time. And, until we heard other school stories, from *so* many people who had a family member with an intellectual disability.)

The private schools (like the Catholic school our friend Lynn had taught in) were rare, and to send a child there a parent had to send their child away to board at the school. We were definitely not going to send our little bitty daughter off to live with strangers. Period! There were few laws on the books that stated to the world that these children had rights, and that they had a right to an education. That is until the law changed. We know many people must have fought for this inclusion. We were just another family who loved their children and wanted inclusion and equality for them. Equality nearly always requires a battle of some kind, but fighting for what is right is a necessity at times. As the parents of a child with a disability we had to learn to pick and choose our battles, to overlook smaller things so we could concentrate on the bigger issues.

One trait Windy developed early on was listening assiduously to us talk, especially if we didn't think she was listening to our conversations. She would prove this repeatedly. (This is a skill she has honed up on to full maturity in her adulthood. At times she has repeated to someone something she has overheard, and even if benignly spoken. Sometimes when it is retold to the party spoken about, it rarely sounds totally benign. (A prime example is the time a friend's husband called us. They were planning last-minute details before a visit to come and see us from another state. During the conversation he mentioned that his wife had gained some weight in the last couple of years, but he added that they had been on a diet and had begun exercising together as a way to get healthier.

That would have been the end of that conversation, *but as life will happen,* later on in the same week, the wife called, and Windy answered the phone first. During their little conversation she told Windy she had gained weight and needed to lose several pounds. Windy innocently agreed, saying, "Yes, I know. I heard my parents talking about it." We hadn't been talking about it. I knew what she meant. She was referring to the phone conversation she had overheard us having with our friend. But Windy's response to her made it sound like her weight had been the topic of a private conversation David and I had about this friend. I was running for the phone as I heard her speaking. Now try to explain something like *that* to a friend. I tried but I don't know if she totally believed me. Windy was just stating a fact and being genuinely sympathetic. It was times like these that could frustrate us to our limit. Then we had to step back and just be glad she could communicate at all.

I'll tell you what's the truth, having her in the back seat of the car all these years sure has helped us to keep our conversations more pure. Consequently we have learned as a family to think and say the best about someone, **or** we say nothing at all. Everyone in the family has become *pretty* good tongue biters, as we have resisted the urge to say something that really didn't need to be said, and REALLY didn't need to be *repeated* in any context! Keeping (or holding) *our* tongues in our mouth *without* the aid of peanut butter is a great lesson for anyone! A **WINDY LIFE LESSON** for sure. It has really helped us keep out of "sticky situations"!

We were settling in to life in a small town. We met most of our neighbors as they drove by and stopped to say hello. One elderly gentleman in particular piqued our interest as we drove by his home every day on our way to town. Mr. Miller was his name. Another neighbor had told us about him. He sat on the front porch of his turn-of-the-century home, day after day, waving each time we passed by. We mentioned that we really needed to stop to speak to him, but it seemed we were always in a hurry, with no extra time to spare as we sped past.

Speaking of sticky situations, our daughter has also been more than adequate in getting *herself* into some situations. Like the time on a beautiful sunny afternoon in the early fall when the children were finally down for a nap, I *thought*. At least they were when I looked in before taking the garbage out back, and then sitting on the back porch step to feed the dog and water the plants near the doorway. We were now the proud owners of two dogs.

The older dog was resting in the yard. That's when I noticed the new puppy was nowhere in sight, but it wasn't cause for alarm. She sometimes hid under the porch on a hot day, so I thought nothing of it. I was enjoying the feeling of the sun on my back and began to plant more flowers. What a beautiful day! Then like a light in my head turned on, I had a suspicion about the missing puppy. It had never attempted to go very far. Mother's intuition? Maybe. I was just feeling much too uneasy to ignore my urge to go look for the pup. "Here, Muppet," I tentatively called out. I got up and walked to the porch overhang. No Muppet. I went inside and headed for the children's bedroom. Davey was sound asleep, but no Muppet inside, *and* no Windy. Just as I suspected. She was not in her bed! She must be hiding somewhere with the puppy, not too unusual a stunt for her to pull. (She was regularly doing things to either make us laugh, or make us think.)

After a quick search, I discovered she wasn't in any of her normal hiding spots. Her favorite spot was a toy cabinet that had two doors on the front. She liked to crawl all the way in and pull the doors nearly shut. She could fold up like a little mouse and hide in some very small places, all the while remaining uncharacteristically quiet and still for several minutes, until we found her. She thought this game was just too funny not to play with Mom and Dad every once in awhile. She was not in the closets or under the beds. I even looked behind shower curtains and behind the window drapes. Several minutes had passed now. Panic began to creep in.

My cries for her became louder, and I woke Davey up. He started looking too. She always came out of hiding for him. As we passed through the living room, out of the corner of my eye, I happened to notice the front door was barely cracked open. The same door that *always* remained locked. The door she had never been able to unlock, must have been opened by none other than, Windy. We didn't ever use the front door. It was opened only for those times when company came up the front walk.

Now I was about to lose it. Our little girl had sneaked outside. She was alone out there somewhere, and we had to find her. Davey and I ran out together. She was not anywhere outside close to the house. We ran to their swing set in the side yard, and the swings were empty and hanging still. We ran back into the house, and I grabbed the car keys off the hook in the hallway and we got in the car. We slowly made our way down the gravel drive and out into the country road, all four car windows rolled down, and we called her name. No answer. *Then*, we passed the first farmhouse on the left, and there on the front steps sat Mr. Miller, Windy, and our new pup.

Apparently our daughter had decided it was high time to meet Mr. Miller, our nearest neighbor. We *all* met him. He was very nice and told her to come back and see him anytime. She always rolled down her car window to yell, "Hi" as we went by from then on, and he would wave emphatically.

David arrived home the same time we did, and he helped me explain to Windy, with Davey standing at her side as her little protector, about how wrong it was, sneaking off, not asking permission, and how scared she had made us when we found she was missing. He then put her in her room to sit in a tiny chair in "time out." What a sad, sad face. When she cried there was not a more pitiful looking child. You wanted to run to her and cuddle her in your arms and wipe away those tears fast. Tears were streaming down, and the bottom lip was primped out so pitifully. Her head was hung down in deep shame. Davey sat on his twin bed in the same room, with tears in his eyes. He knew he wasn't in trouble, but he couldn't stand to see Windy unhappy, or leave her to be all alone if she was in trouble. Good thing the two sets of grandparents weren't around. They wouldn't have stood for this: to see her so sad.

We stood our ground for her sake—anything could have happened to her. She needed to understand the danger she could put herself in. I went in to take Davey by the hand and lead him out of the room. Windy cried even louder. She was feeling the brunt of her punishment. Solitary confinement was at the top of her "dislike intensely list".

David immediately went to the hardware store and came back to put extra bolts on the doors leading outside so neither she nor Davey could open them without us knowing it. It was frightening. We were no longer going to be able to let down our guard completely as she was learning and changing so rapidly now. Could we keep up and even get ahead of her antics? We'd see; we would have to be on our toes. Some comfort was taken in the old adage, "You can't outsmart a fox." *Or,* could she? Hm-m-m. We knew Windy, and we knew she would just take all this on as a challenge—not as a defeat, even though she apologized and said she understood everything we had explained to her.

Time would tell us all just what limits we could impose on her to keep her safe. She was beginning to assert her independence, that trait we had prayed for and worked so hard to help her develop. Was there a "pause" button we could work on? Nope. Didn't think so. She was on the fast track to do everything she could for herself, all the while showing everyone that cute little personality, and there was no stopping her now!

On the weekends we now had some time to go hiking in the nearby Smokies. David would take fallen tree limbs and make hiking sticks for the kids to hold onto as they followed the trails with us. Davey loved to walk with his dad and lead the way for the girls. I walked at a slower pace with Windy because her little short legs could not keep up with her daddy's and her big brother's stride. Inevitable Windy would tire of walking and would threaten to stop walking unless she was picked up and carried. That worked when she was still tiny, but as she grew larger she was too heavy for us to carry very far up the side of a mountain. Plus, we were out there for good exercise and our health. If she was carried, she would miss out on the great benefits of aerobic exercise. I usually wanted to cave in to her pleas that turned into whining. It was easier on me to put her on my back and carry her than to hear her moaning and groaning.

Hiking was fun for us, until the complaints started. David, however, saw these times as a wonderful learning experience for her. He would consistently walk back and gently explain to her how good it was for her legs to walk on her own, and that we would stop at the next turn (or at the next view or at the top) to take a break and get a drink from our water. She challenged him big time. She would defiantly look him in the eyes and say, "Fine. You go. I'm *not* going!" and she would toss her walking stick to the side and sit down in the dirt on the path. The first few times she did this he coaxed her up and on, but when he saw her ultimate motive of being in control of the situation, and of us, he turned me away from her one notable day and led me on down the trail by holding (gently pushing me forward) onto my elbow, after informing Windy that she was welcomed to stay put, but that we were going on because we came to walk as a family, and we were going on to have a good time.

He whispered to me to keep walking for her sake. She had to develop an independence, yet learn there would be times she had to push on through hard times, he explained, or she would never live up to her potential. He also wisely knew that she would have to respect authority and learn to compromise when need be. I needed his strong conviction on being firm with her, even when she was tired, bored, or testing us. My inclination was to turn back and give in to her. Besides, there were black bears out here on the trails! (We had never seen an actual bear on any hike, but it was possible!) Had I given in, it would not have been what was best for her, even though my motherly intentions were good and rooted in love. So also were his intentions, rooted in love, and this is where our difference of opinions, different perspectives, were greatly needed and helpful.

It had become a real test of how far she could push the parental limits, and she was having her version of a temper tantrum. Before anyone becomes alarmed over parents leaving their helpless little child in the dangerous mountains alone, let me inform you that we *never* left her sight, neither did we take our eyes off her. We did walk slowly on ahead. Never in our lives have we walked *that* slowly, before or since. Windy sat in her spot for what seemed like a very long time. When she finally moved, we sighed a big sigh of relief. She slowly stood up, retrieved her stick, and mumbling something under her breath, (glad we don't know what it was she said!) and began to catch up with us.

Then with a new sense of direction and strength, she passed up all three of us, and took the lead. She seemed to tell us by her action that she would stay with this family no matter how frustrating we might be to her at times, but for heaven's sake, move over, and don't get in the way of what she had to do and where she had to go. Case closed!

That particular day marked Windy's newly formed independence, and by golly, she *liked* it! She never offered to "sit" on a hike again, but she did pass us up many more times, and she *always* walks faster when she's in the lead.

A born leader is soon recognizable, and she was beginning to display the traits. We also recognized that she just might leave us behind if *we* didn't stay up, figuratively speaking, despite the fact, that she had Down syndrome, and maybe, just maybe, *because* she had DS. Windy was beginning to recognize that fair or unfair, she had more to prove to the world out there than the rest of us. She took it as a challenge to be met, and not a defeating blow. (Another **WINDY LIFE LESSON** for you and me.)

School started, and I walked Davey into his first real class experience, kindergarten. There was a brave smile and then, when we could no longer see each other, there were tears. I'm talking about me here. Davey was fine. My little fellow was a big boy now. He had always been in my tender care, and now I had handed him over to the educational professionals. Separation anxiety lasted just a little while, and then we both began to enjoy this new found freedom and independence for a few hours. He made new friends quickly and enjoyed school.

He even enjoyed work he brought home. He proudly came in with his first homework, stood up straight, squared his shoulders, and said in his rendition of an older boy, "Dad, I need to go study like you did in school, so please tell Mom and Windy that I'll be busy for a while. You can come and check on me though." David held back a smile and said, "Good boy, son. Go get started, and I'll tell the girls to keep the noise down. I'll be in to see you, and you can show me your homework."

The roles had switched with the one becoming a student as the other began a career. (The two of them spent many an hour over the coming years, on homework assignments. When the task became too grueling, or as an incentive when a large assignment was completed, they always managed to slip away for a little R & R. This took the form of fly fishing, or kicking or throwing around a ball of some type.) Davey was settled in a good school where he could be with friends his own age. Now it was Windy's turn to go to school. It was her time to have the opportunity to be with kids her age and to be an individual.

The big day arrived. The first day of pre-school was fun for her because she liked to be with people. I stayed to watch her participate in the activities and to prompt her in certain situations. She was extremely quiet (I was surprised at that.), but she didn't hesitate to join in with a little coaxing. After the fourth day, her two very kind teachers, Julie Moody and Helen Quarles, felt they would like to have a "go-alone" with her in the group. I felt happy and a bit leery, simultaneously. Would she be too shy? Would they understand her when she spoke? As it turned out, she wasn't (too shy for long), and they could (understand her), most of the time. After a few days the children and teachers became accustomed to her pronunciation, and communication became easier. (On a side note Helen Quarles's son, George, became a well known football coach. Windy has a picture of him helping her carve a pumpkin in that preschool class.)

Some days I went to work at David's office. (We had met a builder, David Hayes, who later became a friend of ours. He helped us remodel an old store, known as the old Butler Store, into a lovely office.) I went to work to help him answer the office phone, made appointments, and was generally there to lend support and talk to his new patients. We met so many wonderful people. The new Dr. Smith was learning how to listen and to help solve the vision problem of each person who came into our office. He set a precedent that he still follows today: he tries to advise and give the care to his patients that he would give to his own family members. He really cares about people, and they know it. Blessings came by way of two very nice ladies, Sue and Patsy, who worked in the office. Both were a little older than us and very capable. They soon had that place running smoothly.

Other blessings came by way of another eye doctor, Jim Crutchfield. On Wednesdays, for over a year, Jim would fly his small plane to Morristown from Tazewell, pick David up and take him to his office to work for him, while Jim took the day off to play golf! David's salary was the way we paid our house payment until his practice built up. God provides in amazing ways!

Windy was accepted as a full-time student after her two-week trial period, and we could finally relax for a while, at least until the next battle came our way. *And* you can count on them coming your way when you are raising a child with a disability. All you want is for them to be given a real chance to be accepted. It's a lot like rowing a boat against the current, upstream. We were learning to enjoy the calm waters, but we weren't foolish enough to throw away the paddles . . . we knew we would need them later on for the rougher waters ahead.

We had real reasons to be apprehensive about her speech then. Her voice was delicate and raspy sounding, and it was hard for people to comprehend all her words. She had learned quite a lot of words out on the playground in Memphis and had expanded her vocabulary, but to our chagrin, one of those words was of all things, "Dumb-ass". "Stupid" wasn't even a word heard, or said, in our home, and *this* word was so much worse and was, of course, one of her personal favorites. One of the older neighborhood boys had called all the kids this word at some time or other, and although we spoke about the inappropriate use of the word, she seemed to be enthralled with the way it trilled off her tongue and out of her mouth.

Fortunately, it was also sort of garbled, and the sounds sorta ran together, and no one but us knew what she was saying. (This may be the only time we were fine with letting her diction slide!) Usually she saved it for just the right time to say, like when a friend pushed her down or grabbed a toy from her hands. That is, until we stopped by one day to say hello to Lonas Tarr, at his and Bill's Chevrolet car lot. Evidently she had reached a new language plateau that day, now forever etched in our memories. When we waved goodbye to Lonas, Windy leaned out the back window and yelled loud and clear, *very* clear, "Bye, dumb-ass!"

She must have wanted to set the relationship out on the right foot and impress him with her speaking skills. Needless to say, we were *mortified*. What kind of family would he think we were? A normal one, probably. Kids do things sometimes that embarrass their parents. Isn't normal what we'd wanted all along? *Well*, we guess so. Normal *can* have its down-side though! Lonas never mentioned it . . . maybe he hadn't heard her for the passing traffic on the four-lane in front of his business. We certainly never mentioned it to him!

Windy and Davey loved school. They were easy to awaken and get rolling in the early mornings. Davey was excelling. He liked reading, music and anything science related. Windy liked crafts and music. Her teachers were pleased with her attention span and alertness, but they observed her at play and wished for her to be more aggressive in defending and taking up for herself. (Her use of the favorite word thing had passed, thank the Lord, and she had become complacent when confronted by a child.) She wouldn't go tell the teachers either. They watched her and tried to explain to her how to get something back or to come and tell one of them. David and I tried to explain. *Then* Davey took over and told her just how to do it. She nodded her head as if to say, "All right, I can do that." She did, too. In a few weeks her teachers said she had learned to hold her own. She was never malicious and never, ever, started trouble, but when it came her way, she stood her ground. She'd really need this one in later years. Another valuable **WINDY LIFE LESSON** was learned by us in the process: when confronting conflict, never be malicious or try to get even—but stand your ground, even if the bully is much bigger!

All too quickly a year passed, and Davey would begin first grade, and Windy would start kindergarten. And we were expecting a new baby. Excited about becoming a father again, David would lay his hands gently on my growing tummy and feel our baby turn over and kick. He was excited over the new little Smith on the way. Davey and Windy were very excited. They kept talking about their baby brother or sister. We all decided we would call him Michael, if we had a boy. We stated our belief to our extended family on this new life God had sent, and we didn't speak of "what if" again. The entire family did a lot of praying for the health of that baby. So did our friends. The ladies in our Sunday school class came over to our house and prayed with me several times. Deirdre and a friend from my Bible study, Marty, prayed daily for me and the baby.

What a fun year to look forward to we thought . . . until I started asking whose room Windy would be in. We had liked Davey's teacher so much. She had a real joy for teaching, and all the children adored her, and we thought she would be a good teacher for Windy too, as she began her education in the public school system. David and I were naturally surprised when the primary school administration told us, "She would not be attending the same school her brother went to: they had a wonderful little class at another school several miles down the road. They were much better prepared and set up to handle the special needs children," they assured us. It was a nice way of saying, "She can't go here, not to this school."

We were shocked. What was wrong with *this* school? Why couldn't she attend just like her brother did before her? (This was just a few years after the federal laws dealing with Education had changed to mainstream students with disabilities, and God bless those who fought for inclusion, and I do mean fought, to have the laws changed.) We found out we had to put her in the small rural school they had "suggested" for her placement. We didn't have a choice on schools it seemed. We thought we had better check out the physical structure of the school, meet the educators, and at least give them a chance to explain their curriculum to us. It might be a blessing in disguise. We had to be willing to look things over.

For a little background history to see what we were up against, and I quote according to facts from the Internet on Wikipedia, the free encyclopedia, "Before the Education for All Handicapped Children Act (EHA) was enacted in 1975, U.S. public schools educated only 1 out of 5 children with disabilities." Many of these children were segregated in special buildings or programs that neither allowed them to interact with non-disabled students nor provided them with even basic academic skills.

Continuing the same source the article says, "The EHA, later named the Individuals with Disabilities

Education Act (IDEA), required schools to provide specialized educational services to children with disabilities. The ultimate goal was to help these students live more independent lives in their communities, primarily by mandating access to the general education standards of the public school system." A lot to quote, I know, but it's necessary for you to understand the barrier that had just recently been pulled down that separated children born with a disability and the opportunity for an education in the public school system in America. Thankfully the wall was down, but the complete inclusion was going to take years. (Windy would attend Farragut High School's *first* Least Restrictive Education (LRE) class, but that was in her future for the fall of 1991. This was her first year of school in 1979. Case in point, it took a LONG time to trickle down in the public school system.

We truly kept an open mind as we took her to visit the classroom the county had set up to comply with the mandate for an education for a child who qualified within the guidelines of "Special Education". We declined from enrolling her, we told those in charge, until we had visited the school. We weren't ready to "sign her up" until we knew the what, the who, and the where of it all. David and I insisted on seeing for ourselves where she would have to ride the bus and how long of a ride it would be just for her to receive her rightful education. We were uneducated about all of these things concerning her rights to an education, but we were learning by default.

We three got in the car and timed the ride to the school, the only place that was ready to educate her. We left home and started driving on the four-lane highway. We drove on for several more miles until we came to a small, older school. We were trying to make the best of the situation. Maybe the special education teachers would be so highly educated that it might be worth the long bus ride for Windy.

Sure she would have to leave the house earlier than we felt was good for her, and she would probably come home pretty tired in the late afternoon we figured. We wanted to meet the teachers and see the classrooms to see firsthand what Windy's days would be like.

That September morning was sunny, but held a promise of a thunderstorm later on, I noted as I glanced up at the graying sky as we were getting out of our car. Windy hopped out of the backseat in eager anticipation. She was more than ready to begin her lessons. We walked in the front door and walked straight into the office where they gave us directions to the Resource room, as it was called then. Back out the front door we went and around to the side of the little building where we stopped at a set of small concrete steps that led down to a door. We stepped out of the warm sunshine and went down into the cool, darker atmosphere. Our hearts were dreading what we would have to face on the other side of that door. This was not a good sign to us.

Inside was a basement classroom with a very dismal atmosphere. A few windows were high up on the wall, yet the students could not see out because they were up so high. We saw two instructors in the room, a young male and a young female, and we introduced ourselves and Windy. They shook our hands and told us to look around. They went back to where they had obviously been seated, on an old plaid sofa that had seen better days, to do what we supposed was making a plan for the day's lessons. There were about ten students in the room. They ranged in age from about six to twelve-years old, and all of them had intellectual disabilities, and some had physical disabilities as well. Most were mobile, but two were in wheelchairs, and one child was lying in a homemade adaptation of a wheelchair that remained in a reclined position. The chair spoke volumes to us as to what great lengths parents were willing to go to in order to help their child attend school. Someone had lovingly constructed a very functional chair for their sweet child to be more comfortable and more mobile.

All the children were, for the most part, eerily silent as they sat at the long, low table without any books or lessons in sight. (We guessed their books for the new curriculum had not arrived yet.) A few coloring books and an assortment of old broken crayons sat in the middle of the table. The children capable of reaching for the crayons were not even bothering to do so. The atmosphere in the room was dreary and cheerless. We hoped they only had to stay in this room for a short period of time.

We asked the teachers how often the students changed classes. We were told that they didn't leave the room very often because it was too hard to get them up the front or the back stairways. The students remained in that room for the entire day, even taking their lunch there, "Because it was too hard to get the wheelchairs up all those steps and still leave someone to supervise the other students in the classroom." They were hopeful this would change soon. We were too, but we chose not to wait for that to happen.

We turned in agony to look at the situation before us where the students were expected to learn. We said a brisk thank you to the teachers, and I took Windy by the hand. Our hearts were hurting for those precious children, who were capable of learning *something* with the right incentives. They deserved at the very least love, kindness, and rooms with a view!

The weather had become suddenly cloudy and overcast. So had our moods. It was as if the pending storm was indicative of our stormy life ahead—in our quest for the best education for our daughter. I went up those basement steps two at a time to keep up with David. "Not my daughter. She will never go here. If we have to move to another town to get her into a good school where she can learn, then we will move. Come on Miss Vicki!" (He sometimes used his nickname for me from the Southern old-fashioned way of the Heady children addressing me in Memphis.) "Get in the car!" *Like I needed instruction on what to do next! As if I would stay*! I thought this silently, but I didn't say anything. I knew better than to comment out loud with a smart remark at the moment. Windy was very quiet, too.

Windy's daddy was upset, and rightly so. It was a social injustice to gather all the children with a mental or physical disability in a bleak environment like that, but definitely not unique to school systems all over the country at the time. Too few special educational funds allotted, schools with no extra rooms to dedicate to Special Ed, and a lack of qualified teachers with Special Educational degrees abounded.

That has changed drastically in Windy's school years and beyond. There are many wonderful teachers now who love these special needs students and spend hour upon hour instructing and encouraging them to learn and to grow in all aspects to improve their lives. There are still areas in our public school system that could stand to be improved in their special education classes, but they are light years away from what it used to be.

For one thing, we expect miracles from overworked educators and from overcrowded Resource Rooms. Hopefully these too, will improve one day. We still have a long way to go, but we have come *so* far.

David quickly began to seek employment in other towns and we decided to move back to our hometown. He had been successful from the beginning; his patient load was busy and he was making a good income for us. But we were willing to leave it all for the sake of our family's future. Some things are worth the sacrifice, and this was one of those things. It was the right thing to do at the right time. If Windy got a quality education, our entire family would have a higher quality of life we believed. Her brother Davey would be happier if she was happier. It was just a fact.

(Just a note to go on record and say it is now a positive fact that Special Education is top notch in Jefferson County and Anderson County, and throughout Tennessee. There are many dedicated and wonderful educators helping all the children with special needs get the best education available. This fact thrills us for the children of the counties, and for their families.)

Sadly, even before our move back home, we discovered Windy might not be attending Davey's school after all, for there was no place for her in the classroom, and no special-education teachers in the elementary schools for her in that county either; it was a blow to us. It was such a simple thing to want out of life. Our daughter could not attend the school of our choice, close to our home. We had assumed everyone would want to take Windy and offer her the best education possible to enable her to reach a greater level of learning.

We had a meeting with the Superintendent of Schools, H.L. (Jody) Morrow. He was the same man who had been David's and my principal in grade school. We remembered he would walk down the school halls either whistling or smoking a fragrant cigar. The two of us had visited his office a few times before this, but admittedly, not as adults, and not when we hadn't been sent there by a teacher for excessive talking or misbehaving. Now it was totally different. This time we were the adults, and we had a request for a child of our own, and the request was: Is there a place for our daughter in Clinton Elementary school?

Jody Morrow was a nice man, a John Wayne type of guy, with a ready smile (nice, under a big, gruff "bark") and he listened to what we had to say, but he was absolutely noncommittal. He did tell us there was a classroom *somewhere* for her in the county, but this particular elementary school had no classroom at the time. "One *could* possibly be started," he stated, "*if* there was a real need recognized by the Board, and *if* the county could get the teachers *and* the funding by the fall." His emphasis was on the "*If*'s" and he asked us to give him time to see what, *if* anything, could be done. We left with his reassuring words ringing in our ears, that he "would let us know, as soon as a decision was made by the local school board." David and I weren't holding our breath, but we felt if anybody could get it done, Mr. Marrow was the man.

Extracurricular activities soon began in full force, and we stayed busy going to soccer practice with Saturday morning games, swimming lessons, and all kinds of outdoor activities. Before we knew it, a new school year was fast approaching, and we had heard no word from our local school. David called to ask, and days later I called to ask—all to no avail. Each time we called to inquire about Windy's placement, the secretary of the Superintendent's office told us that they had no news of a classroom for any Special Education program. We began to wonder if it was God's will for Windy to go to Clinton City Schools. Maybe it was the law for the school to make a place for her, to hire a teacher and teacher's aides, to find a classroom which had handicapped accessibility for classrooms and bathroom facilities, but many things had to come about before it happened. We were sure it was an expensive project and not a quick fix by any means. We assumed that there were things probably taking place behind the scenes that Jody Morrow was not privy to talk about.

School systems were being sued all over the country because of the lack of proper educational classrooms or teachers to educate the many Special Ed students that were now required to attend their local schools. This Least Restrictive Education, allowed the schools to accept students with disabilities, was not endemic to our town's school. It was a law that schools all over the nation were dealing with. It would take a long time to find the funding, implement the programs, educate the teachers, and make a success of it in the educational systems. The needs of the students were as varied as the students' personalities. It was a huge inclusion attempt, and we recognized it was a huge challenge for all involved. But, come on, it was the *right* thing to do.

The long delay in hearing if they had found a place for Windy was sad to us, especially since it was the same county where our parents, grandparents and great grandparents had been educated. (My maternal grandfather had even been the Superintendent of the Anderson County school system during the 50s. None of this mattered if you had a child born with an intellectual disability.) It was another crushing blow . . . our quest for normalcy for our family life could not possibly take place if one of our children could not grow and learn in a good school setting.

It became blatantly obvious that her potential was not going to be reached without total participation on our part. We began looking for a school that *would* accept her. Surprisingly, additional research led us right back to our home turf. We found out that Anderson County had a free-standing school for children with special needs called Daniel Arthur, in Oak Ridge. This was looking like our best choice. (We had heard of it but really didn't know much about it.) We learned it had been established by teachers, principals (mainly a Mr. Steve Brody), and parents of special needs kids in Anderson County, in the 1960s, at a time when these kids were excluded from receiving any formal education. We also learned that the Arthur family had given time and funds to help establish a center in honor of their son, Daniel. The school system later took over the operation of the school as it transitioned from private operation to public.

It *was* a completely separate school though, segregated from the regular students on its own campus. (We didn't like that part.) But there were good parts to like: it turns out that we knew some of the teachers who taught there, excellent educators, and we heard wonderful things about the school from many people as we began to ask questions.

The school was still several miles from where we ultimately ended up living in our new home, but at least not in a basement setting. Each classroom was equipped with modern furniture and books. It was an institution with teachers who really cared about their students and wanted to help them learn all they possibly could. We were impressed on our first visit. We were also told that if she enrolled there, a small, yellow school bus would pick her up at our backdoor and bring her back home every day. And, the time she would spend riding on the bus was very reasonable—no long bus rides all over the county. It sounded promising. (Believe me, we could use promising.)

(Promising to us now are the great educators and programs we have known about through the years. One exciting example is the Cafe Le Reve, started by teacher Sandra Elder, at Maryville High School, in Maryville, TN. The nonprofit restaurant located on the school campus teaches the students in Resource many valuable life-lessons. They learn how to run a business, make change, shop for food, prepare food, and how to serve it properly. They offer delicious, home-cooked meals at a low cost. It's an ingenious idea because everyone involved gets so much out of the experiences they are exposed to. There are now many innovative ideas out there like this in our public schools, but there's always room for more!)

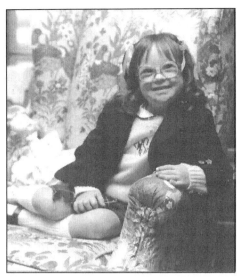

ARC Poster Child

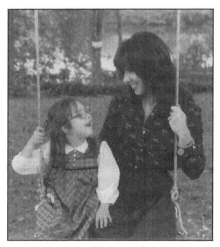

Swinging with Mom

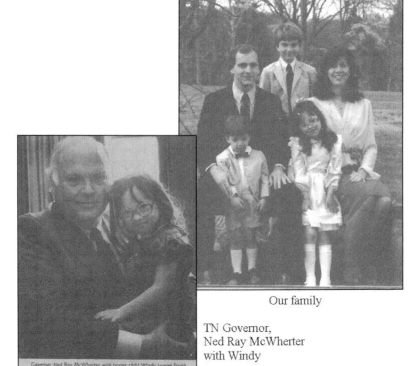

Our family

TN Governor,
Ned Ray McWherter
with Windy

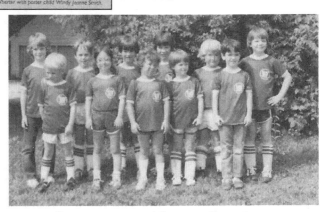

One woman amongst the men—Soccer team

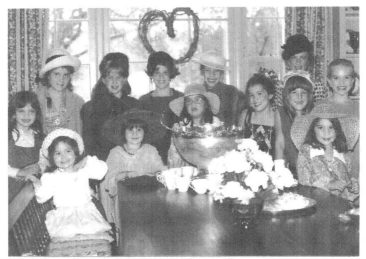
Ladies at "High Tea"

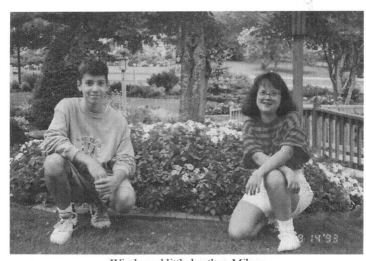
Windy and little brother, Mikey

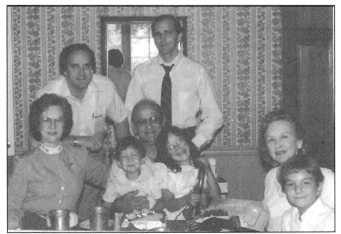
With Nanny, Papaw, Uncle Richard & Aunt Margaret

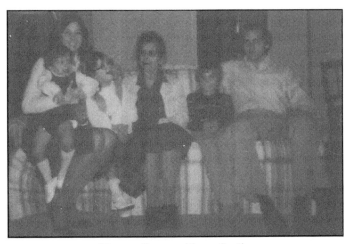
Mamaw Emma with our family

Chapter Eleven
A Little Brother

Once the big decision to move was made, things started rolling rapidly along. David soon had his practice sold to another young Optometrist, and we began the arduous job of packing up. My brother-in-law, Jack, and my dad, had been in practice together for a couple of years and came up to talk to David about joining them in practice there. It all sounded great. We would be moving back home as adults with three children of our own!

(Everyone was excited about us returning home, especially Patsy Wright, a lady who had worked for Mom and Dad as a housekeeper, and who became a sweet friend of us all. She was so glad to get the chance to be near Davey and Windy again, and she fell in love with our baby, Mikey. We were glad to get near her, too. She was a lifesaver to us through the years. We all loved Patsy!)

Michael, our third child, was born seven months before we packed up to move, in 1978. His birth was so different from that of his sister's, five years earlier—we were now so acutely aware of the possibility of giving birth to a child that may have a disability. We decided not to have an amniocentesis done when we found out I was pregnant because we trusted that we would get the baby we were meant to have. Another reason for opting to forgo this testing was because the medical procedure was relatively new at the time, and we were told "it could cause the mother to lose the baby if there were complications, and sometimes there were complications with the procedure." We deemed the risks too great to have it done.

We had trusted God twice before to give us the children we were meant to have, and we trusted Him this time, too—no matter the baby's health or gender. Girl or boy, disability or no, we wanted this baby, and we started praying for him/her every day. Dr. David Rueff, my doctor, patted me on my shoulder and smiled in agreement when I quietly but steadfastly told him our decision. He had given me all our options (The law dictated that healthcare providers had to present all the options, regardless of the physician's personal or religious convictions on the subject.), but he was visibly glad we had made the choice we did.

After our third child's birth, the nurse asked if we had any family in the waiting room that we could show him off to. We told her our parents were out there. We weren't sure if anyone else had been able to come to the hospital. Immediately after we had rejoiced over the birth of our new son, she wrapped him in a small, soft blanket, and handed him to David, who kissed him on his tiny, pink cheek, and then he handed him over to me. Then David leaned down and planted a kiss on my cheek. After allowing us a few intimate moments of checking out his hands and feet, looking into his beautiful dark eyes, (They turned out to be brown like his mama's and siblings.), the nurse wheeled the entire bed to the door leading into the family waiting room, so our parents could see him with their own eyes.

When she pushed that swinging door open, we saw that the room was crowded with nearly every relative we had between us, and several friends too! The room resounded with loud, "Yahoo's", and there were tears of joy as they beheld Mother, Daddy and baby. We were so surprised—we had a "full house"! It was a great feeling to know how much we were loved. David reached down to lift our baby up like a Super Bowl trophy so all of them could see him.

Michael, or Mikey, as we all call him, was someone for Windy to "mother." She and Davey helped teach him to walk and talk, with his lessons beginning as soon as we brought him home. They had waited for years to have a brother or sister, and they didn't want to waste any playtime with him that they could get. They must have figured that the only things holding him back from being a really fun friend was his inability to speak or to move on his own accord. The lessons began from day one.

Windy had to be watched constantly because if you walked out of the room for only a second—even if she looked as if she was occupied with something else—she left *anything* she was doing to run to him. She would immediately and gently roll him over onto his tummy, place her tiny hands under his armpits, and slowly and cautiously drag him forward towards her, hoping to give him a head start on crawling. Davey must have been in charge of diction and grammar . . . because he got up in his brother's face and pronounced words *all* the time. He even tried the peanut butter on the finger trick as his brother got older, and he got bitten for his trouble after the first tooth arrived. (He ditched that lesson after that!)

We found the perfect house down the hill from David's parents, Juanita and Bill, and just across town from mine. It was next door to my first cousins, Judge Buford and Celdon Lewallen, (Because they were my parents' age, I had always thought of them as an aunt and uncle.) and just across from David's aunt and uncle, Jim and Margaret Underwood. After years of living away, it all sounded good to us. The Bond home on Eagle Bend was "For Sale" or so the talk through the grapevine said. (Someone at *"Wednesday Club"* or maybe it was the *"Timely Topics Club"* overheard someone say the house *might* be up for sale. In our town, it meant they could put the "SOLD" sign in the front yard after the meeting. There weren't many choices available, and houses went fast.) When we asked Mrs. Bond about it, she told us to come by and see it.

Mrs. Bond was the cutest little woman in her 80's, who looked like a sweet, little Mrs. Santa Claus. She was petite and wore her white hair on top of her head in a full thick bun. She told us she had been thinking for a long time about going to live with one of her daughters in Atlanta. We were instantly smitten with the house and grounds. We didn't see the tiny outdated master bath with the tiles falling off, we saw the two-acre, manicured lot on the river. We didn't see the only routes to the family room was through the dining room or the laundry room, we saw the eleven foot ceilings, in the lovely wooden-paneled family room, with a wall of high windows looking out onto the water and the huge ancient oak trees. We didn't see the leaky roof that needed to be replaced, we saw the cozy pine kitchen cabinets with a wood-burning fireplace in the kitchen. Blinded by love, we bought it, sans realtor. No one was there to point out the flaws and the necessary repairs to us starry-eyed buyers.

The kids loved the house and spent many hours in the large family room. Davey and Windy's on-going tutoring of their baby brother must have been an advanced Childcare 101 course (They had stored up an amazing amount of training skills from our self-taught, home training and from the CDC sessions!), because Mikey was crawling everywhere on the floor when he was only five months old, and he learned to walk, really to run, at eight months because of their constant coaxing. He also talked in complete sentences before age one. Really! Complete and comprehensive sentences, after repeating words they patiently said over and over and over to him. (Windy had not spent all those hours in early infant stimulation for nothing. She was doing some infant research on her own we suspected!) Mikey would wake up in the mornings in his baby bed, stand holding to the side rail, dressed in a little baby gown, and would yell, "Hey, Mom! I want a bottle. The yellow bottle, not the blue one. Milk, not orange juice, and put a nipple on it!" It was kinda odd, having a little bitty guy yelling specific orders at you, but I must admit, very helpful.

It really was a miracle I carried Mikey to term—because Windy gave us quite a scare on a shopping trip when I was seven months pregnant with him. My sister and I had decided we would drive to a nearby town and buy some clothes for her three children, and for our two, and for the one on the way. When we all piled out of the car onto the sidewalk in front of the large store windows, I hurriedly grabbed hold of Windy's hand and told her to hang on and stay with me. She still had an uncanny way of slipping off and out of sight if you let your guard down for a second.

I was determined that we would have a stress-free shopping trip this time, and that I would set the tone and layout the rules, flat out. Windy hopped out of the back seat, stood up and stretched, and immediately turned her head to stare intently at the mannequins displayed in the windows of the department store where we were going to shop. Stooping down, I placed my face on the same level of her face. Really all I was hoping for was a steady gaze back from her, so I would be assured she understood my desire for appropriate behavior from her.

I took my hand and gently turned her chin in my direction, to make her look me in the eyes. She squirmed a little but she did manage a quick look my way, and she did say, "Yes, Ma'am" so properly, like any Southern Bell would say to her Mama. (I was impressed with her compliancy and good manners and later realized that had been my downfall, because if I had given it much thought I would not have trusted her for a second. The good manners and complyancy were a cover-up for her masterminding a getaway!)

We casually walked through the door of the store, me confidant that I was in total control, she, I now know, confident that if she waited and watched me for the inevitable lapse of my *full* attention, she could make her break for the next escapade she had already formulated in her mind. The stage was set.

The group of us wandered down aisle after aisle of clothing. We would periodically stop to look for a moment at a particular item and then move on to the next piece of clothing that caught our eye. When we got to the baby department, we were all animated over the cute, tiny baby clothes we found. Holding up one thing after another to share oohs and aahs over, I temporarily dropped hold of Windy's hand to lift up the tiniest pair of blue jeans I had ever seen. Everyone was caught up in finding the perfect little outfit for our new addition when I realized that I had not heard Windy's voice in the recent mix of voices. A mom just knows her own child's voice, even in a crowd. I looked down at my side, and there was no sweet Windy waiting obediently.

"Windy?" I said loudly, just in case she was hiding nearby under the nearest clothes racks. "Has anyone seen Windy?" we asked each other. Davey said, "Don't worry, Mom, she couldn't have gone far. She was right here." His voice calmed me, she rarely ventured far from him. He was all of seven years-old, but he was used to cautiously watching out for her. (The responsibility he took upon himself, added to my reliance upon his help in keeping an eye out for his little sister, all made him remarkably responsible for his age.)

We spread out and started looking for her in places we thought she might hide from us. We asked any, and everybody, if they had seen a little, dark-headed girl with pink glasses on, about so high, holding our hands to about three feet off the floor. Everyone we asked shook their heads, No. No one had seen her. How could that be? She had vanished as if into thin air. It was incredible!

In the meantime, my niece, Kristi, had gone to the front door to watch anyone possibly trying to leave with a child that didn't belong with them . . . our Windy to be exact. The store management was quickly informed, and the store was put on instant lock-down. They announced on the intercom that all the exit doors were to be guarded, and no one was to attempt to leave until the missing child was found.

Then all of a sudden, *laughter*, of all things, began at the front of the store and drifted to the back where Davey and I were still frantically looking for her. The words, "We've found her!" were shouted out and repeated by people standing all through the store. Their words echoed back to us. We were joyful over the wonderful news but didn't understand the reason for the laughter penetrating the room.

As we ran closer to the front we found out why there was laughter. Windy had been discovered by a woman shopper, who leaned into one of the display windows to take a closer look at an outfit on a mannequin, and she was startled to find that a little mannequin with a large brimmed hat over its head and covering its face had *moved!* Evidently, Windy had immediately taken off for that window the moment I let go of her hand! She must have planned out every detail of her escape beforehand, and had wasted no time in carrying it out. (We knew she was smart, but ingenious was becoming a word we used more frequently to describe her antics.) She had stood quite still and silent in the display window for a good five to six minutes! What a ham!

We were all so relieved to find her safe, and we hugged her tightly. Then I made darn sure she understood that there were consequences for running away. I told her we would talk more about it when we got home. We had entertained the people in the store enough for one afternoon. It was time to go home! I took her hand and we walked out of the store. Once outside I began to settle down and the fear and trembling subsided. "Try to look on the bright side, try to look on the bright side," I kept saying to myself as we all piled back into the car and drove off.

Windy was safe, thank the good Lord, but she could put herself in harm's way if she kept this behavior up. She would have to learn the "rules" of behavior out there in society, just like we all had to learn. *Give us insight, God, please give us insight on how to teach her this skill.*

As the three kids grew up, they became buddies. Windy became close to both boys, and they were crazy about their sister. They treated her as an equal, no two ways about it. Windy's brothers gave her no special treatment—she was always invited to tag along, and she was always included as one of the gang, but they expected her to pull her own weight, and to behave. She learned many valuable lessons from them: she learned to hold her own by watching our boys, she learned to be gentle, but determined. We noticed that she *always* tried her best at everything she did, and she was very competitive because she always tried to keep up with her brothers. She even beat them on an occasion, if she got the chance: in a foot race, in a card game, in a video game. It was always sweet for David and me to watch when she won something because our sons showed their true hearts . . . they were just as pleased to witness her victories as she was thrilled to experience the victories. It was the old "student teaching the teacher a thing or two." Her teachers in these cases were her brothers.

Living in our old hometown had some great benefits for all of us. Our driveway connected to a road that made a circle in front of all the homes built in the 1950s, and '60s. The kids could ride their bikes and Big Wheels all around that circle to their hearts' content. There wasn't much traffic on the roadway, and the inhabitants of those houses were always on the lookout for kids on the move. Our Smith kids, the new kids on the block, were the only children living on the circle now, except for the Cutshall kids: Bret and Reed, at the end of the cul-de-sac, up the hill. (Their parents, Judy and Dwayne, stopped in to tell us how *happy* they were that another family had moved in near them. I loved Judy from the minute I met her—when she met Windy, she immediately asked me if she could come for a play-date with her daughter.)

Judy and Dwayne became our good friends, and later became more like a big brother and sister to David and me. They gave us advice on many things: on home remodeling, showed us how to tile a bathroom, gave us quick lessons on how to stop water leaks, and how to handle emergency ceiling repairs. Plus, they were ever-ready helpers once when a little toddler boy (ours) spilled a gallon of wall-paint on the kitchen floor, and in his excitement he grabbed for his sister's plastic shopping cart she had left nearby, to make pretty bright stripes around and around the island, and down the carpeted hallway into his room. Don't ask. We cleaned it all up, but it took a while!)

We sort of invaded the peaceful neighborhood. The senior neighbors had been able to drive out of their driveways for years without having to think of children playing in the road. Now they had to be cautious not only for children but also for abandoned toys, groups of kids, and dogs chasing after kids. We liked thinking of it as breathing life back into the old neighborhood. (Some undoubtedly thought of all that liveliness and noise as life-disrupting.) Well, it *was* loud and lively, but at least we did bring laughter and merriment back in a big way—and and our kids enjoyed living there.

We all liked living back home next to the Holley family: Margaret and Charlotte, childhood friends of our parents. Charlotte and her husband, Harlan, lived on one side near us, and Margaret lived on the other side, with their elderly parents. They were constantly entertained by our kids, as they were always ringing their door bells, attempting to sell them old used magazines, flowers they had just picked, or pencil drawings of their recent art work. They also asked if it was a good time to visit with Mr. and Mrs. Holley, who were in their late 80's. (Dave and his younger siblings have always had a heart for older people.) They graciously invited our kids in, and they even purchased many of their items for sale . . . they were always kind to the friendly Smith kids.

A big bonus and contribution to our children's fun childhoods were the members of the Hicks Family. There were ten children in their family, and they lived directly across the main street from our house. There was Michael, Robby, John, Laura, Kathy, Mary Ann, Liz, Susie, Danny and later, Sarah. Dr. Bill was a pediatrician and Jan, his wife, was an attorney, and the assistant DA of the county. They were a large, multi-racial, Catholic family. (They adopted the first five children when they were just babies, and then after a few years, had five birth children.) They were wonderful, loving kids. Sure, at times, there were squabbles and disagreements between brothers and sisters, and between the Hick kids and the Smith kids, but they seemed to really enjoy being with each other. Diversity and acceptance of people with slightly different heritages, skin pigmentations, and intellectual disabilities was no big deal for any of the thirteen of them.

The first time we met them, there were only nine Hick kids, the youngest had not been born yet. They were out playing in their estate-sized yard when they heard our kids in the big front yard playing football with our good old Springer Spaniel, Lady. Lady would bark loudly at the words "Hut, hut, hut!" as they hiked the ball from the quarterback to the receiver. Then she would run with whoever had the ball to the goalposts for the winning points. Football was her favorite sport. Fritzy, the Hick's little black dog, came running over to find out where the barking and the sound of kids at play was coming from. The Hick's kids followed their dog and came running into our yard.

As the children mingled with our kids they began talking and introducing themselves. I had been sitting in the swing on the front porch watching my kids enjoy the lush, green grass. Dave was trying to teach Mikey, just toddler age, and Windy how to play as a team. There was a very small team, but the crew heading their way would make two teams! And they were all ages and heights. Mikey and Windy would be able to stay out there and play ball, too. That was great!

When I saw kids heading toward my kids, I got up slowly to walk towards the gathering group. I wanted to meet *them,* and I wanted to see their reaction to Windy . . . when they realized she had Down syndrome. It was just such a natural thing for me to do, I didn't think much about it. I just knew it was coming, this moment of "are we going to play with this kid or ignore her." That attitude of getting ignored worked with some children, but not with Windy. She wouldn't allow them to ignore her for long. *She* was always aware of these moments, too. I watched for her calculated looks as she sized up the group.

I moved up closer because I knew that it was imperative for these new kids to know that she could fit right in with them as they played together. The sooner they knew that, the better off things would be for everybody. Sure enough—it didn't take long . . . one of the older boys looked over at Windy. Here it comes, I thought to myself, *"God, give me the right words to say here!"* The boy had noticed Windy couldn't enunciate as well as her big brother did, and so he asked in a loud voice, "How come your sister can't talk so good? Is she a retard or something?" (Kids are experts at picking up on differences and calling someone out on that difference, even if it hurts feelings.)

"No, she is not!" Dave (now called Dave, because he no longer wanted to be called Davey) shouted back quickly, "She's smarter than you are, I bet ya'. You just have to listen carefully to know what she's saying!" (He hated that "R" word. He was trying to get rid of that horrible word from people's vocabulary before his sister ever did!)

I didn't want Dave to get into a fight because he felt he had to defend her every time they met someone new. I knew he would try to protect her, even if the kids were older and larger than he was. Love *is* blind! There had to be a better way! I looked at Windy, and I could tell she was in the process of deciding whether to cry about his stinging remark (because she was obviously hurt by the derogatory word), or was she going to get a running-start and attempt to beat the "holy crap" out of the bigger boy? I knew the tell-tale signs of her indecisiveness in a situation like this. I also knew her tenacity. She may have looked like a helpless, frail, little girly-girl, but what *they* didn't know yet was this: she was a wiry, strong-willed, rambunctious tomboy, who could hold her own in a good fight. It was time I tried another tactic for the sake of everybody.

I stepped in among them, "Hey, kids, I'm the Smith kids' mom. You can call me, Miss Vicki (Jason Heady's name for me in the 70s, and it had stuck.). It's great to meet you all. Thanks for coming to visit us. This is Dave, Windy and Mikey. Then I asked them to tell me their names. They quickly called out their names, and we all laughed together. "Give us a little time, and we'll remember your names. And by the way, Windy will remember your names, too. She'll know all of you soon. She's really very smart, just like her big brother Dave said. She *loves* to play with other kids, and be outside with them. She just happens to have something called Down syndrome. We don't ever use that *other* word I just heard spoken, and I *never* want to hear it again in this yard, or anyplace else, for that matter! Down syndrome is just what God allowed Windy to have when she was born."

I had a captive audience now; they were smart kids, too! "She can learn and grow just like you all, but she does take a little more time to learn *some* things, and we could sure use your help. Would you all help her to learn to play your games and talk plain like you do?" I was appealing to their sense of compassion and righteousness now. This had to work on two levels. If our daughter was going to make friends and fit in with her peers, as well as with her brothers' peers, these potentially new friends needed to know the facts about Down syndrome. Knowing the truth from the beginning would give them a basis of understanding about a disability they probably hadn't known about before now. Then, I knew I had to let kids be kids and allow them to assimilate and observe. They were bound to see how much Windy was just a kid—more like them, than not. I had learned that once children recognized the facts, and got to know Windy better, they usually became quite accepting of her and quickly forgot any differences they initially perceived.

"I'll bet you could teach her things faster than I have been able to," I encouragingly stated. I knew what I said to be true: kids learn quicker from other kids. I had seen it proven, time after time in our own "home laboratory." Another observation I had also seen was how quickly children find something different about another child, and begin to pick on them about a given area. They think they can draw attention away from the rest of the group, usually to hide their own feelings of inadequacies or weaknesses. Sometimes I had seen kids become lifelong friends after they acknowledge an obvious difference, and then start a friendship based on the things they *do* find in common. Kids are so open and honest with each other. They tend to rally very quickly to a proper plea for helping someone who needs help and support. I have also found that to be true! I smiled at the children gathered in our yard, and I waited for the answers I was hoping for.

"Sure, we'll help her!" came the happy affirmative answers from each kid there. Then they all joined in the pickup football game and started playing ball together. Even Mikey and their two younger sisters were included and watched out for as they toddled around the yard. I was really impressed with that. Not all kids would have tolerated, or been as gentle to the younger ones like this group of kids were. This was a good sign that they were all going to be great companions for each other. I walked back to sit on the porch swing, to give them some distance from an adult standing over them. It was, in an effect, my way of conveying to the Hick kids that I trusted them—that I knew they were going to be kind to our Windy. I really did believe they would indeed help her grow and learn in the future as they became friends.

After about twenty minutes of play, I heard Dave say, "Hey, she's not a baby. You can treat her like a normal kid, you know!" With that he ran after his sister, took the ball from her (the other kids had allowed her to steal away the ball in an easy surrender), and he explained the rules of the game to her. He told her if she took the ball again, someone would run after her to get the ball. She told him she was ready to play fairly.

They *had* been babying her on the field of play and had not tried to tackle her, even when she stole the ball away. After Dave gave them the word, they started treating her like one of the gang, and she benefited from their normal treatment, and so did they. They all learned from each other. The girls taught her so many jump rope rhymes, chants, dances, board games, and card games that were great for her to learn. The games required her to think fast, and to remember some elaborate sequences. The Hick girls were delighted she could grasp and memorize so quickly. (So were we! She could clap, snap, high five and jump with the best of them in no time.) Several times the Hick family had them over to spend the night in their big, old home their parents had bought from the Kincaid family.

Among the gigantic boxwood shrubbery, a large, stone, two-story enclosed gazebo stood sentinel in the backyard. That old gazebo became a place where they held many a fun picnic. All the children walked to ballgames together, played in both our yards, went to the city pool to swim, and generally became fast friends for years. (Our Dave and John Hicks are still good friends and John keeps Windy abreast of his siblings' welfare. Windy loves to hear all about what they're doing now.)

Matt Lusk, Mark Kreis and his sister and brother, Holly and Ben Gamble, Jenky and Molly Bostic, Susie and Scott Caldwell, Deaver, Andy, Luke, and Kate Shattuck, Jody and Elizabeth Pryse, Amber and Andrea Stults, Chris Wright, Marty Hennessee, and Megan and Rob Harmening were more neighbor kids from around town or from just down the stately, tree-lined Eagle Bend Road, who came to play. Many of their parents had been friends of ours in grade school. They all joined in and accepted Windy, and her brothers, as friends. (Windy, Mike and Dave like to reminisce sometimes over those fun-filled days, and when they do, they all start telling stories and have the best time laughing together.)

All the kids learned an invaluable lesson by being around Windy, and one I hope they never forgot: all of God's people are due respect and kindness and love. It was to be a lesson the Hicks family needed to learn because the tenth child for their family was a girl, Sarah, who was born with Down syndrome, only a few years later. They all loved our Windy and treated her like a sister. When Sarah came along, a special sister, just like their buddy, Windy, they knew what to expect . . . a sister who wanted to be treated as normal! They loved her from the beginning. As soon as they could, they all began to teach their sister so she could reach *her* fullest potential. It was so sweet to see them be so tender and caring with her. They brought her over to our house the minute their mom allowed them to, so Windy could get to know her.

I took our kids to Dr. Hicks, and we looked to him for medical advice and for the general well-being of their health. He was a wealth of information and topics. He always had an intelligent and studied answer for all of our questions. He was always on call for them, ready for any stitches or medical help they might need at night or on the weekends. (There were a few of those moments through the six years we lived there.) That was an awesome comfort to us.

When his daughter, Sarah, was born, we reversed roles. He would call *me* with questions, and for answers to certain situations in raising a child born with DS. All of a sudden I was the professional. He and Jan had always been very kind to Windy and had treated her as a normal child. I assured them that they were more than ready to tackle this huge undertaking. I also advised them that it would take lots of prayers and patience, but we knew she was going to be a blessing to them! And, Sarah has certainly been a blessing to every one of them.

> David and I have now talked to hundreds of couples who have been faced with the challenge of raising a child with a disability. Mikey and Dave have spoken with many, many people who have a family member with a disability. We didn't know God was giving us a ministry along with a baby daughter. Having the opportunity to speak to, and encourage others, has been a blessing to us.
>
> When God gives you a seemingly impossible task in life to do (at least it seems to be so in the beginning) you

usually focus so much on your own circumstances that you fail to see (or, at first, even care to see) how what you're going through will enable you to help other people going through the same, or very similar circumstances. Our prayers back when Windy was small, were about God helping us. Now they are mostly about helping us help others. He turned our pain into others' gain. We like to counsel and give hope, real hope, to those who feel there is no hope. When they hear about our Windy—they find hope.

Everyone can share their life story to help others in their walk. Everyone has a unique life story, and we can use our experiences to give encouragement and counsel to others. We don't know who gets more out of it though, the one doing the counseling or the one receiving it. It's probably a tie!

During this time, we began attending a church in Knoxville called Cedar Springs Presbyterian Church (CSPC). We first found out about the church through the Tarr family, who didn't even attend church there.

Not long after we moved, the Tarrs came to our house to eat dinner with us. They had gladly accepted our invitation, but with the stipulation that they had to leave early, early enough to get to a church service. They had already arranged to go hear some special speakers at a church in Knoxville called Cedar Springs on that date. They told us the speakers were Francis and Edith Schaeffer, from an organization called L'Abri. David and I had never heard of them, but we could tell Deirdre and Bill were very excited about going to hear them speak.

During our dinner together they invited us to accompany them. We decided it was worth the trouble to find a baby-sitter last minute, and to go with them. (K.K., a sweet family friend of ours, came to watch our kids so we could take off in a hurry! Being back on home turf gave us an abundance of wonderful people to call on in a pinch. Beth Ann Bevins, Stacey Burger, Fleta Riggs, Maude Riggs, Mrs. Bunch, my niece, Kristi, and my sister-in-law, Teresa (Nolan), Shelia. They all were so good to our kids on the days I had to work or on our date nights.)

Thank goodness we made the effort. It turned out to be a huge blessing in many ways. We were to find out that night that Dr. Schaffer was considered the leading theologian in the *world* at the time!

David and I sat in amazement as we heard the things he and his wife spoke about. They spoke about babies born with disabilities, and Down syndrome in particular. (The Tarrs had not known the subject of their talks that night!) They told why they believed God wanted these children to have a chance to live productive lives. They were saying things out loud, to a packed crowd what we had never heard anyone say from a pulpit, but we had lived out. David and I went back to hear them every night they were there, and we got the opportunity to speak to the Schaeffers after the last service, on the last night of the conference. They encouraged us in a mighty way.

We felt that if a church was bold enough to have the Schaeffers come and speak, then it was the right church for us. The Tarrs didn't know to what depth their invitation to join them would lead to. It seemed like a last minute invitation (to them and to us) but we later believed it had been planned out in detail beforehand, another Divine Appointment.

Cedar Springs became our home church. It was growing so fast, so many people were joining the membership and visiting each Sunday, and we were only one of many young families eager to hear the word preached by Pastor Don Hoke, the head pastor. (He had been a friend of Billy Graham's, and one of Billy's grandsons, Tullian, would come to join the staff of the church for a while.) He and his wife, Martha, were such wonderful people, and it was wonderful just to be with them and hear them impart their godly wisdom in their unique way.

Pastor Hoke baptized Windy and Mikey in Fort Loudon Lake a few years later. Windy was always delighted to see him, and when she spotted him in church or out in town somewhere, she never failed to go running up to him to give him a big ol' hug. Miss Martha, his wife, told me on several occasions how much those hugs meant to him because, "He is probably perceived to be a somewhat subdued and reserved man. It causes people to give Don a respectable space, so subsequently he is not hugged a lot." Since people generally reframed from hugging him, Martha always loved to see Windy approaching because she knew she was bound to see her give him a hug. She said he really needed those hugs.

It was just another way God allowed Windy to use her loving spirit to bless others, even if that person was a well-known person, or not. They are all the same to her—she loves everyone, and loves to give them hugs.

There are *many* lessons Windy has taught us. One of them is: material things are not as important as people. Windy tested her grandmother to the max on this. My mom, Flo, showed her true colors one day when Windy was about three. It's no secret Flo loved fine things. She loved to decorate their home, and sometimes other people's homes, and Dad was always happy to show their visitors what she had done to make their house more beautiful. She also loved to put on a party and bring out the lovely china, silver and crystal she had collected over time. She was also our family's "Miss Manners". Emily Post's book on proper etiquette was *always* within easy reach of Mom. The boys in the family always knew to take their hats off in the house *and* in a restaurant. It would never do to keep it on and tempt fate or Gaymom's comments. (The name Gaymom, her grandchildren's name for her was descriptive of her always happy, always buoyant spirit. It suited her to a "T".)

On the day Mom was tested to the nth degree, she and I were busy talking. Windy had quietly wandered from the living-room, where she was playing with her small little dolls (her people, she called them), right into Gaymom's dining-room (which had two doorways leading into it from two different rooms). The room was a "no-no" and totally off-limits to the small children always running about on their visits. There was too much in there that they might get hurt on, or too much they might hurt in there! The large, shiny, crystal, hanging chandelier, beaming tiny dancing rainbows on the walls, had to have been an enticer for our little toddler. She was always trying to con us into taking her in there or begging us to let her touch all the pretty things she observed from a distance on most of her visits. We always obliged.

Windy must have walked around to the door farthest from us and poked around until she found some interesting looking Styrofoam boxes on the oak floor. Mom and I were sitting in the den looking at some new decorating magazines she had just received in the mail when we began to hear a faint, strangely beautiful, musical sound: a different note ringing ever so quietly, and then a faint glass-breaking sound would follow. It took us a second to realize that it was coming from the room next to us . . . the "off limits' room." We jumped up and ran in the direction of the noise.

We found the source of the sound. There was Windy, seated on the floor with her little bottom crouched back on the heels of her feet, holding onto the stem of a small crystal goblet like it was a drum stick, hitting each beautiful goblet, lined up next to each other in that box. With each contact of glass to glass, the sound of a musical note was made by her efforts, and then she hit each piece just a tiny bit harder—till it shattered the glass to pieces.

It took four times for us to hear the mysterious, musical, then breakage sounds, before our brains could process the reason behind the sounds. The glass was ever so delicate, and it was a blessing she hadn't been cut. Mom was horrified. She had just ordered the "Eleanor" style cut-crystal to complete her set. She looked at Windy and then at the broken shards before her, all the while Windy remained perfectly still; head and eyes downcast. I hurriedly crossed (leaped) over the carpet and helped her to release the glass stem, now void of its upper half, still gripped in her hand, and to help her step away from the box with the broken glasses. She had managed to do a couple hundred dollars worth of damage in a short time.

When Windy stood up, she saw her grandmother's stricken face. Gaymom was startled at how quickly she had done the deed, and how badly she *could* have been hurt—all while we were so close in proximity to her. Windy, remorseful, went running over and hugged her grandmother's legs and said, "I so sorry! I so sorry!" She hadn't done it to be naughty. She had been fascinated with the sounds. She also knew she had broken a rule or two. Gaymom picked her up and held her close. She explained how she could have been hurt and explained to her that she should always ask if she wanted to do something, and to ask her mom or an adult *first*. Most importantly she told her that she did forgive her. I was so proud of my mother. She showed great love and dignity that day. She also proved she *was* a very fine lady. You can't find that loving reaction in any book of manners. It came straight from the heart! Gaymom proved she cared more for her precious granddaughter than anything she owned. She really loved Windy with all her heart.

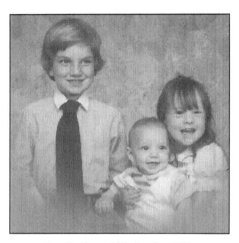

Proud of new little brother Mikey

Chapter Twelve
Daniel Arthur School Years

On the first day of school at Daniel Arthur, I walked with Windy out our back door to the bus waiting in our driveway. She got to the open bus door and started to climb up the high steps (so very high for such short, little legs). All of a sudden two older boys scampered out of the bus and introduced themselves to us. Then they gingerly picked her up and lifted her up those big steps. Two wonderful friends and protectors walked into Windy's life that day. Their names were Tony, a tall, stocky Caucasian boy, and Billy, a shorter, slighter-built African-American boy. They became her self-appointed bodyguards while traveling to and from school, and even at school in the halls or on the playground. They were always available if their services as protectors were ever needed. Each morning one of the guys would get off the bus, carry Windy on, and then they would place her in a seat, up near the bus driver.

David and I were touched by their kindness, but we didn't want to impose upon them, and we wanted them to know that Windy was capable of stepping up and getting on the bus all on her own. I walked out to the bus parked in our driveway early one morning and greeted the boys as they bounded down the steps and onto the asphalt.

"Good morning guys! I want to tell you how much Windy's dad and I appreciate your help getting Windy on the bus every day, but really, she can climb up and get on all by herself now. You all don't have to get out and go to all that trouble."

"Oh, Mrs. Smith, it's no trouble, we *want* to do this!" Tony said, with no hesitation.

"And, we love Windy, and we want to help her," Billy said in his shy, quiet manner. "She's so little and she takes such small steps. She *needs* us."

I was stunned by their sincerity and sheer goodness. If helping our daughter every morning helped them to feel more needed, then who was I to tell them, No?

"Okay, then. Thanks, so much for your help. Those *are* big old steps, and you know she *could* fall. Both of you all are really a *big* help to her. Thank you, guys, again, and I hope you have a great day at school," I said to them, as I saw them straighten up to their full height, and square up their shoulders, as if they were proud of the fact that were perfectly able to meet the challenges of helping little damsels in distress head-on.

They picked Windy up, and they boarded the bus. I watched as they put her in a seat, then they headed to the back of the bus where the older kids rode. It pulled out of the drive and rolled down the street and out of sight.

I stood in the same spot for a few minutes quite humbled. Those boys were eagerly willing to help someone they thought needed them, and they refused to see their own disabilities as a reason to deny that help. Throughout the next few years, they never quit taking care of Windy. They graduated from the school, and Windy finally had to get up on the bus on her own accord. When they left, she missed her friends and their kindness to her. From time to time she remembers them in her prayers, and every time she does—I cry.

> How many of us are willing to sacrifice our own true comfort for the sake of a friend? Maybe you will be more inclined to be a better friend to someone in your life, now that you have read of Billy and Tony. Please, go do

something nice for someone, and come back to read this book later. You'll feel better about yourself, and your friends will feel really good, because someone took the time to show them real kindness and true friendship. (And yes, a family member qualifies as a friend!)

The school was an answer to prayer for us at the time. Windy had access to a fine education via the exceptional educators. You can mandate the law, but you can't mandate love for the students. The principal, Steve Brody, and the teachers who taught there, loved the students and their profession—or they wouldn't have been there. It was obvious they cared.

Daniel Arthur had another Clinton boy enrolled there by the name of Freddy Fagan. He has been a resident of the town all his life, for 60 some years now. The people of the town have looked after him, fed him, clothed him, given him rides to ballgames and other events, and have shown him respect and love for many years. They have even named a street after him, and one of the former teachers at Clinton High School has written a book about Freddy's life. It tells you a whole lot about the town and its people. Windy still calls it *her* hometown. She loves it there, and she loves many of the people who also call it home.

The school proved to be a wonderful learning experience for Windy for the six years she attended. It was small enough to get one-on-one instruction, and yet big enough for her to walk the halls and get to know many other students and teachers. She was *not* shy about stopping by someone else's classroom to say hello to someone she already knew or wanted to know. The mere fact that she was only supposed to be going to the bathroom and coming right back made for some trouble for her with her teachers sometimes though.

Everyone there knew Windy, and she made a point to know everyone. There were some students just learning to walk and to be mobile on their own. Most were larger in stature and taller than she was. On her bathroom breaks, she would take her time getting back to her classroom and instead help some friends on the way. She would stand at the end of the long hallway and shout out words of encouragement to her friends' struggling commitment to become mobile. On more than a few occasions the teachers went to get her out of class, to allow her to wave and dance around, a small distance from the person learning to take those steps, because she was such a great encourager. She was so profuse in her praise and affection for them as they made their way forward.

She even helped kids in her own room. Her teachers told us when she would get her school work done, she would quietly get up and go over to another student's desk and place her small hand over their hand as they held their pencil, and say, "Hold it this way. You can write it easy this way!" She always wanted to help when she saw a need, and the wonderful thing is, she didn't then, neither, does she now, deliberate too long on whether she should, or shouldn't offer help. She just offers—if she is turned down she is not hurt, and she doesn't reflect on the rejection.

Another **WINDY LIFE LESSON** for us: she sees a need, and wants to take an active part in meeting that need. Already at a young age she was stepping into a leadership role. We could see her transforming from a child with a disability into a person who had the discernment to develop her abilities, and right before our very eyes. And she was becoming someone who knew how to encourage others to see their own abilities! It had been our dream for her from the time of her birth, and now it was becoming her own dream. *It was obvious to us* *that God was directing her steps, not for us, but for her, and for His glory!*

She was blessed to have several great teachers while she was at the school who were as adamant as we were that she would learn to read and write. Mrs. Juanita Gulley and Mrs. Bertie Bostic were great blessings to our family. They worked tirelessly to instill good manners and at the same time teach the children they were capable of learning—all the while pushing "the line" past the limits where they had been told to expect it to be. The dedicated teachers walked and looked over the shoulders of each of their students, as the kids copiously wrote the alphabet and the numerals. Talk about the patience of Job! At times they sat the students on their laps where they could look at the pages and words and correct and guide them to read in a warm, secure environment. These conscientious teachers made herculean efforts to ensure the students placed in their care had the optimum learning experiences.

In this loving and organized atmosphere the children prospered and blossomed. I was so thrilled to know some teachers were still around who cared enough to instruct in such a gentle patient manner. Windy excelled. She brought home her own little individually styled books, books her teachers had constructed themselves with words they knew she recognized and would swiftly catch her attention. We read to her every day, and then we had her read back to us. (I read until I was hoarse some evenings. I wasn't about to give up on my dream for her to read on her own.) She also worked diligently on her writing skills, as she copiously wrote the alphabet, over and over, on her wide-spaced, lined notebook sheets. Just when we would all get frustrated—she, from writing, and we, from helping with homework and not seeing much progress—she would suddenly learn something new, like a light bulb turning on, and she would make a gigantic leap forward.

The electricity was present all along, we realized, we just have to know "where and how to click it on" so to speak. Those teachers knew from their years of experience, how to help the kids find that switch. Most importantly, they knew each child's progress would be dictated by the child. They were not frustrated by a certain time frame, neither did they set a time limit for any of their students. Goals, yes, but it was not looked upon as failure if those goals had to be moved forward a bit. They taught us, in due time, everyone could learn. They were proving it to be so in their everyday classrooms. Their teaching attitudes and beliefs in a solid education for kids who had disabilities were paying off.

After school hours we were busy going to all our children's activities. Windy played soccer and took ballet. She loved participating in both. She was a delicate, feminine, little girl that adored good competition. She had turned into a very competitive player! She was a friend to everybody . . . *until* she was on the playing field, and then look out! She would maneuver around you before you knew what had happened to you. And she was pleased with herself!

Not long after we moved she asked if *she* could play soccer. Both of her brothers had joined a team. Why not? So what if there was not one other girl on any of the teams. (Not only were we having to overcome the barriers of intellectual disabilities, we were having to tackle the barriers of being a female and wanting to play sports in a traditionally male-dominated game!) She asked me why she couldn't play. I didn't have a good answer for her, so instead I took her to ask someone directly about it. I took her to meet a coach face to face. We wanted to hear just why our daughter couldn't play with everyone else. So what if she had been born with an intellectual disability? She knew when to kick and run. She knew how to score. I braced myself for a winning sales pitch. (I had begun to feel like I was Windy's Agent. I represented a winner here, I just had to help others recognize she deserved a chance. A real chance. That was all we were asking for.) If he had said no, I would not have pushed the issue. There were other sports we could interest her in.

I went up to Dave's coach at his next practice and asked if she could play on the team. We didn't know him personally, but we knew some of his family members. He kindly stopped what he was doing to really listen to me, and then turned to look at tiny, little Windy and asked her, "Can you kick the ball?" "Oh, yes, I can!" she affirmed, not wavering from his stare. She had the confidence to do this. She wanted to play on a real team more than just about anything at the time. She didn't look at me, but my question to the man had instilled in her the bravado she was displaying to him. She stood tall, as tall as thirty-nine inches can look. "Then get in there and show me," he commanded. "OK!" she hollered back at him, and off she went. God bless him for giving her a chance to prove herself capable of playing on his team! In just minutes her determination on the field was obvious to him, and to everybody else on the sidelines.

As far as we know, she was the *first* girl to play on a soccer team in the county. Girls didn't play on a "boys" soccer team back then. Windy was proving to be a leader, and she was certainly leading the girls in sports in 1979-1980. Being the only girl didn't bother her one bit. She liked it! She was used to hanging out with two brothers. When another girl joined the team a few weeks later, Windy was all for it!

Those kids on her new team were great with her. They learned she was just "one of them," and they accepted her fully. David and my hearts were elated. Our daughter was playing a team sport! The sky was the limit now! We were seeing her develop way past what we had first been told she could ever do. It was especially gratifying to her. Davey and Mikey were proud of their sister, and it helped them to see their peers accept her. (Thank heavens for sports and for volunteers who are willing to give of their time to coach sports. A big thanks to all you who coach out there! Please keep it up! The kids need you! Don't ever doubt the worth of your presence on the field, on the court, or in their lives. The games eventually come to an end, but the good influence a great coach can have on the kid's life lasts a lifetime!)

It wasn't long before acquaintances of ours, Doug and Billie Fain, who were members of The Arc (I refuse to use the name it was then known by, Windy insists I do *not* use it.) suggested we send a picture of Windy in for a contest being held statewide, in their search of a Poster Child for the organization. They told us, "We think Windy is darling. If more people could get a chance to see her picture, we think it would be encouraging to other parents, especially the parents of a new born baby with disabilities."

We sent in a very cute picture of her leaning on a white fence in our backyard, dressed in a red dress with a white pinafore and another one with her leaning against a two hundred year-old tree wearing a little blue plaid skirt, a yellow sweater monogrammed with her initials in navy blue, and a little navy blue blazer to complete the outfit. She stood with her arms folded, smiling out at the world with joy and confidence. And, guess what? She won! As a result she had her picture placed on several TV ads for The Arc group statewide, and she got to meet the Governor of Tennessee, Lamar Alexander.

On two different occasions, she was introduced to the House by our high school friend, Tennessee Representative Tom Wheeler, where she received a standing ovation, toured the Capital on a private tour, stood in the Governor's office with him for photo-ops, and even surprised us (and the governor) by running over to sit in his chair behind his big desk. She sat way back in the seat, and crossed her arms behind her head. Then she leaned forward and placed her elbows on his desk, resting her chin on her fists, observing the room from his personal vantage point. Always a ham, she had the whole room laughing when Governor Alexander jokingly said, "She looks really comfortable in that chair and looks like she is trying to take my place!" It wasn't *just* a joke to her, she seemed to like all that political stuff already.

Later that year she made several Public Service Announcements for The TN-Arc for television, with the Spokesperson for the group, Honey Alexander. Honey, is the wife of the Governor. All this at the tender age of seven! Both her brothers went with her on trips, and they were amazed at the fun things they got to do—all because of some contest she had won. We had several fun-filled weekends in Nashville because she won that contest and the local Arc membership increased tremendously for the next few years.

Chapter Thirteen
A Change of Direction

By the end of Windy's sixth year at Daniel Arthur, the county school board decided it would make a super place for the teenage kids to go who had been suspended for an assortment of reasons from the schools across the county. They needed to be out of their regular classrooms for a "season," but they still needed a place to attend classes and continue their education uninterrupted. This meant they were expected to ride the small school buses to and from school with all the kids who had a myriad of disabilities. They were responsible for finding someplace for the other students to go to school while being suspended from their previous schools, and Daniel Arthur was a county school with space available to house them and the instructors required to teach them.

Yes, there were other factors involved in the decision to open a school to enable the students to continue to receive an education without too much interruption. We too, were in agreement with that: troubled kids needed supervised instruction while receiving an education. We wanted the kids who had been expelled to get help in all areas, educational and otherwise, just not at the sacrifice of our kids with special needs and their education.

It all turned out for the best because the public schools in Anderson County were gearing up to make the final leap into integrating the children with special needs with the regular students, in the regular classrooms. There were just some unanticipated awkward and potentially dangerous moments in the "between times" of the transition. Transporting the students proved fertile ground for some of those precise moments.

The transporting of these new "alternative students" with the existing students who rode the school buses was a whole *other* issue. The buses were all small, yellow minibuses, and they transported the students with special needs, in the care of one adult driver per bus, and she or he, had an all-consuming job of driving them to and from the school. Some drivers had to help some of the children get up the steep steps and *into* the bus, not to mention those who had to have their wheelchairs loaded in as well. The drivers had to be able to trust that the boarded students behaved, sitting still in their seats, while they helped load a student at the different scheduled stops. (David and I had always been so impressed with how well the kids behaved while the other kids came aboard.)

The idea of putting these two groups of kids together on a bus that spring term, without extra chaperoning and proper supervision for the students who were *already* being disciplined for their disruptive behavior, was a nutty idea, and proved too much for the drivers *and* the kids with the disabilities. (DUH!) This "merging" had not been in effect for long when "a situation" arose involving *our* family.

We were called to the school one morning because petite Windy had been caught on the bus ride to school with a lit cigarette in her hand. They even told us what brand the confiscated cigarette was: a Camel. We had had enough! It was the last straw for us. We could see that these bus rides were going to get real "bumpy."

We didn't smoke, and she had no access to cigarettes in our home. It sounded suspicious—someone else had been involved in this. (Even if she *had* wanted to smoke, I personally think she would have attached a long, black cigarette holder to it for exaggerated effect. Maybe a Virginia Slim? Now, if they had told us she had done *that,* we might have been a little more suspicious that it *had* been her idea!) David and I got in the car and drove immediately to the school where they had the suspects detained in the principal's outer office. Windy was sitting in a big wooden chair with her short, little skinny legs swinging in the air—she couldn't touch the floor yet. She wasn't upset over the ordeal at *all*. That was a huge clue to us that she knew she was in the right on this thing. (As she grew older, and wiser, she became more incensed by injustice and flagrant lying.)

The older boys seated across the room from her were slouched back in their chairs, with a "devil-may-care" attitude. We took a seat beside her, and instead of talking to our daughter about the incident, David began talking to the boys—and consequently found out the truth. David had casually asked one of the guys if he could bum a smoke from them, and the "said" brand was offered up. Surprise! After our investigation, the cigarette brand was found to be the same exact brand in the pocket of one of the new, older guys, who had ridden the bus that day. (David's own boyhood had prepared him for situations like this, and he put his experiences to good use!) The rest of the story came out. Someone thought it would be real funny to give Windy a "smoke," they said, since she was so friendly, and (already) they could tell she was such a clown! It didn't take a professional detective to deduct the truth. It didn't seem to bother them at all that they had been found out. They told the whole story and laughed as they told it. Windy wasn't angry at them for getting her into trouble, I noticed. She sat trying to hide a smile as they spoke about the incident. She thought it had been funny, too!

The principal heard the confession through his open office door, and he immediately walked into the waiting area and gave Windy and us his apologies and dismissed her. Then we walked her to her classroom. We told her we would talk about it when she got home from school, and I told her I would be there to pick her up. No more bus rides for her. It hadn't been a huge offense, but truthfully, something worse could possible happen in the future. After all, these "new students" had been expelled for various reasons, none of them good things. David and I felt all this had been a sign of things to come. A warning, so to speak. You could say, a "smoke-signal" warning us of possible impending danger ahead.

So many things had changed in the last two years at the school, and some of the teachers we had known had already retired or had left to teach in other schools. Change was again in the air for our family.

Consequently, and because of the laws mandated from the federal government in the areas of Least Restrictive Environments (LRE classes), all the county schools began classrooms for the children with disabilities, who lived within a set radius of each of the school zones. In other words: kids with disabilities now had the opportunity to attend the school closest to their home. Finally! A victory for true equality.

The self-contained school had not been a perfect environment, because it segregated the regular classes from the special education classes. The LRE classes would not be without its share of equally trying problems for the students and adults, but at least it was a gigantic step in the right direction. (No situation is ever the perfect situation for every student or every teacher.) We knew it was time to find another school for Windy. She had absorbed all the good she possibly could from Daniel Arthur School. It was time to set up a meeting with those in charge, at the school closest to our home. Hopefully, there would be no more long bus rides, and no more quotes said to us like this one, "There *is* no place for her in her brothers' school." We would see. One thing was certain: we weren't naive anymore about the schooling issue for our daughter. We had received our own education about the laws concerning her education.[5] It was change for a good reason. Windy was living on the cutting-edge of Special Educational history.

Lord, here we go again . . . we can't see that next step. This is so unlike our own childhood. We attended the same schools our parents did, sometimes even had the same teachers they had. Where do we go from here as a family? We're listening, God. And, we know You know this, but we don't have much time to make this major decision. You know what Windy needs, and you know what Dave and Mikey need. Please show us soon. In the meantime, let us grow to be better people in the waiting. Amen.

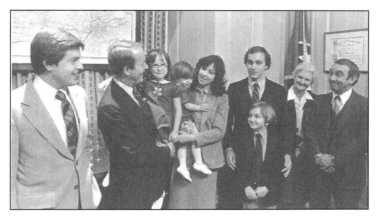

Windy in Governor Lamar Alexander's office with
TN Rep. Tom Wheeler

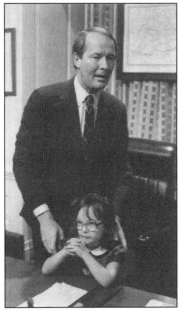

Right after making a beeline for the
Governor's chair

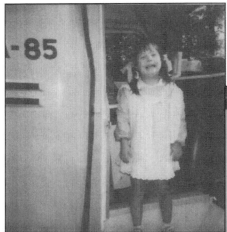

First bus ride to school

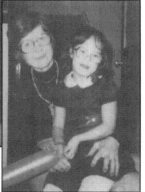

With beloved teacher, Mrs. Gulley

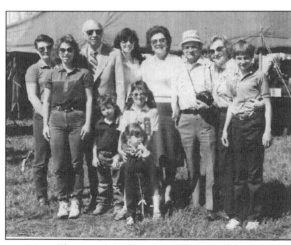

At Area Five Special Olympics and some of the family

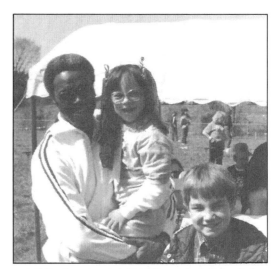

With Olympic Medalist Winner, Ralph Boston

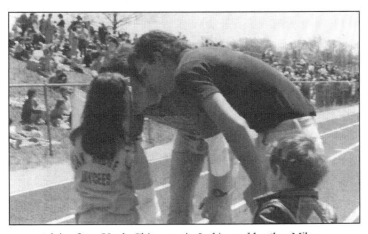

Advice from Uncle Chip, cousin Jackie, and brother Mikey

Chapter Fourteen
Attending C.A.K. with Her Brothers

We became excited over the possibility of all our children attending the same school district in the same block. Mikey was starting first grade in the fall. Dave would be old enough to attend the middle school right next door to the primary school. David and I met this challenge of finding a school with prayer and determination—we were ready to find equality out there for our girl. This time we had the law of the land on our side. We just didn't know where she belonged, where she could get the best education available for her.

Interestingly, a relatively new private school called Christian Academy of Knoxville (CAK) had opened a few years before and had just moved to a new campus in West Knoxville. They had started to advertise their grades, first through the senior year of high school, on a local Christian radio station, WRJZ. It sounded so good that we decided to visit the school campus with the encouragement of a new friend, Tracy Rice, who already had three children enrolled there.

While we were looking for a new direction for Windy's continuing education, Tracy convinced us to go for a visit to CAK. She had only good things to say about the teachers and their curriculum. She looked at our oldest son one day, so handsome in his shirt and tie, just coming home from a choir performance, and said, "Your Dave is such a gentleman, and a very nice kid. He needs to be at CAK for his high school years. Mikey and Windy would love it, too!" She began to tell me all about the school, their mission, and their encouragement of parental involvement. She had included Windy as if her inclusion was a perfectly normal thing to do. It made perfect sense to us. *Maybe* we had a chance to enroll them in the same school after all, just not in this hometown of ours. It was a few miles away. It would mean I would have to drive them to school about twenty-five minutes away. It would be more inconvenient, but it was well worth exploring the possibility. So with David's encouragement, I dialed the school's number to make an appointment to meet with the Headmaster, Mr. Carl Swindell, and with the Assistant Headmaster, Mrs. Jane Williams.

Here was another step in our life that had not been on our radar. "Well, we'll go see what they have to say, and we'll walk around the campus and get a feel for our next step," David said to me. Who would have thought our quest for Windy to have a new classroom would lead to a new school for all of our children?

No commitments yet, we would have to pray for real clarity on this. Would our boys want to leave their friends and the familiar? Would it be a good decision? I had loved waking up in the small town, hearing the weather and traffic reports in Knoxville, and reveling in the fact that none of that was a factor in getting our boys back and forth to school. There was that old "comfort zone-stretching thing" again. Darn it!

Our family decided together that this new school was awesome, once we had visited and met some families who helped start the school. We enrolled all of our kids and they were accepted. Windy adored all the children in her and Mikey's new classrooms. She was older than all the children in the first grade, but she was the same size in stature, and probably on the same level in her reading and writing skills. When we took her in for testing that was required for grade placement by the school, Mr. Swindell had suggested we place her in the first grade, so she would get the fundamentals and foundations of the curriculum of the Abaca system they taught. She was now academically behind her peers, and we felt she needed all the review she could get. We had seen her hit many plateaus as she learned new things. Sometimes she learned something immediately, and at other times, she seemed to be unable to grasp something, and then all of a sudden she would make huge strides in her understanding. David and I wanted her to read with comprehension and to write with purpose. First grade was a good fit for her to begin in this situation. She was so little and petite, she would fit right in. And, if it all worked out, how great would it be for the children to learn what another child, someone born with an intellectual disability, was like. They could gain insight, compassion and understanding for others that they wouldn't have had otherwise.

She was the *first full-time* Special Ed student with an intellectual disability CAK had ever accepted. First is something she, and we, have learned to accept as her role in life. Hey, somebody has to be the first, right? Being the first is usually never an easy or sometimes not a readily accepted position to be in. She has shouldered this great responsibility with bravery, dignity and determination. I guess you can surmise by now that we loved CAK from our very first visit! Mikey and Dave ran all over the school with kids their age, who came to show them around. Nice kids that seemed to care about making real friends with the new kids. The boys were as excited as Windy had been. *Thank you Lord!*

She had learned to read and write by sight reading, and now that would be reinforced by learning to read phonetically. We all agreed that she would be okay restarting the first grade class, but there was one hitch—would Mikey be okay with his sister in his same grade, or would it be creating problems for our family, instead of solving some? We had talked to him privately before we enrolled them. We had sensitively explained the whole situation and talked over some possible scenarios that might take place with kids on the playground or in the classroom. Although he was only six years-old at the time, he said, "Of course, I want my sister with me at school. I don't want to go there if she's not going to go there! You don't understand,

Dave and I love her so much that the kids will love her, too!" Our youngest son said this with such a look of sincerity and love in his dark brown eyes that David and I were sure (even though he was very young) that he was ready to accept the challenge of attending school with his big sis. We didn't tell him, but we had talked it over with the headmaster and principal, and if things didn't work out, after a trial period, we were prepared to find another school for her. We wanted him to find his place in this new school, regardless of where his sister attended. Windy's brothers deserved a great education, also!

And, you know what? He and Dave *were* right about the other kids' total suppport of their sister. Those children in the two classes were some of the nicest, kindest children we had ever known. Was it because they had been briefed by the teachers and their parents? Was it because of our boys' attitudes and total acceptance of their sister? Was it because of Windy's own attitude and sweet personality? Or, was it because of a Divine intervention? We believe it was *"All of the above."* The children picked up on the way our Michael and Dave spoke and behaved with Windy. They saw their teachers treat her as a full, equal member of the student body. They saw her as having to follow the same rules and regulations as they did, and they also saw her being reprimanded, the same as they were when she broke a school rule or misbehaved in class. True equality was all we had ever asked for. CAK was all about equality. God paved the way.

We were all excited over the new school situation that year. Dave was in the eighth grade and Mikey was placed in one of the first grade classes, while their sister was placed in another. The two first grades had separate rooms, yet the two classes spent many hours together in Band (where she learned to play the flute like her Mama), Chorus, Art, and Physical Education, and of course, playtime on the playground. They shared friendships, and in the beginning everyone watched how Mikey treated his sister. He acted like you would expect a boy to act toward his sister: he was cordial toward her most of the time, but ignored her the rest of the time. He played ball of some type at every opportunity and chased girls with his large circle of friends, who were boys. Windy, with a large group of girls, was playing ball, playing "house", and chasing the boys back into their forts.

During recess one day, in the third year of their attendance there, a new girl was introduced to the kids on the playground by the teachers. Bonnie (not her real name) was a shy little girl. She had recently been adopted by a sweet Christian family in hopes that they could help her overcome her horrendous childhood, which included being abused. Her new mother related to us years later how she had looked anxiously on, a few feet back from the group, as Bonnie looked down at her feet and refused to look up at all the new, curious little faces standing in front of her. The silence was deafening for a *long* moment, then Windy stepped out of the crowd, walked over, and reached out and grabbed Bonnie's hand. "Come on, Bonnie," she said with great dignity, "You're on *my* team." All the girls ran after them to continue their game of tag on the school yard playground.

In an instant Windy had accepted and included the 'new' girl, and the rest followed along. (Over twenty years later that mother is still grateful for Windy's loving attitude, and says she will never forget how kind Windy was to her daughter, or the way she accepted her right *where* and *who* her daughter was at the moment.) Our daughter was a catalyst in introducing Bonnie to the other girls in the class. Another **WINDY LIFE LESSON**: Look around you and see if there is someone who needs you to come along beside them and befriend them, just the way they are right now! Never mind what others think. Doing the right thing is never wrong!

David and I met and made many friends among the parents of the students of CAK. I knew our children would make friends fast, but it was also fun for us, as adults. A real bonus I hadn't really expected. Wilson and Nancy Ritchie befriended us and had us to dinner several times. David and Wilson became running buddies. (Wilson later gave us a generous gift of a large weight machine. We kept it in our garage, and all five of us used it for years. It was a God-send to us. Windy still exercises because of the habits we instilled in her by using that home gym.) JoAnn and Lenny Simpson, and Nancy Cochran and her husband, Tom, became fast friends.

I have never seen such acceptance from a group of kids. They all bonded, despite their differences, and became close friends. They were so nice to Windy. Many of them became a peer tutor to her later on, taking the extra time to help her understand the work assignments. She came to love them all. Ellen Cochran, Tracy Dry, Sarah Byerley, Celeste and Jennifer Simpson, Wendy Griz, Tori McLean, Katherine Parker, Emily Brewer, Erin Russell, Frannie Bowman, Kim Sherrill, Julie Benner, Amy Stooksbury, Allison Dorian, Kelly Crawley, Amanda Travis, Jenny Swindell and Sarah Rice are just some of the girlfriends who befriended her. Friends mean so much to Windy, and to us, because we are grateful for those who love her as a true "BFF" friend.

There were many birthday parties that she was invited to. (Her "Party Girl" rep was being "written in stone"!) She enjoyed being with others and celebrating life. She still does, and her joyous attitude just makes you have a better time!) She made friends with her brothers' friends. Eric Cochran, Jonathan Albright, Curt Wright, Phillip Smith, Chad Blowers, Josh Hinman, Derek Griz, Jeff Phillips, B. Jones, Jamie Swindell, Seth, David, and Paul Bowman, Willie Guzman, Dean Rice, Austin Parsons, and many more became familiar with the feisty little sister of the Smith boys! Some of those friends she still sees on occasion, some she hears from on Facebook, and some send her greetings by way of her brothers, when they hear from them.

There were other friends she met during this period in her life at other places outside of school, Jennifer, Kristen and Amy Palumbo, became dear friends, and David Jay and Carrie Osborne went with her to be volunteers in Nashville at the State Special Olympics for several years.

Kellie Thomas, at gymnastics, and Laura Hill, in Clinton, became close friends. These two girls had also been born with Down syndrome. David and I are grateful for all these kids who grew up with her. We're grateful for their assistance in helping her grow into the incredible woman she has become. Part of her successful development was because of each person mentioned, and because of their complete and loving acceptance of her!

Living in our old hometown for six years had been a decision we never regretted, but as sure as we had been about our timing then, we now knew it was time to move. Our new church was thirty miles away, and our children's new school was twenty-five miles away. David's new office was near the church, and it was time to move nearer to it all and shorten our commute. Between work and school and after-school activities, we were spending too much time on the road. Dave was in the Ensemble choir and was on the CAK soccer team, and we had many practices and games to attend. Windy had started classes in gymnastics, and Mikey got a lead part in a school play. On top of that we were all involved with church activities. Some nights we were getting home very late and homework was done in the car or at David's office—not the best of circumstances for any of us. Dinner needed to be cooked and on the table so we could enjoy being a family together. If we were going to have three kids enrolled in a private school, we would have to adhere to a strict budget since David had just begun his solo practice in Knoxville. We couldn't afford a house so we decided to rent.

We took a weekend to drive around the city and check out the neighborhoods. West Knoxville was just beginning to grow explosively at the time, and homes for rent in close proximity to the school were hard to come by. One particular neighborhood was a little too close for us. The houses were on smaller lots and built close together; it felt claustrophobic after living on two acres. The lack of old growth trees screamed "too new" to us as we drove by the little trees planted in the tiny front yards. I told David that we could never live in *that* place, in *that* neighborhood. Well, guess where the *only* nice house in our price range happened to be when the real estate agent called us the following Monday morning? You guessed it, in *that* very neighborhood. Once again, God knew best. It was located near every place we had to be each day. A "no brainer." David called our agent back in a hurry and told her we *wanted* to rent the house. We packed up our belongings and furniture to move West . . . to West Knoxville, that is.

We moved into that newer rental house, and it was like living in a vacation house after living in an older home that had to have something repaired *all* the time. All the plumbing worked at the same time, and there were no leaks in the roof, and the yard could be mowed in about twenty minutes! The boys had their own rooms for the first time, and Windy had a room across from ours. I had no idea that life could feel this freeing and fun. We spent many happy hours together in the first-floor family room watching ballgames and movies. Even our Springer Spaniel, Lady, liked the new house!

Our children quickly made friends with Laxmi Krishnamurphy and other children in the neighborhood, and there were a lot of children available to play, at any given time. They made lemonade and sold it in a stand they had spent hours making with the Ashworth boys, Stephen and Matthew. They went fishing with David in a pond filled with fish, a short bicycle ride away. They jogged with us on the streets.

After getting settled in for about two months, we had the pleasant surprise of a phone call saying Windy had been chosen to be a participant in the upcoming 1986 International Special Olympics, to be held in South Bend, Indiana, on the campus of Notre Dame. It was such a great honor to represent the state of Tennessee in Gymnastics. Competition was going to be stiff: seventy-four countries would be represented, and all fifty states. This was a *big* deal!

Windy and I started exercising by walking and running, up and down the many hills in our area, and we stepped up the gymnastic lessons with specific routines to practice. When I couldn't go with her on her daily jaunts, Mikey and Dave talked her into jogging or fast walking with them. We were all looking forward to the "Biggest" Special Olympic Games there are. Whether we could attend with her or not was another thing. It was far from home, and the games lasted ten days. It looked pretty doubtful that we would get to go, but we kept hoping that when the time drew closer we could come up with a solution.

In the meantime, another big surprise came our way when our friend, Sam Brown, called us one day to tell us he was coming to Knoxville to practice Orthopedic Surgery, and that he and his wife, Rose, had bought a new house. When he said the name of the same neighborhood we were living in, we knew instantly one of the reasons why God had allowed us to move to that particular place. Their new house was only *two* streets over from the home we'd rented! David and I had prayed for Sam for a long time. Now we' could finally spend some quality time with him and Rose. Sam and David and another friend, Pete Graves, began jogging together and

Sam really began to allow Jesus to control his life and future plans from then on. This move hadn't been our plan. We just had to be willing to go where He led.

Family life soon took center stage as we settled down to the most "normal" life we had ever had. Christian Academy of Knoxville (CAK) turned out to be even better than we had anticipated. What a joy it was for us to drop our children off at the same school and to know that they were instilling the same principles that we were at home. It was not a perfect school with perfect teachers, but we weren't sending perfect kids from perfect parents either! The education they were receiving was super, and they were also required to memorize Bible verses each week and to recite them in front of the class. The Christian education they were receiving was priceless to us. Windy seemed to jump at the chance to memorize Scripture, stand before her peers, and recite from memory. After dinner she would pore over her Bible assignments at one end our long, pine, harvest dining table, while one brother spread his books at the other end, and another brother worked at the middle of the table.

Most all of our kids' teachers were wonderful. Two of Windy's first teachers were Betsy Thomas and Mrs. Ann Sullivan. All of her teachers were very patient and kind to her, but they expected her to complete the school work. We loved that about them. Windy did, too!

Homework was tedious for Windy because she wrote slowly and read slowly, but she always *enjoyed* the discipline and hours spent in her brothers' company doing the same things they were doing. Her competitive spirit always rose to the challenge, and she conquered her assignments. It was hard for her, but even harder for us to witness as we saw the long hours it took for her to complete each task. She didn't complain, not once. She wanted so badly to be treated normally, and she was willing to do whatever it took to fit in.

She loved school, and she woke up early each morning to get ready without any prompting from us. She was dressed and in the kitchen for breakfast usually before her brothers were up. She was harder to get into bed (she is still a night owl to this day!), and she'd lay awake for awhile every night before she fell asleep. When she did go to sleep, she slept very lightly, the slightest noise awakened her. She would sing quietly or talk to herself in a whisper sometimes until she fell asleep. Always the next morning she was up "with the chickens." (As an adult, she now has no trouble 'sleeping in,' although it is rare that she gets a chance to.)

There are so many things that our kids remember from their school days, but one incident in school can still send our boys into hysterics as they recount the story of their sister and her interpretation of a particular subject.

When Windy and Mikey got to the sixth grade, their teachers gathered all the sixth graders together for a sex education class that was mandated by the state. Being a Christian school, they hoped to be delicate in their terminology, and still teach the students what they were required to learn. After some introduction to the subject, one of the teachers began to describe inappropriate behavior, and she gave the example of when someone touches themselves in private places in front of others. She was trying to warn them of a "flasher" who might try to expose him or herself in indecent ways. She said this was *never* acceptable behavior, and if this ever happened, the child should go tell another adult immediately or to scream for help.

Windy, being totally unaware of the real meaning the teacher was trying to instill, innocently raised her hand. "Yes, Windy," the teacher said.

"I just want to say my Dad does that all the time. So do my brothers and their friends. All guys do it, especially if they're playing ball. It's disgusting and gross!"

She was talking about how a man has to "adjust things," from time to time. She was right; we had witnessed it taking place on many a basketball court, football field, and baseball mound—in real life or on a televised game. She was finally getting to voice her disgust with this male behavior. The class knew what Windy had really meant, but they laughed uncontrollably anyway. All the nervousness over the dreaded Sex-Ed class had been blasted away by her funny take and description. She sat smiling at the hilarious thing she must have said to make them laugh this hard! Somewhat aghast, the teacher rapped her pencil on the table several times to make the class come to order. It took a long time to calm them down. Windy had stolen the show.

The teacher made the proper distinctions and continued on. She had definitely lightened the mood for the classroom kids though. That story still gives our boys and their friends a big laugh! Oh, well! What can I say here, Windy has undoubtedly brought joy and laughter into our lives in unexpected ways! Enough said. Next subject!

Special Olympics Meets were always grand times for Windy and for our family. Windy excelled at running dashes. All that friendly competition playing in the yard with her brothers paid off in the Olympics. She has oodles of medals and ribbons in her closet to prove she can run like the wind. Besides running, she enjoyed competing in many other events, and she tried her best in all of them. She was also on a basketball team while attending Daniel Arthur School and she loved the field events, as well. (Gymnastics participation came later on in her teen years.)

Dave and Mikey *always* went as her volunteers to be huggers at the end of the events. They wouldn't have missed going and volunteering for anything. They loved going for Windy, as well as for all the other participants. David and I think they looked forward to the big yearly games as much as their sister did. Throughout each and every year, of the fifteen or more years they went with her, they always took friends of theirs to help volunteer with them. And, I do mean *many* friends. Dave and Mikey would get permission to take whole classrooms of students.

Christian Academy of Knoxville had never sent student volunteers to any Special Olympics Games before our boys took them with them. (Neither had Farragut High School, until we got permission to take a group to be volunteers with us.) Most of the students in these two schools had never been around anyone with a disability, except Windy, whom they all adored, and it was such a wonderful introduction to so many kids with special needs. Admirable traits could be found in any given event. They observed the limitations of movements, physical strength and intellectual disabilities, but the most impressive thing was the will to succeed and win. It was life changing for everyone who came to watch.

Our boys played a huge role in introducing many of their classmates to an entire segment of the population most of them were previously unaware of, people who need our help and compassion. They also showed them that these kids with special needs were really just kids like they all were, with the same feelings and desires and dreams. They soon discovered new truths about these kids with special needs, and everybody benefited from knowing each other.

Dave had learned all about having a sister with Down syndrome from his toddler years, and Mikey had been born into the family dynamics. Because of our boys, their peers learned the invaluable lessons of making friends with those who were born with intellectual and developmental disabilities. They learned to volunteer for the athletes, and to pray for them, and for their families, continuing well after the Games were over.

David's family members and my family members always attended the local Area Five Special Olympics and were great supporters, always spurring our girl on. Each Opening Ceremony they would release the beautiful Homing Pigeons into the sky, and we watched them circle the field and then fly away. That's when my sister and I would lose it, since we couldn't hold back the tears. It was such a touching moment to see the athletes marching onto the field, ready for competition, and reciting the Oath that Eunice Kennedy Shriver had recited at the very first Special Olympics in 1968.

We got to meet her in 1987 at the International Special Olympics at Notre Dame and thank her for all she had done for all people with disabilities. It was an honor for us. She had a heart for people with special needs because of her sibling, Rosemary, who was born with intellectual disabilities. She started Special Olympics in honor of her. They had well-known brothers, former President John F. Kennedy, former Senator Robert Kennedy and former Senator Ted Kennedy. Having a sibling who was born with a disability had certainly influenced that family in a great way!

The Oath is repeated aloud by every one of the participants at every opening ceremony, all over the world. It says: "Let me win, but if I cannot win, let me be brave in the attempt." Then the words, "Let the games begin!" resonate over the crowded stadiums, and a great cheer rises up from the voices of the participants and from the audience! The words always grab at my heart.

It was in these deeply felt moments that my heart would ache, privately and silently. I felt the pangs of those first few days of her birth once again. I had to face afresh the fact that she would never be normal. It was an undeniable fact, and her participation in the Special Olympics was a reminder to *me* that Windy had been born with Down syndrome, and it was a disability that was *never* going to disappear, or go away. It was also a reminder of God's Grace . . . here she was, alive just like we had prayed for, and healthy and ready to compete. What a wonderful venue the Olympics were for her to participate in. She was *always* brave in her attempt. She could have been born with so much more debilitating disabilities. We saw so many blessings all around us! *I had to hold my head up and look at those birds in the sky. If You watch over the sparrow, a tiny, little bird . . . I know You are watching over us Lord. Take this sorrow I feel at the moment and let me see the BIG picture. I'm looking up, Lord, I'm looking up!* Before the last bird was out of sight, I was always ready. I had to be brave in the attempt at life, too! . . . *Let the Games begin!*

It was so uplifting to see the students in regular classrooms taking the time out to be huggers and volunteers for the games. We were impressed with the character and integrity of these student volunteers, and with the kindness and consideration they showed for the participants. I can think of only one altercation that took place in over twelve years.

Some kids had stopped by to watch the events during class changes one year during the Games. I was walking by a group of teenage boys, trying to get to the other side to watch Windy in her long-jump competition, when I overheard them talking. They were gathered in a loose huddle and were laughing and placing bets on the participants. I stopped in my tracks to listen. I heard one boy say, "I'll put ten dollars on the tall retard in the bright blue shorts!" as he slapped a ten dollar bill in the outstretched hand of the obvious ring leader of the group. Their group grew bigger as more boys joined them to put down their bets, pull out their dollar bills, and call out more derogatory descriptions of their "picks"—followed by loud, rude laughter. I couldn't just walk on by. My "mama bear" instincts took over! I marched up to the boys and elbowed my way into their circle. No one stopped me.

"Stop this insanity!" I yelled, as I smacked at the money in the boy's hand, the one in charge of holding the money. I took them all completely by surprise. (My reaction even caught *me* off guard! I hadn't stopped to think this through!) The dollar bills fell to the ground, and strangely enough no one moved a muscle to retrieve them. In fact, they became completely still and silent, as they stared at me. What kind of nutty woman was standing in their midst? They didn't know if I was an undercover cop or a teacher on a mission! It would have really frightened them to know I was just a Mother! (Everyone knows mama bears are easily provoked if potential harm is near, and they are the most dangerous when they believe their babies are threatened. This was threatening, inappropriate behavior towards my child, and all the other children out there. I had the utmost respect for the Athletes out there, and I could not tolerate this belittling of their lives.)

"How could you all *do* such a thing? Betting on these kids and making fun of those who are out there trying their best? *They* have more guts than *you* do! You all should be ashamed of yourselves. God has given you strong bodies and sound minds, and *this* is what you choose to do with *your* blessings? You should be volunteering to be helping those kids out there like your peers are. If you don't have the decency to help them, then get your butts back in school, or I'm going to tell your Principal about this, and I can pick your faces out of a line up," I said as I deliberately looked in their eyes around that circle. About this time a police officer came up to me to ask if there was a problem. There were several police on duty to help with the security and extra traffic because of all the buses that carried the athletes from the area schools. I know I was speaking *a little* loudly. I didn't care. I was in 'Mother protection mode,' and I was livid. I felt righteous indignation for all those participants. I had to come to their rescue, I had to stand up for the dignity of their precious lives.

"No, sir, not *now*. In fact, these guys have graciously donated some funds on behalf of Special Olympics!" I said, as I bent down to pick up the fallen bills. Not *one* boy said anything in protest. They actual stood quite still as I stood back up and said brightly, "Thanks boys, and I'll expect you all to sign up next year to help these kids out. These kids need all the volunteers they can get!" I walked away briskly and went straight to the Head table set up on the field where the Olympic Staff had been placed. I thrust the money in the donation box. They stood watching me. (I guess they wanted to be sure I wasn't a thief with a great little way of making some extra cash—by pretending to be outraged, and then pocketing the winnings!)

They turned to go back to class; one boy even waved a slight bye to me, albeit hesitatingly, more down by his side rather than up high in the air. Still, it was a show of acknowledgement, as if to show me he was sorry. I raised my hand to wave back. They were just teenagers. We have all done dumb and irreverent things when we were young and just learning what it was like to be an individual, too afraid to stick out and be too obviously different from our circle of friends.

Hurtful fun is never *really* fun, and it is always *most* hurtful to the one doing it, whether you realize it at the time, or not. For sure, you can learn a good lesson to make you a better person, a kinder gentler person, good coming from a bad experience. The most important thing of all is learning that God forgives us for all our mistakes. God *is* Love. He instructs us in the right way to live and treat others. He forgives us when we ask Him to, and He gently picks us up, dusts us off, and then urges us to go out into the hurting world and share the Good News to *all* people.

Those high school boys betting at the Special Olympics didn't realize the depth of their behavior. I prayed for God to allow them to be able to "see" all people as He sees them, and to learn what it is like to follow Him as they grew to manhood. And, I forgave them. In my humility I saw myself—how I had been before Jesus took full control of my life. They had many hard life lessons to learn ahead of them. I could only pray they learned them sooner, rather than later, in life. My heart went out to them.

Windy heard about this happening when some of the teachers were talking about it a few days later. Now we know it was one more thing she filed in the back of her mind that would come out one day . . . another good reason to change the name of a committee she would be asked to serve on.

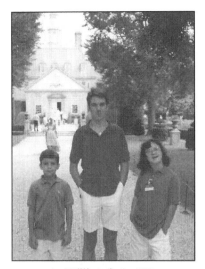
Williamsburg, VA

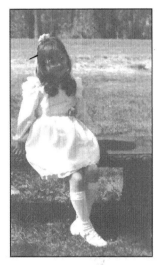
Spring Beauty

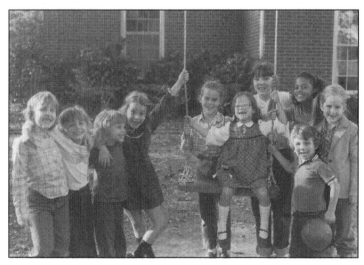
Birthday party fun

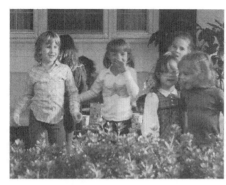
Telling Secrets

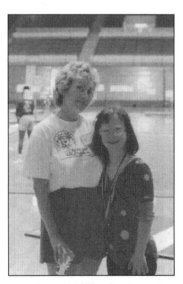

With special friend and coach,
Alice Gregory

Dave and Mikey at Special Olympics for
their sister at Notre Dame

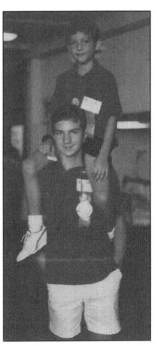

Her greatest cheerleaders at
the games and in life

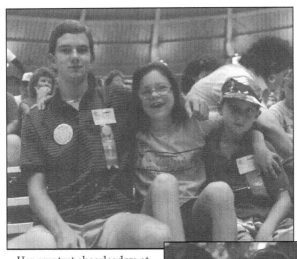

Olympic Medalist winner,
Flo Jo

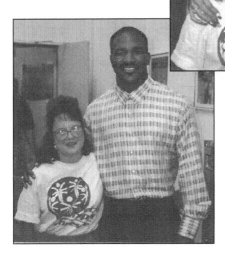

World Champion Boxer,
Evander Holyfield

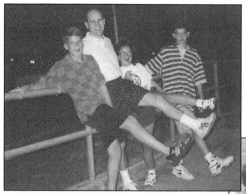

Friend Joseph Moore with Windy and family at Special Olympics

With Daddy after her big gymnastics win

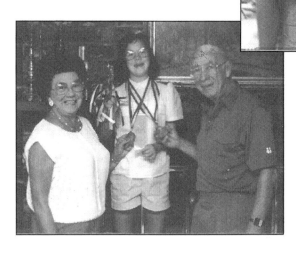

Showing Gaymom and Poppie her medals

Chapter Fifteen
Making Friends and Influencing People

Notre Dame was the site of nine of the most glorious days for our family. All five of us experienced unbelievable moments of happiness and wonderful memories. One memory we have is of an Amish family gathering we were invited to. It was quite unusual for anyone outside of their religion to be invited to a private function, and it happened without any preplanning.

Families in South Bend, Indiana, and the surrounding areas, opened their homes to family members of the athletes, graciously providing rooms for them to stay while attending the games. Our host family was the Sowers, Dale and Ginny. They were a wonderful Christian couple, who became dear friends of ours. They opened up their home and their hearts to us. They didn't miss any event Windy was competing in, and they were kind and accommodating to our boys. They fed us, drove us to events, and even gave us a car to drive while we were there.

The Sowers had a friend, Pauline, who had been raised Amish, but was now of the Mennonite faith. She knew all the good places to eat and shop since she had many family members in the area, and she offered to guide us on a day trip to see the beautiful farms, and to taste the delicious food in the Amish community of Shipshewana. Windy could not go with us because of her scheduled practices, but we wanted our sons to see this part of America. Having Pauline with us gave us real insight into the Amish lifestyle.

Our hosts took us for lunch to a wonderful restaurant with farm-to-table cooking. While we were there Pauline recognized some cousins that she had not seen in several years. After going over to talk to them, she came back to us with an invitation to visit a real

Amish farm. The Sowers told us of the rarity of this opportunity and encouraged us to go. We couldn't pass up the opportunity, so we took our new friend to her cousins' reunion about five miles from where we were.

Our visit turned out to be an amazing adventure. Pauline's large family had gathered for this celebration from several hundred miles away, all by horse and buggy. Thrilled to see Pauline, they allowed us a glimpse into their lives that day. We got to see how they lived because they invited us into their barns and home. The man of the house even gave us a ride in his new horse-drawn buggy. Afterwards we ate cookies and fresh squeezed lemonade on colorful quilts spread out under massive shade trees in the front yard of her family's old large white farmhouse.

All the women were dressed in their best dresses (Pauline explained to us), and the men were dressed in black pants and white shirts. Some of the older men even had on black suit jackets, despite the hot day. They all seemed to be enjoying a rare day off from work and visiting with each other at the large (and I mean very large) family gathering they were celebrating. The men, chatting in groups of eight to ten, were standing along the perimeter of the yard. The women were visiting in large groups gathered in the middle of the lawn and in the kitchen. There were children of all ages everywhere you looked. Many of the relations had not seen each other for many years. Some had come from long distances to get to this central location. Pauline said she was blessed to see many family members she had not seen for a very long time. They seemed sincerely glad to see her. They treated us with kindness, but were somewhat guarded with us. We felt honored that they would include us at all. The children were very friendly and came over to whisk Davey and Mikey away to join them in their games of tag.

We stayed about an hour. The women asked us into the house, and we got to see how they had cooked a huge dinner for all the company in the wood-burning oven. The bread smelled heavenly. There were a dozen loaves lined up on the counter, and they cut us a slice to sample, but first they spread some fresh strawberry jam on top.

About the time we were getting ready to leave (and when we thought the gathering couldn't get much bigger), another young family arrived with seven, beautiful blonde-headed children that scrambled out as soon as their dad had stopped the horses. The young mom climbed down with a toddler in her arms. Pauline let out a small," OH!" and ran to hug a niece she hadn't seen since she was five years-old, now a mom. I took one look in their direction, and I knew the toddler had been born with Down syndrome. I got David's attention so he would look at the cute, little blonde girl, too.

I waited until they had all greeted each other, and then I slipped over to talk to the little girl the mom had just put down to sit and watch the other children at play. All the kids spoke in Dutch to one another, and I didn't know any Dutch, but I knew a smile and sweet words could be understood by anyone. Sure enough, she smiled back at me, and her mother smiled at me and seemed so grateful that I would pick her out of a group to speak to. No language barrier here! I then told her mom, going to sit next to her (she spoke perfect English) that I had a daughter who was thirteen, and that she had been born with Down syndrome.

"Oh, *please*, tell me, when did your daughter learn to talk? And did she learn to read and to write? Does she run and play with your other children?" Her questions came tumbling out, despite the frowns I noticed she was getting from the older males in the group, who were quietly staring at us, a few yards away. I don't think they wanted her to be in such a personal conversation with a stranger, especially not with someone who was not one of their own. She ignored the stares. So did I.

We talked about Windy's development, and I encouraged her to allow her daughter to try things for herself, to ask her siblings to let her do things on her own. They might be "babying her" and really holding her back, I gently explained. I could already see that happening, the way her brothers and sisters kept coming to check on her, the way they hung around her, as we spoke. I also noted the darling little girl was very happy and content to have them wait on her "hand and foot." She didn't have to try to reach out for a dropped doll, someone scrambled to retrieve it for her. She sat there grinning. I could see she had the system figured out! In her favor, too!

The young mom's eyes flashed as I recounted Windy's determination and achievements. I suggested she raise her just like she was raising her other children, and to be careful not to spoil her, or to let the others spoil her. I encouraged her to teach her, allowing her to learn like the rest of her siblings. I also told her about Windy's faith in God, about our faith in God. I told her to pray for His guidance about how to teach her. These were obviously the words she had longed to hear for her daughter, and it was coming from someone her people called "the English"! We hugged and teared up over our shared bond. We might have been from two different worlds, but God had united us for a reason. I think she had more hope than she ever thought was possible for herself, and for her daughter.

Our hug was a lovely ending to a lovely day . . . and then I did something outlandish, at least to the Amish . . . I plopped down to have a seat on the ground, put my hand into my shoulder bag, and drew out a folded newspaper to show her a picture of our child. (It was the only picture I had of her that day.) Windy had made the front page of the Chicago Tribune Sports section just that morning!

It took up an entire half a page. (We had been told by someone yelling out to us from a crowed sidewalk on our way to breakfast that morning, "Hey, Tennessee! Go buy a Chicago Tribune and check out Windy's picture!" We went to find a newspaper stand and bought several copies.)

I carefully unfolded the paper and there Windy stood on that sports section's front page in living color, wearing her gymnastic leotard in red, white, and blue, and posing with her Bronze Medal. I was proud of my girl! I wanted this young mother to see how pretty our daughter was, and to give her reassurance that her daughter would grow up to be lovely. Windy looked so beautiful, so triumphant after her great win, captured for all the world to see by some photographer who had been captivated by her winning smile and grace.

The mom looked down at the newspaper page I had spread out on the quilt, and she hid a slight smile with her hand. Then surprisingly *every* man standing in the yard silently came closer to lean in over our heads, to look at the picture. It was a bit claustrophobic for a few tense moments. I didn't know if they were going to start shouting at me, or if they might grab the paper. I had not intended to offend, only to encourage. I didn't know much about the Amish, but I had always believed them to be a gentle people. For those few anxious moments I really hoped it was true!

Not *one* word was spoken in our presence about the picture, or about our daughter. There was complete, utter silence. The woman and men had all stopped conversing. They may not want to have pictures taken of themselves, but they didn't mind looking at one of someone else! It was a strange moment, but one we won't forget. I'll bet they haven't forgotten either.

Everyone took turns looking, and then they all backed off and walked away. I stood up, looked around quickly for David and the boys, and folded my paper and put it back in my bag. The mom and I hugged again and I watched her take a quick look to be sure she was not being watched, and she bent her head down close to my ear and said, "Thank you!" She smiled slightly as she dipped her head down and then scooped up her baby in her arms, and followed the rest of the ladies into the house to begin preparations for the large dinner they were going to have—but not before I placed a quick kiss on her daughter's cheek! Her mama smiled a smile that could have lit up the sky. Nothing like a mama's love!

Later, David and I discussed whether they came to look out of curiosity, just to see what a girl of thirteen who had been born with Down syndrome would look like, or if they were looking to reaffirm how strange we all were out in the world. We'll never know, but we do know that the little girl's daddy, grandfather, and uncles were the first to come and have a look (Pauline told us on the ride back). The child's family had been the most curious.

Hope comes in mysterious ways, and on that day I had been the mysterious way it had come to a young Amish mother in the middle of a heat wave, on a summer's day in the middle of Indiana. Our Windy had made another front page and had made someone's day in the bargain. Probably someone's life, too! That little Amish girl was going to learn everything her brothers and sisters were learning. Her mom would see to it. I recognized "the look" in her eyes as she gazed at her daughter while I spoke to her. I had only confirmed to her what was already in her heart.

David and I went sight-seeing one other day, but our two boys never left Notre Dame Campus. They refused to go. Dave said, "Dad, Mikey and I have decided these kids *need* us, and we can't leave them." Mikey stood beside his big brother and said, "Yeah,

Dad, we're staying here with the kids!" They had volunteered and signed up to be huggers and escorts for the USA team members, with the Civitan Club Volunteers, and were having a blast! God love 'em! Dedicated to helping those with disabilities, they were developing a strong moral character they would have the rest of their lives. We were so proud of them. They deserved Gold Medals for *their* fierce interest and concern for other people. They were young boys, but already proving to be far more mature than other kids their ages in many ways.

I wrote an article which was published in October 1987, and placed on the front page of CAK's newsletter. You get a real feel for the ten days in Indiana when you read it over. (Please excuse the use of the word handicapped instead of disabilities, but it was the most commonly used word at the time to describe those who were born with a disability.) Below is the article in its entirety:

A VERY SPECIAL GIRL

International Special Olympics . . . what exactly is so special about the event held every four years? The children and adults involved are no more special to God than any of us in His eyes. They do, however, have special needs in that they are all intellectually, and many physically disabled, as well. God has allowed these precious people to come into our lives, and if we allow, to teach us so much about real priorities in life, unconditional love, forgiving hearts, and true faith and hope. They are a people set apart because their success isn't measured by the world's standards.

This summer Windy Smith, a student at C.A.K., had the privilege of being chosen to participate in the 1987 International Summer Special Olympic Games held at the

University of Notre Dame in South Bend, Indiana. She represented the state of Tennessee and our school in gymnastics. She won a Bronze (and later a Silver) medal in floor exercise, a Bronze medal in beam exercise, and 6th place in the Ribbon routines.

(The entire family went down on the floor to encourage her before she was introduced. Her turn was quickly approaching. Dave and Mikey hugged her and told her to "get out there and show them how it's done!" She hugged them and smiled confidently back at them, as she said, "I will. Don't worry!" Then I got to hug her and gave her a kiss on the top of her head, and told her that I was so proud of her and to do her best. Then her dad hugged her tightly, and she looked up at him and asked, "Dad, if I get a medal will you get me a cone of ice cream?" He replied, "You win and I'll get you two scoops!" "Wow! Okay!" she replied, as she gave him a high five. Her Coach, Miss Alice, came to retrieve her, and we went to be seated near her starting point.

All of a sudden her name was called out over the intercom. "Next will be Windy Smith, from Knoxville, Tennessee, representing the USA, performing her floor routine!" She stepped out, turned to look up in the audience to her dad, lifted up two fingers, shook her head 'no', then raised three fingers up to him, and nodded her head. She then walked out confidently, presented to the crowd with her right arm up in the air. Her music, the theme song from the movie, *Chariots of Fire,* began, and she completed a fabulous routine, almost flawless. That little dickens had negotiated with her dad for a triple cone on the spot. Her dad had been on the spot . . . and she was fully aware of the fact! By the way, before the day was over, she enjoyed a giant cone of frozen delight—three scoops! She had sure earned it!

The Chicago Tribune (Sports Page) ran two, color feature photos of her. She was one of 44,700 athletes from around the world. (What are the odds of anyone noticing our girl and putting her picture in the paper? And, twice already? You do the math. We couldn't have made it happen. She couldn't have made it happen.) There were also 20,000 volunteers from Civitan International, the Junior League, area churches, and many other clubs and individuals, including many entertainers and sports figures that came to visit with the participants on the fields, courts, and floors of the events. People such as Whitney Houston (who sang for them), Spud Webb, Patrick Ewing, Don Johnson, Barbara Mandrell, and Susan St. James, Arnold Schwarzenegger, and many more came to speak to and visit with the athletes.

Windy's parents and her brothers, Dave and Mikey, attended the nine-day games and events hosted by the Kennedy family, and brought back a lifetime of memories. Describing the trip, her parents said, "We laughed awhile and cried awhile and laughed again." It was an emotional time seeing the athletes perform and exert their best. At first glance it may have, by the world's standards, seemed an impossible feat, but they were doing the impossible. Take for example, the twenty-three year-old male gymnast, who was deaf. He would need total concentration to do a simple, small leap in the air because he also had cerebral palsy. After each move, the crowd would leap to their feet and cheer him on, and he would look up and smile a sweet, thankful smile that left not a dry eye in the stands. The audience's tears came from the depth of emotion he elicited from them. He showed the on-lookers such an awesome, strong display of determination and courage that you could not watch without feeling strong emotions.

Another example of the games is the sixteen year-old track runner, who sprang out ahead of his competitors only to stop seconds before he crossed the finish line to encourage and cheer them on to victory. All the athletes performed their routines or sports and then cheered on their competition as if they were part of the "old home team!"

One black girl from Africa, about twelve years of age, walked by Michael, and in response to his smile, reached out her hand, gently touched his check and smiled. Reaching across the miles of her homeland and across the races and the handicaps, she was communicating love—a love much like the love of Jesus Christ, who is the Savior of all—all races, all nations, all people, great or small.

May we all learn to reach out beyond our pasts, our backgrounds, our weaknesses, and reach toward one another through the love of Christ. Hopefully, we can say someday in our lives that we have laughed and cried and laughed again. In our joys and in our sorrows, and in the sharing of each other's joys and sorrows, may we find that true joy that is (found) in Him (Romans 12:15). Life is tough many times, yet God calls us to perform our best in all things "...*as if for the Lord.*" (Colossians 3:23). We are also to build each other up and to encourage one another, just like the athletes did for each other, and as the Bible tells us in 1 Thessalonians. 5:11: And when things look impossible by the world's standards, we are to strive as if it *were* possible because *"all things are possible with God."* (Matthew 19:26)

Below is a summary from one of her many CAK teacher-parent evaluation meetings, dated 1988. We kept it because it truly sums up her character at the time.

> "Windy is no problem in the classroom. She keeps busy with her work. She has a sweet spirit and evidences a strong Christian testimony. Dr. and Mrs. Smith are encouraged with the exposure to C.A.K. academics and for the Christian education she is receiving. Mrs. E. and Mrs. D. desire that Windy make gains this year, but they feel inadequate in regards to giving Windy individual attention and quality of time in teaching her. "Teachers and parents are to be encouraged with the progress Windy is making, and for the good influence they are having in her life," Mrs. Smith told us. We teachers feel her personality and positive abilities are outshining her inabilities. In summary, her teachers and her parents are satisfied with the results."

We could see Windy becoming more sure of herself, more confident in her own decision making process. The class work was a struggle, as we assumed it would be. CAK was known as a difficult school with loads of homework for the students to do. Homework was always tough for her to complete.

Many a night, David, I, or one of her brothers, sat with her, while she diligently and slowly finished up an assignment. She was motivated, almost self-driven to a fault, to do what the teachers had asked of her, and to do what her peers were doing in class. It was painful to watch at times, but very rewarding, too. Windy is a person who takes pride in whatever she does, and she wanted so badly to be like everyone else. Even when we tried to encourage her to take a break or to go at her own pace, she stayed with it. Seeing her efforts, her perseverance, made all of us try all the harder in our own situations. A **WINDY LIFE LESSON** to carry with us throughout our lives.

The Smith kids went to school at CAK for six years. Dave graduated from there in 1990, and Windy and Mikey completed the sixth grade. At the end of that sixth school year, the principal set up a meeting to inform us "that they could no longer see to her educational needs in ways they thought were most beneficial for her." In other words, they had no special education classes or instructors for older, special education students at the time. I was frustrated and sad, but knew it was only a matter of time until we heard those words.

It was disheartening because we felt that of all places, a Christian school should embrace and help educate someone who needed extra help and special care. (But, we understood their reasoning and knew they were really interested in her future.) We had prayed for many years that new classes would be started there just for these kids. It was a matter of funding, and the extra funds were just not there. She would have to go to a public school. Most public schools were prepared to help educate kids with special needs now. Hard to accept at first, but it worked out the way the Lord meant for it to be. Our new search led us to the high school just down the road from our new home. We went to look it over and were impressed with what we saw, and with the plans we heard about for the new class just beginning in the fall for special needs kids. It turned out to be a really great thing for Windy!

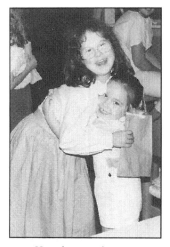
Hugging cousin Joey

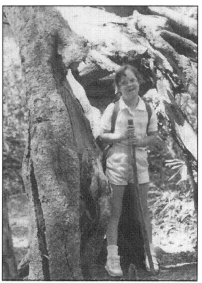
Hiking the Smokies

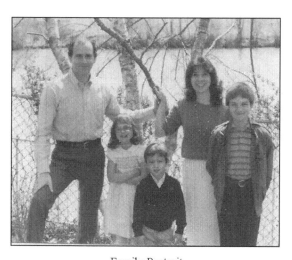
Family Portrait

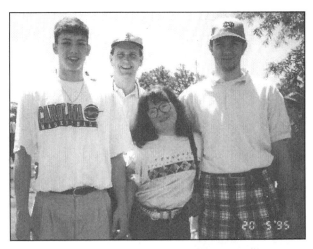

At Vanderbilt for Special Olympics with dad and brothers

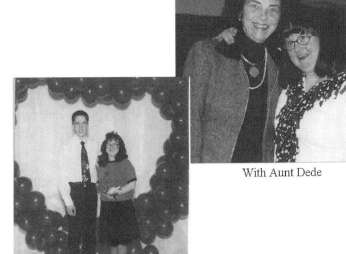

With Aunt Dede

At a dance with friend, Dan

Chapter Sixteen
Farragut High Living

Windy was excited about attending a real high school with kids nearer her age. She was going to be a freshman, and her younger brother was going to go to seventh grade. Instead of being in the same grade, she would be two years ahead of him now! She was very pleased with that scenario. (When Mikey found out they didn't have a place for his sister at C.A.K., he informed us that it would be a good time for him to change schools, too. He said he wasn't going to stay where she couldn't stay. Did I mention all our children are somewhat determined?) So we went with him to visit Farragut Middle School, and he liked what *he* saw. He was ready for the switch. He had great grades and was a good student, and he was so outgoing we knew he would be just fine. Their big brother was going away to college. We knew Dave was going to be fine, too!

We were a little leery of their sister's future in a public school setting, however. She had always gone to smaller schools. Windy wasn't leery, she was excited about the change, just the opposite of what I thought she would be when I broke the news to her. (For the first time, her big brother would not be around for her to lean on.) We guessed she realized it was an opportunity to stretch her wings in a large school, and she would have the opportunity to make even more friends. And finally, she could again bask in the important position of being Mikey's *big* sister. High time! In high school! This was going to be *High* living to her, for sure!

Our new neighbor, Jean Hill, worked at the school and couldn't say enough nice things about the school or the teachers. She stood and told us great things about Farragut schools, out in our yard in Fox Den subdivision, where we had just moved before the new school year started. Jean, her husband, Steve, and their daughter,

Meredith, "sang the praises" of FHS to us. She also assured us that Windy would get along just fine in the new LRE room she would be assigned to. She said it was a great group of kids that attended school there, who lived in the surrounding neighborhoods, and that they would be kind to Windy and to the other students who would be in her classes. (She was one hundred percent correct! There were, again, some of the nicest kids we ever met going to that school and living in our neighborhood!)

All our other new neighbors came over to welcome us to our new house. They came to meet us bearing homemade casseroles, cakes, cookies, and friendship. Kitty and Alan Holman, and their four kids: Haley, Scott, William, and Charlie, was the second family we met. (Kitty's mom, Flo, had grown up near my mom, Flo, and we didn't even know each other until that day!) Other neighbors came. Julia and Mike Fleming and their daughter, Emily (Windy loved them from the first, and to her delight, Julia turned out to be a sister of the famous movie star and model, Andie McDowell.), Richard and Vickie Smith and their son, Barry, and Janet and Rocky Good with their two kids, Ryan and Emily, came to welcome us to our new home. Kari Hill (now Mikey's wife!) and her friends: Kristen Cook (Doty), Courtney Zacheretti (Hammett) and her sister, Kat (Spottswood), and the Weissinger sisters were to befriend Windy. Brian and Jason Key, Stephen O'Connor, John Wisnowski, Drew Burnette, David Wood, Matt Maples, Matt Kerr, and Cory Mayfield got to know her and became her good buddies.

We also met Darren Rothenberg, from down the street (who went on to play football for Vanderbilt). Jamie Conway, or J.D., as he is known now, and Darren became Windy's "honorary brothers." (Windy still keeps up with J. D. and his girlfriend, Sally Long. J.D. is a veterinarian out West, but we make a point to see him a couple of times a year. Darren and his family get to see her every once in a while.) These two guys were Mikey's best friends, but they learned to love and protect his sister. During those good old times, I cooked many meals, many big meals, so I could feed them when they came to stay with us. We felt blessed to have met so many great young kids, and to have settled into such a friendly neighborhood. It was a wonderful place to raise children. Windy also became good friends with Addie Rouse, Rachel Wood and Andrea Maples, students at Farragut High, who later volunteered to be peer-tutors to her, and to her friends in Special Ed.

She liked her new teachers, Sue Clark, Kathy Burke, and Donna Connors and a special coach, John Heatherly. She loved being able "to change classes with the masses." When the bell rang, she quickly learned to pass down a crowded hallway to get to class, and still manage to speak to students she had made friends with. We shouldn't have wasted any time worrying if our daughter would be intimidated by the sheer number of students, or if she would be bothered by the process of changing classes. Nope! We shouldn't have wasted a minute of concern on her. We were to find out Windy had found her place in the world as an out-going teenager, and she was, "Happy, Happy, Happy, Happy!"

By the time she had attended high school for several months, she was getting into all kinds of trouble with notes she was writing to the boys she had crushes on (So very well written, I must say!), and for notes she wrote on behalf of friends who couldn't write as well, who had crushes of their own to be declared. She would transcribe a note (make that *many* notes) and then have the friend sign it. I was given a couple of the confiscated notes by a teacher. We were impressed. She was a *great* writer! (Maybe not the reaction the teacher had been expecting from me.) I had been called into the Principal's office for a little friendly chat about her transcribed missives, i.e. notes to B-O-Y-S. It was sort of bittersweet for me. Yes, Windy was in a little bit of trouble at school, BUT she was in a *normal* high school, acting like a *normal* high schooler. I outwardly (and quickly) agreed to her educator's idea of an after-school detention to help curb her note passing in class. Inwardly, I was really pretty pleased—Windy *could* write and reason with the best of them. *You go, girl! Just not during class.*

Over the next few years we sold a house, built a new one two doors down from our old one, and Windy never complained one time about change. Of course, it didn't hurt that she had the largest closet in the house, and a big bedroom thrown in for good measure. The wall color? *Windy's Bubblegum Pink.* That's the color the paint store wrote on the cans. She had critiqued the color mixture until it had been pronounced perfect by her, and we have used it in every room she has had since. (We flipped houses to supplement our income before there were TV shows about it. Plus, David and I love the whole process from design to building, and I love to decorate. And Windy has always been a happy volunteer helper and gives her valued opinions in each situation.)

She and I spent some quality time together during those years. We would leave the guys to their televised ballgames, and have some mother-daughter bonding, as we watched the *Anne of Avonlea* TV series. Those hours of lying across her twin beds and watching this program in her room were fun times. She loved the fact that I would put aside all pressing matters to join her. Being the mama of boys kept me busy going to their events, practices, games, cooking, washing clothes, all the things that a mother has to do. But one night a week was our time, and she would shut her door and make a point of locking us in—No Boys Allowed! At least for an hour.

For the most part, her whole high school experience was fantastic. She was in the very first LRE class—Least Restricted Class, which Farragut High School ever had. No one could speculate on how the student body would accept these students with disabilities as they took classes together for the first year. The educators warned us about this when we went to her enrollment appointment.

No one had guessed it would go as smoothly as it went. It was a blessed experience for all concerned. The students with the disabilities learned so much as life expanded for them in education and social skills they had never had access to before. The "regular" students learned how to accept and befriend people with disabilities and learned that these students were more like them than they had expected. The teachers were surprised just how eager the new students were to learn, and found they were celebrating right along with the students when they grasped a new idea or concept. Everyone benefited from the experience.

We met some of the mothers and dads of the kids in Farragut's LRE class, and in the other high schools in the Knoxville area. We liked what we saw: they loved their children and wanted the best for them, and they, like us, had worked for years to help their child develop to his/her fullest potential. Belinda was the name of a girl Windy met and became best friends with. Belinda's mom, Shirley Noonan, was as proud as she could be of her lovely daughter (one of four children in her family). Sue and Steve felt the same about their darling daughter, Heather. She also met two girls named Peggy Nenninger and Michael Kelly who had loving, supportive families. It proved to us that there were many families out there who were also loving and raising their kids right along with their siblings. It was so encouraging to us!

Windy has always believed in herself, even on those rare days when she was made fun of by other kids, and could have been hurt or could have been made to feel inadequate. She knew deep inside that she was made to excel, and the courageous spirit she displays and her generous and loving heart seem to literally draw people to her. I told her she was a child of God. (I had whispered these words to her, that Jesus loves her. Even when she was a newborn. I have been blessed to whisper these truths in the ears of *each* of our children and to *each* of our grandchildren. I treasure those moments in my memory.) She chose to take the facts and soar with them. She knows where her true worth comes from. She has never allowed adversity to 'shake her to the core.' She stops to think about difficult things, and then she looks for a bright side to help her over the hurdle. This next story of her quick adjustment to new and sometimes "iffy" situations could teach us all a thing or two.

One evening, after Windy had been going to her new school for about two months, the five of us were gathered at the dinner table, and David turned and asked her how things were going at the high school. She replied, "Great! I love it." She continued to eat. He then asked her, "Does anyone ever say anything unkind to you?"

She stopped eating, put down her fork, pushed her eyeglasses back up on her nose with one finger, and looked him squarely in the eyes, and said, "Dad, does it really matter?"

"Does it matter to *you*? Does it ever hurt your feelings? Make you sad?" he queried back.

"No, Dad, it never does hurt my feelings, and it doesn't happen *much*. Everybody likes me a lot. I'm popular with everybody because I like *everybody*." She said it matter of factually, sans conceit, or fake bravado. She smiled sweetly at her father, and then picked up her fork, looked at her food, and continued her meal. David and the boys and I looked around at each other sort of momentarily stunned, and then we all smiled, and I distinctly remember Mike and Dave letting out pretty big belly laughs over that one. They more like exploded into laughter.

"There's your answer to that question, Dad!" Dave said to David.

"Yes, son, that's that. Now, please pass me the bread, and we'll change the subject. How was your day, Vicki?" he said in as serious a voice as he could muster, trying most unsuccessfully to hide a smile.

At that, Windy smiled into her plate and did a quick bob of her head as if to say, "Subject Closed." This was definitely a **WINDY LIFE LESSON** . . . people will sometimes say things that could hurt us, yet we have the option of allowing it to penetrate our hearts, or to 'move on.' Windy always moves on—but usually not without saying a prayer for that person. Really, she does. She has the discernment to know that ugliness comes from deep within a person who needs God's love and grace. She lives out the grace part and lets God be God. We all have learned truer grace for having known our Windy. Sure we taught her this "leaning on our faith thing", but she had to grow up and reject, or accept it for herself. She is a shining example of showing grace towards other people. We need to pray for those who say or do hurtful things—and then just leave the rest up to Him.

Now in high school, Windy learned many things, and she taught many things. She taught everyone she knew how important her birthday was to her, and believe me she knew many, many people in a short amount of time. Her friends were so kind to her as they put her birthday announcements on the radio every year she was in school! They even announced it over the intercom for everybody to hear. She also received cards, gifts and entire cakes on her big day. She was treated normally most of the time, and she was treated like a princess, at certain times, on her birthdays especially!

Her senior year she was nominated by the entire student body to run for Homecoming Queen. (Her daddy escorted her out onto the football field at halftime. His smile was as wide and as proud as his daughter's!) She sang in the Ensemble Choir (She met a girl named, Kari there and said that she was the girl for her brother! Kari became Mikey's wife, seven years later.), danced with all the cutest guys at the dances (Some asked her to dance, and others she asked to dance.), and everybody knew and loved her from the most popular to the not so popular.

She was a friend to everyone. She sees no color or race distinction and wrote to an African-American friend one time, "Hearts are all the same color, that's the way God sees us." (Her words make us wonder again about who *really* has the disability.) The kids adored her because of her cute sense of humor, and they loved the way she could sum up a situation in just a few words. They thought she was hilarious, and she was—and is!

We have been very conscious of her weight and tried to teach her to eat healthy. She knows how to select the right foods, but she has a real sweet tooth. She and her dad have had several talks about eating for your health, for a healthy weight, and a healthy heart. We were so afraid she would develop a heart condition or gain an enormous amount of weight as she grew older. So many people with Down syndrome seem to gain weigh so easily as they become older and less active. All this to say, she knew from a young age how to have a healthy life style.

Eating healthy was on David's mind when we picked Windy up from another camp, this one sponsored by *Joni and Friends*, one of Joni Eareckson Tada's camp for kids with disabilities. After we had loaded her suitcases into the car, she got in the back seat behind her dad, who was driving. As we started out the camp gate David asked her, teasingly, if she had eaten any fattening food while she had been there. She quickly leaned forward, without *one* moment's hesitation, rubbed the top of his bald spot, and asked, "Did you grow any hair while I was gone?" She grinned sheepishly and leaned back in her seat with her arms folded as if she had accomplished her goal. We were too tickled to continue the food issue. That's just what she had in mind all along: her version of "beat the parents at their own game"!

Windy had enjoyed a Tumbling Class held at the Civic Center so much that we hoped to enroll her in a gymnastics class in Knoxville at the Academy of Gymnastics that was located off Dutchtown Road. We passed by it every day. Once again, the situation required an explanation. (If you think these sounds like a broken record, I'm sorry, but you should have tried living it. It wasn't easy, but somebody had to do it, and I was usually that someone.) I went to the front office and asked if I could speak to the owner of the gym. I told them that Windy had Down syndrome, and then I had to explain to them just what Down syndrome was. I told them she really wanted to take gymnastics, and I assured them that she was capable of becoming a viable member of a class.

I left an "out" for them, and said if they ever thought it best that she quit the class, we would leave as friends. One of the coaches, "Miss Alice," happened to be on break at the time and was sitting there in the office, and she listened to me with empathy. She immediately volunteered to take her in one of her after-school classes. But she admitted she had never taught a child with an intellectual disability. She said she thought she would be interested in trying.

The gym personnel gave her the go-ahead, and Windy joined in a regular class for a while. Then, when special training and long routines had to be learned for Special Olympic competition, Alice began a class exclusively for that. That's about the time Alice asked someone to leave the class . . . and that someone was me. I had been there from the beginning: watching, making suggestions to the coach, and to my daughter, so they would get as much as they could out of the hour of class. Then the two of them bonded, passed me by, and relegated me to the sidelines. I was ecstatic. This gymnastic deal was going to work out.

Word got out that a Special Education class was offered at the Academy of Gymnastics, and the class started to grow quickly. We met outgoing Beth, a tall, pretty, athletic blonde girl who came to join the class, and quiet, darling little Emily who loved gymnastics, too. Windy's friend Heather, a cute, petite brunette stole Miss Alice's heart the minute she met her. Another beautiful girl, Michele, joined them and livened up the group even more. Kelly, a pretty girl, a few years older than the rest of the girls, demonstrated to them gracefulness and skill. Miss Alice now had a full class of young ladies eager to get the most out of their hour under her instruction.

Alice turned out to be an answer to prayer. She was so good with the girls. She expected a lot out of them from the get-go, no coddling and low expectations from her—she expected their best, and they complied. They learned so much from her. She learned so much from them, she told me, more than once. Windy adored her and so did the other girls in her class. Alice went with us to competition for several years at the State level in Nashville, at Vanderbilt, and went on to the International games as a coach, and she loved *every* second of it.

She said she was the one, who was blessed by being in the office the day Windy and I stopped by to see about classes offered for people with disabilities. Windy and her friends (and all the families) think we all were the ones blessed. Either way, God knew the perfect timing. (And, the perfect person to be their gymnastic coach!)

After Windy won the International Bronze medals, a huge color poster of her was hung in the gym, on a large wall for several years. Alice, and the other ladies who worked there, had the photograph enlarged into a poster, framed it, and hung it up to surprise Windy. They were so proud of her. Younger gymnasts would pass her, look up at the poster, then at her, and ask for her autograph. You would have smiled to have seen how she glowed at being someone the younger girls could look up to. I know we did our fair share of smiling as we looked on. It was so sweet.

There in that very gym I had quietly asked if they would give our daughter a chance to participate in their gymnastic classes, and Windy had carried it to a level I hadn't known was possible for her to achieve. There have been so many "Wow!" moments in her life that David and I really believe God has orchestrated it all. Someone who doesn't believe in God might say it has all been chance. They could say it—but then they would have to look at the odds here. Maybe luck, or some other "cosmic force" they might think could have been the driving force behind the wondrous events in her life, but this many? No way. Her life is Divinely engineered. We just hope you see the hand of God in it all. We hope you receive a blessing for your own life as you read about hers. He's been there all along, making clear the path she should take, and we are so grateful for His love for our daughter. He's there for you and your family, too. No matter where you all are. That's the real hope.

If, as they say, life is grand, if you can count on more than one hand, people you consider to be special, true friends, who care about you, then Windy's life is grand indeed, because she can count good friends on both hands, her toes, and then some. (We lost count of the many friends who came by to wish her well when she became ill one time. We were astonished at the outpouring of love and kindness we witnessed during that time.

At age thirteen, she became deathly ill . . . turns out she had to have an emergency appendectomy, but not before a long day of tests and prayers. Dr. Brown saved her life after exploratory surgery. She wouldn't complain about the terrible pain she was having because she didn't want to miss bowling in Special Olympics that morning. She was stoic when the doctors probed and prodded her abdomen. Always as a toddler when she fell off a swing or fell running on pavement, it took her longer than a normal response to feel the pain. She had a delayed response and also has a high tolerance for pain. Not a good combination when a serious illness is the issue!

She made it through surgery just fine, but the recuperation was a long, painstakingly long, process. She nearly fainted every time I put her in the shower to wash the large open wound on her tummy. I would get woozy and almost pass out when I looked at her tummy. I hurt for her. We learned to look up (Shouldn't we always heed this procedure?), keep our eyes up away from the hurt place, the two of us, as I held her steady when she stepped over the side of the tub and into the stream of clean water needed to cleanse and promote healing from the inside out. The wound was deep and raw, but with time and the proper care, it began to close up.

She had so many visitors at Parkwest Hospital where she spent the next ten days. The nurses told us they had never seen more visitors and friends come to one room for all the days of her stay. Bobby and Pat Scott, and their son Benson, brought her a small pin in the shape of an angel. Bobby leaned down to kiss her head and told her, "We brought you an angel pin because you're everybody's little angel." All those visitors with sincere concern and gifts that filled her room was proof enough to us that she had shown love and had received love back. It was evident to us that she had already been a wonderful influence in many people's lives. Her 13th birthday was a divine milestone in her life and ours.

While Windy was still in FHS, we got tickets to take her to hear Bryan Duncan, the Christian singer/songwriter. We had time to go eat before the concert, and she told us *Buddy's Bar-B-Q* was where she wanted to go. It's a local chain that makes great barbecue, but we were sort of surprised by her choice, since we thought she would have picked another restaurant for her big night out. Something more 'fancy'. David consented and drove to the Buddy's closest to us, and we got out and walked in. Guess who was in line to order his own dinner? None other than Mr. Bryan Duncan himself! Windy left us and walked straight up to him and told him she was so excited about getting to hear him in concert. He was very sweet to speak with her for a few minutes, and as he left he waved and said he would see her soon.

David and I assumed he was just saying he knew she was going to be out in the audience at his performance. We thought it was nice that he kindly remembered to say goodbye to her. She grinned 'from ear to ear.' When we arrived at the church where he was singing, we found some great seats in the middle, four rows from the front, where she could easily see the stage. She had barely settled in her seat when she excused herself to go to the bathroom, which was right out the side door. I felt it was safe for her to go alone. I hated to get up and ask everyone in our row, already seated, to excuse me again since we had just come by to find our seats. One person going was enough disturbance. "Please hurry back. You don't want to miss a note," I said to her back, as she prepared to go.

After about ten minutes I realized she had been gone longer than I had expected. I knew I had no choice but to step out and disturb all the people who sat between me and the aisle. So, I did. There was no Windy in the bathroom, in the foyer or hallway of the church. Back down the row I went, back to our seats to tell David I couldn't find her. The room was filled with people we knew and who knew her. He said to relax, she was fine and could take care of herself. That's the part that bothered me . . . had she found a friend and gone to sit with them? Should I get back up to go search? People will think I have a *problem*. Well, I did. Just not a bladder problem . . . I had a problem with my daughter. My daughter had given me "the slip".

I was relieved to see her finally coming back though the door that I had been anxiously watching. It had taken her sixteen minutes. I watched as she said politely, "Excuse me," as she slowly made her way down the row of seated people and back to us.

"What took you so long?" I whispered. I was ticked off.

"I've been talking to Bryan," she explained excitedly. (*Bryan who*?) "At Buddy's, he asked me to come backstage to meet him and his band before he sang. He is so nice, and so are the members of his band. I told him I would be praying for him. He thanked me and said he needed prayers." She smiled happily and settled back to watch the show about to begin.

Here I had been worrying about her safety and well-being, and she had been backstage hobnobbing with the 'star' of the show. Why hadn't she told us? Because she knew I wouldn't have let her disturb the man. Yes, that's definitely why. And, yes, to tell him that she would be in prayer for him, probably encouraged him, now that I think of it. God circumvents mothers' best laid plans and advice sometimes. I was glad . . . now I didn't have to be so hard on myself to be the perfect mom . . . because there's no such thing. I was proving that on a weekly basis. I was again cognizant of the fact that our girl had a mind of her own . . . and a mind stayed on Christ. It might make me a bit uncomfortable at times, this independent spirit she had, but I had to admit, she could be right about many things, too!

I settled back to watch the show with the knowledge that there was *always* a story behind the show. She is irrepressible!

The concert was a blessing to us all. Bryan sang his song, *"Nothing But Blue Skies Now",* and I smiled through the whole song. I had heard this song coming from Windy's room, several days prior to the concert.

> *Yes, God, You have brought beautiful blue skies into our lives with Windy. There have been storms, some difficult ones, but there have been beautiful blue skies along the way also. Thank You, for the relief the blue skies always bring.*

CSPC, Cedar Springs Presbyterian Church, youth group was such a God-send for our children when they became teenagers. When Dave was a teen he had loved gathering with friends and attending the various functions. Now, Windy and Mikey loved the fun outings since they got old enough to join. Most of their events were fun-filled times, and the kids grew spiritually. All the trips turned out well except for one of them. It didn't go too well. Not the wonderful blue skies this time.

The year Windy turned seventeen, she and Mikey got to attend a long weekend trip with the group. They had a new youth pastor, Jim, who was going along, so the kids could get to know him. Jim was a handsome dude. We saw him standing on the sidewalk as everyone was loading their suitcases in the outside bins of the bus. So many kids signed up to go that the church had to rent a bus the size of a greyhound bus to transport the large group and all their gear for the camp.

The cute new leader was a fact not missed by my daughter. She must have been smitten the moment he addressed the kids for the first time. From the moment they arrived at camp things must have gone downhill for her. Knowing none of this, David and I were feeling good about the trip.

It was a thrilling thing for us to know that our children would be having a great time and that we would have a whole weekend alone! We knew they were in good hands with Lucinda, Alan, Jim and the other chaperones, and Windy was happily included in the group. We were grateful for that *and* for the awesome leaders.

Parents can play while the kids are away—so we relaxed, went to dinner and a movie, and the unusually quiet house was bearable, since we knew it was only temporary. So was the peace we were feeling. Temporary, it turns out. Trouble was brewing, and we didn't know it.

Almost in the first few minutes after they arrived back to the church parking lot, I could tell Windy had probably gotten into some kind of trouble on the trip. *Something* hadn't gone right. She hugged me with a lack of real enthusiasm, and then left me to go over and grab her bags as they were being lined up on the sidewalk for ownership distribution. Mikey was enthusiastically talking with friends and saying his goodbyes. Windy began hugging friends and saying her own goodbyes. But I had that old, sick sinking feeling in the pit of my stomach as I waited to help them load their stuff in the car. Who was I going to talk with about "this something" soon to be revealed?

Sure enough, before I got in our car, one of the leaders asked me to please come by and talk to them before I left. I walked slowly toward the office with Windy by my side. I insisted she go with me. Whatever this was, she was going to have to "face-the-music" *with* me at some point. (I knew it wasn't about Mikey, because he looked tired, but content. Windy looked tired, and more than a little downcast. That's why I just knew to ask *her* to go with me. This was about her no doubt.)

She sat outside the door of the room they had told me to go to, while I entered to face the group alone. Three of the leaders, sitting in a loose semi-circle in folding chairs, told me they had enjoyed having Windy on the trip, but they felt like I needed to know how she had flirted with the new youth minister. They used kind words to describe the way Windy had acted around Jim. (They were really concerned about her behavior and wanted to help her. I knew that it was because they cared for her that they were taking the time to meet with me. I also knew they had all they could handle with the other teens in the youth group, understandably, and I was sorry Windy had taken up even more of their time. They were all volunteers with a heart for the youth, and our family was grateful for them. But I also felt our daughter needed a place to belong, too.)

They said she had followed him around the camp, hung around and waited for him to finish eating his meals, so she could walk with him, and the other people he was with, to the different events. It was obvious to everyone that he was her new crush. (*Now* I knew about it, too. Hadn't heard it before.) They were perplexed about how to handle the situation. When I asked what they had said to her, they said they didn't know what to say to her. They asked if I had any suggestions.

I suddenly asked them if Jim was married. (I didn't know him. I had only seen him boarding the bus.) They answered, "Yes." I asked them if they had told my daughter that he was married? Then I asked if his wife had attended the weekend getaway, and they said, "No." And then I suddenly realized Windy didn't know there was a "Mrs. Jim."

"Well," I said, "that's the answer. All we have to do is tell her he is already married. You just treat her as you would anyone else. You just need to explain what's appropriate and what's not appropriate. That's what we do. That's what we've always done. Just treat her as you would anyone else. She'll understand." I went over to the door and asked Windy to step in. She walked in very slowly. She wasn't looking forward to this interview. I don't think the leaders were either. They weren't trying to hurt her by telling on her. I understood that, but we had to fix this quickly.

I asked Windy if she had followed Jim around on the trip. She didn't try to deny it. She looked up and said, "Yes." (Bless her, she wasn't going to try to worm her way out of this. She was painfully honest about it. My heart ached for her.) I then asked her if she knew Jim had a wife, that he was a married man?

"Married? No, I did *not!*" she said with complete disgust in her voice, and she seemed to recoil with the revolting words. (No one had mentioned that fact *and* she had seen no woman with him. Probably this was her reasoning during the trip . . . "No girlfriend about? Cute new guy—he appeared to be "available." Why not place yourself where he couldn't help but notice you in a crowd of pretty girls?)

Our audience was satisfied with the evidence. The thought had never occurred to them to explain his marital status to her. They had "handled her with kid gloves." Plain talk was what she really needed. Her communication skills were well-honed. She has high morals and good common sense. Normal behavior was what we expected from her. A crush was normal. A crush on a married man was not normal, nor accepted behavior in our family. End of discussion. End of crush.

She never mentioned Jim again. She flirted with boys nearer her age, had fun on other church trips, and never got into that kind of "trouble" again. However, we never relaxed totally when she was away again. Even her church group was not completely ready to handle kids with disabilities. Still, it made me sad, for her, and for us. She needed a break from us, and we needed some real down time. It didn't happen for us until she joined the Sunday school class at Concord First Baptist several years after this incident. Everyone in the class has a disability and she could be herself and let down any guard.

It wasn't a perfect situation either. She was used to a lot of freedom as she moved from class to class in high school, and was considered a young adult. Now she was back into a more structured setting, and a more rigid format of "following the leaders." The good outweighed the bad. She was caught in between—this feeling of being treated like a child and as an adult, simultaneously. At home we were having the same experiences, as we attempted to make adjustments, as she grew up and grew wiser.

There will be times we need to step in and advise and implement instruction or help. Other times we need to stand by and watch our grown kids make their own decisions, tiny ones as well as large ones, so they can experience consequences, successes and failures. David and I have learned that we could help them mature emotionally as we allow them the opportunity to show and implement independence. Of course the scope and degree of the disability of the individual will dictate the necessity to step in and make the most of these decisions for our grown kids. Most parents know their child's needs. Years of care have honed our instincts and skills as we lovingly raised a special needs person. There is a fine line we must walk in the area of sensitivity to their feelings, while keeping their best interests at heart as we help them develop mental reasoning, cognitive thinking, and personal preferences. We want Windy to feel like she is an adult, yet she still needs our protection and guidance in some areas.

She hears frequently from dear friends like, Cat Zacharetti (Spottswood), Beka Moore (Axon), and Margaret Moore (Gill), Amy Palumbo, and Kristen Palumbo. Their ongoing friendships are dear to her. She also hears from family, via text messages. Her cousins, Emmalee, Molli, Lenzi, Sara, Joni and Joey periodically keep her updated with pictures and news, also. She is thrilled at each contact. With all this technology so easy to use we have to try to keep it in balance.

Sometimes this precarious balancing act causes all of us to lose patience, perspective, and our sense of humor. (Like too much texting or too many phone calls.) When any of these things occur, our family knows to interpret it as a sign to slow down, reevaluate the specific cause of irritation, and to get feedback from each other on how to make our lives better (more cooperative for all parties concerned). We try to see it as a great time to implement new ideas or new house rules.

We try to cover all the basics but there are things that slide past us under the radar. Just the other night we discovered she texted a childhood friend, now an attorney in Kentucky, at just around midnight, to ask her about a famous homemade doughnut shop she had just heard about on the Food Network show, *Diners, Drive-Ins, and Dives*. Sorry! (Nothing like going to a professional for some good advice, right?) Lights-out is another one of those rules that has changed over the years. School and work dictate certain timeframes. Days off and vacation days, dictate others. We have generally allowed Windy to set her own rules here. She has always used great common sense in this area of her life . . . unless a great Disney movie is on (or a movie starring Zac Efron!) into the wee hours. On those mornings-after, she really drags her feet!

David and I don't think all this is a very big deal. We love having our daughter living with us, and we make it work for each of us. Our living arrangement works for us. Windy is able to be as independent as is possible and still live with her parents. She gets to be with her entire family at various times, and she gets to travel to many places with us. She experiences an entire array of options that wouldn't be available to her if she lived away from us. It's the way we all choose to live. Even if that means remaining vigilant as we try to keep up with her!

Each family unit is uniquely different, and each must decide what's best for their family.

Nancy is the friend who opened my eyes to the fact that Windy was one step ahead of David and me, all the time. Once I admitted my fatigue to her because I told her, "It took all I could do to try to stay ahead of what Windy might do or say," and suddenly Nancy died laughing.

"What's so funny?" I asked, a bit miffed that she wasn't sensitively agreeing with me.

"You lost that contest a *long* time ago!" she said, between bouts of continued laughter. Well, it was as if Nancy had thrown cold water on me. Reality struck me hard. I *had* lost that contest a long time ago, and I just hadn't let myself acknowledge the fact. Windy had figured out how to control *some* of her life, with a mom who prided herself on being in control! Funny, Nancy! But I had to admit to her, and to myself, that it *was* true!

A great example of *trying* to keep ahead of Windy is this one: We were in Oak Ridge for a Special Olympics swimming competition. We had all arrived at the Civic Center to watch. Windy and her class had ridden the bus earlier that morning. I just knew she would look so cute in her new red, white, and blue one-piece swimsuit I had bought for her swimming meet. It had taken some searching to find the perfect suit, but we had done it. She and I had packed her gym bag the night before, so she would be ready to go.

David, Dave, and Mikey and I filed in with the several hundred spectators and found great seats in the bleachers overlooking the pool. From up there we could watch her as she came in the side door. Sure enough, she entered in with her teammates as they all walked out in their matching sweats. They gathered at one side of the pool and began to take their sweat suit jackets off.

I gasped out loud . . . so loud David grabbed my arm as he thought something was wrong with me. There was something wrong, but not with me, it was with Windy . . . something was wrong with her bathing suit. She stood there in her cute yellow polka dot two-piece bathing suit, the one she wore to lay out in the sun, in the privacy of our back yard. The bottom half was fine for wearing in public, it had a cute skirt attached to it. It was the top that I was concerned over. It didn't have any straps. All I could see in my mind's eye was her leaning over the edge of the pool in a diving position with a little top on! And just what if it didn't *stay* on? This was no place for a strapless bathing suit. "I'll be right back!" I told David as I literally bounced out of my seat, scrambled down the bleacher steps, and ran over to her group. I wasn't going to tell her Dad yet. (He's a 'fixer', and this was out of his territory. He couldn't fix this.) This was a Mama's job!

I ran up to her. "Okay, I'm not mad at you, I want you to know that, but I want you to put that jacket back on fast! Tell me, where is your new one-piece suit?" I asked her as I stood in front of her, trying to shield her from everyone's eyes. As we talked, we managed to make a quick move out into the nearby hall. I knew I had to shield my daughter from an impending disaster.

"At home, Mom. There are so many cute guys here, and my friends are here from school to see me swim. My one-piece didn't look as good on me," she confessed to me. Her words came tumbling out. She looked like any other teenager would look, standing there pleading with her mom for understanding. My heart *understood* her reasoning. She only wanted to be like all the rest of her friends she went to the pool with, she just wanted to fit in. She knew she was here at an event that only some of her friends could participate in, and she was acutely aware that her friends from school were there to see the events, and that they might think she had a disability. It hurt her deeply to have someone think she needed more help than others, that she was different from them. I could see the pain in her eyes as she explained her reason why she had made her choice of swimsuits.

"Well, we'll talk later about that. Right now you have to swim, and swim to win, okay? Where is your strap that goes around your neck?" I knew we had to do first things first. (Plus, I *wanted* her to do her best. She was a good swimmer. She wanted to be here competing. Now it was my job to see that she had a chance to be the best athlete she could be.)

"Gone. Lost. I couldn't find it this morning." She admitted her mistake, looking so defeated. I could just see her in my mind's eye going through her dresser drawers searching for the strap with me hollering in the background for her to hurry and come and get in the car so I could get her to school before the bus took off for Special Olympics! It made me feel sad for her. I bit my lip and held back the tears. If I started to cry I knew she would too, so I got hold of my emotions. We had a dilemma to solve.

"Well, now what?" I asked her. We both stood bewildered. Then it hit me, as I dejectedly looked to the ground, and *then*, focused on my tennis shoes. "Here you go!" I said as I quickly kicked off my right shoe and started unlacing it, as I spoke. "This will work! It's *got* to work!"

Off came the shoelace, and I threaded it into the two tabs of cloth on either side of her top where the missing strap had been. I tied her up, and she was off to swim. Forget famous brand running shoes making you a champion—we had been saved by good old Keds, with old-fashioned laces!

What girl doesn't want to look her best poolside? Her daddy used to be a Life Guard at our community pool, and I was reminded of my own vanity. I had wanted to look as cute as I could for David and the boys at the pool. My daughter was as normal as apple pie when it came to boys. Normal was what David and I had aimed for.

Big lesson learned by Mom—check suitcase or book bag before we leave the house. It will make for a smoother day—and I will probably be able to walk more naturally and at a faster pace when we attend sporting events, without my foot coming out of my shoe with every step I take!

Windy's outgoing personality has paid off big time for her. She has usually been the one picked out from a crowd to be the person interviewed for a newspaper article or put on a televised interview whether she is participating in a sporting event in Special Olympics or attending an important function. (When in high school, she was asked to do a televised public service announcement with some of her friends and with UT's head football coach, Phillip Fulmer for the United Way. Windy even got to be on a TV program, exercising with Missy Kane, a local celebrity athlete and TV personality.) Her cute vivaciousness, and her ever-ready smile are a huge reason, but it is so much deeper than that. We think it's because she has a Divine calling, and she gives "100 percent, 24/7" in everything she does.

Sometimes you just have to be around her for a few moments to recognize this fact. David and the boys and I have seen this innumerable times. When it happens, the scenario is almost always predictable. We are in a group of people with Windy in the background, not actually being noticed, when someone, usually out of kindness, turns to ask her a question, and as Windy begins to answer, we witness the person being drawn to her sweet voice, her wonderful "Windy" fragrance, and to the sincerity in her speech, as she looks directly into their eyes. Before you know it, they are turning their backs on us and chatting away with her like long lost friends.

A few of these special moments come readily to mind. Once, a couple of years after Windy had graduated high school, we were sitting beside a friend's pool enjoying a visit and a chat with her. It was one hot summer day and some University of Tennessee male students stopped by to look at some heavy porch furniture they had promised her husband they would move to another spot on another level of the decking. With them was our friend's nephew. The four buddies were walk-ons for UT's football team, hopefuls for the upcoming fall season team. After casual and quick introductions, they began talking to us about their aspirations to make the team, and to meet some of the well-known players who were on the team at the time.

The name Jason Price, one of the players, was mentioned, and Windy spoke up, and said, "I know Jason. He's a good friend of mine. I've known him for years. He is my neighbor." Later Benson Scott's name came up. He was quarterback and a placekick holder for extra points and field goals at UT, and son of Bobby Scott, who had played quarterback for UT and was the backup quarterback (behind Archie Manning) for the New Orleans Saints. Windy said, "Benson is one of my *best* friends. We went to high school together." The guys glanced over at her, seemed to sum up that she had some kind of disability, and not too unkindly, just matter of factly, they disregarded her comments and went on talking about practices and football tryouts. Several more names were mentioned in their conversation, and Windy would interject comments, not braggingly, simply stating facts, such as, "I like him a lot. He's really nice!" or "That guy really likes to teach kids to swim. He taught my friends to swim at camp this summer."

Slowly, as they continued talking to the adults, the boys began to look over at her and to pay attention to what she had to say. Her comments were timely, and very informative about the different players' personalities—the same players they admired and hoped to meet and get to know. It was becoming obvious that this girl really knew some of these very players that they had a sort of hero worship thing going on, and she might, just maybe, tell them something that would be helpful in linking someone up in a conversation when they got to go to an upcoming practice, or when they ate at the training table with them. One guy asked her how she knew all those team members, and she proceeded to tell them that she had been friends with several players at Farragut High School, and some of the others had befriended her when they came every year to a camp she attended for "special" people.

Before they left, she had given them tidbits of stories of interest that they took back with them to initiate conversation with their local sports heroes. They gave her hugs and high fives and left happy, all because a cute, high school girl had looked their way—and after some reluctance, they took notice. Don't think Windy didn't bask in this consideration. She was all charm and smiles. Her flirty little personality had come out full force.

Her beautiful character is just so evident, so free of malice, cynicism, and prejudices. She is like a breath of fresh air to a world gasping for one little intake of unpolluted oxygen in our treatment of others. This kind of pure love and faith is impossible to hide, and others are drawn to it as a moth to light.

Just like all of us—when we put away our preconceived feelings and prejudices, and allow Christ's love to shine through—not always an easy thing to do. It takes a concentrated effort. Every day we are to delve into the Scriptures to have His mind, as our own mind is renewed and transformed, day by day, situation by situation, to see ourselves and others as He views them.

This way of life seems to come more easily for Windy and for her friends that are born with Down syndrome, or other intellectual disabilities. It's as if their filtering systems are so much purer than the rest of us. They don't carry around a lot of junk in their minds to weigh them down and hold them back from enjoying life to the max, and enjoying other people's lives. They have normal feelings, sure they do, they get upset with family members or friends over petty misunderstandings like the rest of us. But we are always so touched at how quickly and sincerely they forgive each other and themselves, and they don't dwell on the negatives for days (or years) later. It's not that they forget, believe me, her memory is like an elephant's when she feels she must remind someone about a past mishap. She will only bring up something if she thinks it must be said to help the person do better or to prevent them from making another mistake.

She and her friends chose not to live with regrets from the past. How beautiful a lesson is that for every one of us? She and her buddies can say things or do things that hurt each others' feelings; they are just like the norm in that respect. They just make up quicker, and don't hold grudges. And they have likes and dislikes in food, clothing, hobbies and in people, just like all other people.

Windy will let it be known that she disagrees from time to time. She doesn't go skipping along Pollyanna style without a profound thought in her head. She is quite profound. As her brothers say, "She's a genius, Mom! I've never known anybody like her!"

A prime example of her insight: Once, UT had a basketball coach who did not have a great rep as a kind, sweet talking kind of guy. He hadn't been there too long, and he wasn't going to be there too much longer we had heard through the sports grapevine. Windy had heard things from the news and from some people who knew the man. She had heard the rumors out there that he was leaving. We had to be at the UT Arena for some gymnastic function and happened to pass the current coach in a hallway with no one else around. As we walked, I saw the Coach approaching and I thought to myself, "Oh-oh! What is she going to say?" I just knew she'd say something. Windy looked right at him, and said, "Hey" and then said his first name. He said, "Hi" back as he walked on by. No one else was around, but he didn't take any time out of his agenda to stop and talk to her.

"Honey, you should have said, 'Hi, Coach', and not used his first name. You don't know him. You should show some respect for the Coach."

"Oh, no, I shouldn't! He shouldn't be Coach to the guys. They need a *nice* man to lead them. He doesn't need to use bad words to make them do what he wants them to do. I'm not calling *him* Coach!" And with that she walked faster, so I couldn't give a comeback to her comment. She needn't have worried, I didn't have one. She was "right-on" with what she had said. See, Windy **can** always capture a situation in a very few words. This was another fine example. Right?

We are proud of the way our daughter usually handles herself. Sure she can have her moments, but she is really a very loving and kind person. Any small part we have been allowed to play in her overall development has been a privilege and an honor to help her enhance what God had already placed in her heart from her birth. (That goes for our sons as well, we are honored to have been the ones to raise them!)

We have learned to roll with the punches through the years. I have tried to be prepared for the unexpected, but Windy has surprised even me, her Mom, many times. And I do mean it when I say I have *tried* to be prepared for what she may do or say. You know what they say about "the best laid plans of men and mice"!

I try to look at all angles of a situation and try to prepare her or myself for anything that might come up. I underestimate her at times. My mind can't think of everything! The following story is a prime example of what I'm talking about.

During her junior year of high school we were invited by a friend to attend a special program at a church in Franklin, Tennessee. The guest speaker was going to be Chris Burke, a young man in his twenties at the time, who was born with Down syndrome. He was a popular television star on a very popular series entitled, *"Life Goes On."* It ran on ABC network from 1989 to 1993, with nightly reruns available for several years after. It had been a wonderful presentation of a family with three teenage children. Kellie Martin, a favorite actress of Windy's, played the sister of Chris's character, Corky, on the show. (To Windy's delight, Kellie went on to star in another of her favorite shows—the televised series called *"Christy" that* was filmed in our Smokies.) Corky and his "TV sister" attended a public high school together in the series, and America embraced the show, especially the endearing "Corky."

All of the teenagers we knew watched the show, and I'm sure it paved a very positive way for Windy's future high school days. In that first LRE class she took the school by storm. She didn't just try to fit in . . . she embraced her new friendships and make a difference in their lives. She didn't go on her way quietly—she made a point to say, "Hello" every day, in a big way. Everybody knew Windy. She was living the real life role of "Corky" in her own school, but it was even better in real life! Teachers and students first met Windy in 1992, and they got to know her friendly, outgoing, sincere personality, and they came to love her! (That says a lot about the character of her friends and teachers!)

She would go to the lunchroom on her lunch break, and she would look up friends specifically to ask them how they were doing, and to give out hugs and high-five's. People would open up to her, and share what was happening in their lives. She was a great listener and had great advice to give out. Others befriended her because they liked her and cherished her friendship. Haley Holman (Evans), who lived just across the street, and Addie (Rouse), were the names of two girlfriends she met and grew close to. She never hesitated to tell them she would pray for them. She prayed every night and kept a running list of friends' names that she wrote out herself on a piece of notebook paper. (She had to have their help in spelling their names, but she didn't need any help in remembering to pray. Who doesn't need a friend like that? No wonder she was so popular! She cared for others deeply.)

Windy and her friends never missed an episode of *"Life Goes On,"* and taped it if they had to be gone for some reason for their own high school functions. Susan Nichols and Tony DeFranco were two of her best friends in the LRE room. The girl friends giggled together on the phone as they watched the show at their respective houses. When I say Windy was thrilled with the invite to meet Chris in person, it's an understatement. Someone in Nashville had sent Windy an invitation to come and hear Chris Burke speak and sing at a church in the area.

"Mom, I need to go find a cute new dress, and could you do my makeup for me?" were her words to me as the date of Chris's arrival to Knoxville approached.

"Sure, I will," I said as I got caught up in her excitement. My daughter was going to meet her TV heartthrob, face to face! I was going to help her be ready for this special, special meeting.

In my most fearful moments, way back in her toddler days, as I contemplated her future teen years, I had no idea another television show (The first one being the

Sesame Street program with the young boy with Down syndrome, who appeared as a regular when she and Dave were younger.) would help our daughter be more accepted and cared for as a teenager. But, you know what? Looking back, now I know He was making her path easier than we could have imagined. It was not just good timing, it was *perfect* timing for Windy! Yes, we can even thank God for a TV show sometimes in our lives!

Well, Windy showed up at the church where Chris Burke was a special guest speaker, a few weeks later. She wore a darling, light blue denim dress, and her long, shoulder-length hair, makeup, and pink nails were done to her satisfaction. She didn't hesitate to walk up to Chris, shake his hand, and ask for a picture with him. Her dad was standing right where she had asked him to stand with the camera ready. He snapped several poses, and then got a few impromptu shots of them as they conversed. They seemed to really enjoy talking to each other. Joe and John, his singing partners and traveling companions, and business partners at the time, came up and introduced themselves. Before you knew it, Windy was asking them to come to Knoxville to speak and perform in our area. Her idea caught us off-guard, but Joe and John were so supportive of the idea that we readily agreed that it was a great idea.

By the time we left, we had worked out a time they could all come and stay at our home for a week. She had asked, and they had accepted! Had she been planning this all the way down to Nashville? Probably.

David and I talked almost non-stop on the three-hour ride home, trying to figure out how it had all happened so quickly. Windy couldn't wait to get back to Farragut and tell everyone about her future visitor. Believe me, when he did get to visit, he had a great fanfare from the kids at Farragut High and from The Sonshine Class at Concord First Baptist Church. They had had ample time to prepare for him. The girls had seen to that.

Windy invited her friend Susan over to meet Chris and have dinner at our house, on the day of his arrival. Susan came dressed-up for the event. She looked so cute. Dave was away at college but was coming in for "The Visit." Mikey was at ball practice, but was coming home to meet and visit with Chris as soon as practice was over.

Windy and I set the dining room table, using her choice of china, and we even had fresh flowers for the centerpiece on the table. Soft music was playing in the background, and I felt we looked completely ready for company, and I felt like I had thought of everything . . . I hadn't though. All the while I was tooling around in the kitchen the last twenty minutes or so, I could hear the girls laughing and talking excitedly. Sure, why not? This was big time happenings. I would holler up and check on them from time to time. Windy's bedroom door was at the top of our kitchen's back stairway, and each time I yelled to her, Windy would open the door slightly and say politely, "We're fine, Mom! Are they here yet?"

Finally I yelled up the wooden steps to say they *were* here. She and Susan squealed with glee and then hurried down the front steps to our foyer and the front door. I went to the door to open it and greeted Chris with a hug. I welcomed Chris, Joe and John DeMasi to our home. Chris hugged me back and then walked in and started towards Windy, to hug her. She walked towards him and put out her arms to receive his friendly hug.

That's when I noticed her *hair*. Evidently she had sneaked out my sharpest scissors I kept in a drawer in our Master bath, taken them to her room, via the front steps, and had whacked off a hunk of hair in front of both of her ears! In her excitement before his arrival, she had tried to give herself a sexier hair cut. I knew what she had been thinking without even asking her. I *know* my daughter, I just *didn't* know *when* she might try something daring. I knew I could walk into her bathroom and see several inches of her beautiful, long, shiny dark hair on the pale-pink tiled floor! *Then* I looked closer at Susan, who was hugging Chris now. Her hair was looking really cute, but a good bit shorter all over than when her mother had dropped her off at our house two hours before! What would her mother think? What in the *world* was I going to tell her mother? *Help me Lord. Please help me with this one!*

If I had said one word, only *one*, it would have embarrassed the girls. They had done this to be more grown up, more sophisticated, and it would have blown the whole thing for them. This was a big night in their lives. I acted as if nothing was out of the ordinary, and we got our guests settled in, and had a lovely dinner. Windy had outdone herself this time, though. I would have never, *ever* thought she would have done extreme makeovers before her prominent guest arrived.

I acted like I hadn't noticed. *Hadn't noticed!* I *was* stunned beyond words. (I proved *I* could act that night, because that *entire* evening I ignored the obvious, since it was not the proper time, or place, to talk about the new "Do's." All I could think of was—the show must go on—and life! Ha!

Here is another good **WINDY LIFE LESSON** . . . only this one *she* learned . . . and learned the hard way. Maybe it will help you avoid the same mistake . . . Don't do something crazy to get yourself noticed by someone else . . . even someone who is *very* popular. Just be yourself. And, oh yeah, she also learned . . . hair can take a *long* time to grow back when cut really short. Until it grew back, we had to do all kinds of fancy things so no one could tell it had been chopped off at the ears.

That week was one for the books. Susan's mom was *very* gracious. Maybe she knew her daughter had cut Windy's hair? I will probably never know. No one's talking. It just made a great story funnier. (Funny now, only because we look back at it from this side of the occurrence!)

Chris was very gracious to visit with Windy's friends and handed out autographs like a true pro. He was a typical STAR—he would listen to the person speaking to him, all the while scanning the room for other adoring fans. He was in his element in a group of people waiting to speak to him and get his autograph. He had wonderful manners and was at ease in new surroundings.

Windy and Chris went to a movie at our neighborhood theatre. The film *Grease* was showing. She was beyond happy! An evening out with the star of her dreams! This was exciting stuff! Chris wanted to be sure she understood he had a girl back home in New York City, but that he would love to escort her to the movie. Now Windy was the one not listening fully to what was being said . . . she was convinced he was going to fall in love with her, and take her to New York with him. (We had visited there for Mikey's Farragut Middle School's seventh grade trip. His teacher Patti Rader, had invited us to join them, and I think Windy had been trying to get back there ever since. She loves to shop and was in her element in the Big Apple! Why not dream of going back?)

Chris and Windy had a great time, and they talked from the time her dad dropped them off until the time he picked them up. Gosh, sometimes life is so fun and so surprising isn't it? We were beginning to realize God was answering our daughter's prayers in amazing ways. She had delighted herself in the Lord—and He was giving her the desires of her heart.

Delight yourself in the Lord, and he will give you the desires of your heart. (Psalm 37:4)

A big surprise occurred for Chris before he left Knoxville. We had asked our three guests to go to church with us. When we arrived early, before the second service began, we found seats in the middle section, on the main floor of the large sanctuary. Chris took a seat, and then almost immediately he stood up and began to wave, and call out a girl's name.

Windy and all the rest of us looked at him in a questioning way, and then we saw a beautiful young mother, walking in with her children, only two rows in front of us. The sight of her had caught Chris' attention—he recognized her in an instant. She turned to look in his direction, and she recognized him. She left the pew where she was just going to sit, and he left his seat. They embraced each other heartily in the aisle, as if neither one could believe their eyes.

She came over to tell us the whole story. They had grown up right next door to each other in a New York City apartment building. Their families had been good friends, and they had not seen each other in several years! What were the odds on that? She and Chris in Knoxville, at the exact same time, and at the exact same place, to see each other *that* Sunday morning, or they would never have seen each other.

Chris was ecstatic and hugged her goodbye one last time before they parted for who knows how many more years? He whispered to me as he sat back down, "I was supposed to be here, wasn't I?" I nodded in the affirmative as I smiled back at him. We were all blessed that Sunday morning, by the message given by John Wood, our new pastor, and by that happy reunion of old friends.

This is another story of Chris's visit to Tennessee, and in the theme of "The show must go on!" This time it was a show preparing to go on, just about the time we were passing by the auditorium. David and I had driven Chris, Windy, and our boys to the cities of Gatlinburg and Pigeon Forge, for a day of fun and sight-seeing. (Dave and Mikey appeared to enjoy Chris's company almost as much as Windy did. Chris knew many entertaining stories about the stars he had worked with, and he had a great sense of humor.)

On our drive home it was just beginning to get dark, and all the lights of Pigeon Forge and Sevierville were lighting up the dusk. It's quite an impressive sight. Chris suddenly noticed a large bright sign, with the words LEE GREENWOOD in brilliant colored, giant letters. "I *love* that guy! I love his music! I've met many stars, but I have *never* met him. I didn't know he performed up here. I love his song *God Bless the USA!*"

"Would you *like* to meet him, Chris?" I heard my husband ask him, as I watched him steer the car into the far left lane for a quick U-turn. I looked over at David as if to say, "Are you *crazy. We* don't know him! How can *you* introduce *him* to Chris?" Windy (the apple in this case) didn't fall far from the tree. They are *both* full of fun surprises. This was going to be an adventure!

David found an empty parking space at the large entertainment theatre, and he told Chris, and Chris only, to get out of the car. He said their chances of getting in would be far better with just the two of them. (As opposed to someone at the gate allowing a group of six in without tickets. We could see his point.) Disappointed, Windy reluctantly agreed to remain seated. We waited in the car for their return. They were gone a good twenty minutes or more. When they did get back to the car, Chris high-fived David, and thanked him by saying it had been "Awesome"! David was grinning as much as Chris was.

They buckled their seat belts, and David started the car. David began telling us how he had explained their situation to the man at the entrance door, and they had been escorted immediately to the star's private dressing room door. The door attendant said he recognized "Corky" and wanted to take him to meet Lee. There in the private setting, they had a one-on-one introduction, star to star. Lee was very kind to the young star. He, too, recognized Chris, and then he asked if he could introduce him to the packed house before he began singing. Chris gave a resounding, "Yes!" Since it was time for Lee to take center stage, he went on as planned, and then had Chris walk out as he announced him as their honored guest of the evening! Chris ate up the attention and loved the standing ovation he received. It was music to his ears from one of *his* favorite stars! A star he could say he had met in person now!

Windy (and her family) had managed to show Chris Burke a good time, with God's intervention, and in His perfect timing. We were able to bless someone whose portrayal of a character in a TV series had helped our daughter, and her friends with disabilities, become more socially accepted. Besides that, Windy got to dream of movie stars and possible trips back to New York City, for the next few weeks! Dreams *are* the stuff that keeps us going!

Windy attended many regular classes at Farragut High besides her resource room curriculum. She took biology in Mr. Fergeson's class. She adored him as an instructor and loved learning anything about science and biology. Only once did she come home complaining. She said, "We did a really disgusting thing to a frog today!"

"You did," her dad asked, "like what?"

As she answered she curled up her little nose, made a face, and said, "We had to cut it up! Yuk!"

"Well, did you stop dissecting yours when you found out that was what you had to do?" he asked her, thinking she probably had, due to her reaction to her lab assignment.

"No, Dad, I didn't. I want to make an 'A' in the class. You *have* to complete your assignments."

"Good for you, Girl! I bet you'll do really well in Mr. F's class." She did do well. Her teacher expected her to do as much as she could, and then some. He was a great teacher, and she learned so much in his class.

Then she enrolled in an art class (signed up for it every year she was there in school). She was very creative and enjoyed every second of her art classes. She had two art teachers during her high school years, and they were very complimentary of her artistic ability. They were always showing us works of art she had done.

Some things she learned outside the classroom. We had *never* heard her say a cuss word, not *one* since she has become an adult. (Not counting the word she shouted to our friend Lonas that time when she was four!) While attending high school, she heard *many* choice words. We know she did. I asked her about the language she heard in the crowed hallways of her school. She didn't deny it. She replied, "I hear bad words, but I don't ever say those things!" I assured her that I knew for a fact she didn't.

One day, when she was a junior, I remember her completely exasperated over something, and she was exasperated with me. (As only a mother and daughter can do to one another on occasion.) I remember she said, "Mom, you really piss me off!" It was the closest she ever came to a cuss word. She kept profusely apologizing that night for it and told me she would never say the word again, and we both apologized to each other, and that was that. She has never again come close to saying anything like that to me or anyone else. *Ever.*

What a **WINDY LIFE LESSON**! She is truly a woman of her word. Can you imagine the integrity that displays in her life and what it means to us as her parents? Humbling. Truly humbling.

On a somewhat funny note, concerning cussing, she has *alluded* to a cuss word. When our son Dave once told us about a girl he was being "torn up inside over" and had been for a considerable length of time, she took our family from dead serious to hilarious in seconds. We were all hoping he would move on—make the best of a sad situation. We were riding along in the car and Dave was talking *and* talking about his lost love and asking our advice on what he should say to her. She had acted cruelly to him and had not been even close to being kind. It was pretty obvious to everyone in the family what he should do, but we knew it had to be his decision.

Windy had listened silently for the almost hour-long conversation and finally, apparently not able to remain silent any longer she said, "Excuse me, Dave, but you just need to tell her what Rhett Butler told Scarlet at the end of the movie (*Gone With The Wind*) and get on with your life!" He died laughing, and said, "You're probably right there, little Sis. It's time I gave up and got on with my life! Leave it to you to capture a moment and sum up a situation in a heartbeat! Windy, Windy, you're a wonder!" She had been able to break his chain of sadness and started him on the road to recovery in one fell swoop.

Our daughter wanted to learn to drive in high school. Most of her friends were learning, but she was very nervous over it because she couldn't help thinking of her Uncle Chip, who had died in a car wreck early one morning, as he was driving his two, beloved little daughters to school one beautiful, fall October day. We weren't over the heartbreak. (Still aren't. We trust the Lord on this one, but we still miss him so.) Windy wanted to drive like her brothers did, so despite her fears, she kept after me to go with her to get her license.

I caved at her vocal pleas to "just let me try it" and asked her teacher if it was even possible. She came back with the answer Windy wanted to hear, "Yes", but there are stipulations. She would have to take an agility test to first check her responses, or response timing, to see if she could stop a car "on a dime", to determine if she was capable of making the right decisions while driving out on the road. Her teacher had checked into the possibility and had found a testing instrument at Tennessee's School for the Deaf across town. She made an appointment for her, and I was ready to let the results of the testing tell us if she would be a good driver. 'Lo and Behold', she not only passed the testing, she beat a teacher's score, who had taken it along with her. Looks like we were going to have to put her in the driver's seat in the family car, in a secluded parking lot somewhere, and let her try to drive.

I waited for a Saturday when the huge parking lots were empty, and we traded seats. After adjusting her seat and mirrors, she eased it out of the parking space, and we went for a very slow drive around the lot. She has always had great coordination and is a great backseat passenger in that she watches out instinctively for anyone who is driving her about. She has helped her Dad, brothers, and me as she looks for a clear time for us to pull out onto the highway, telling us to slow down or stop at changing traffic lights, to anticipate a turn ahead. We shouldn't have been so surprised that she was also a good driver herself.

Now this presented a whole new set of circumstances (and to a mom . . . problems). Would she pass her driver's license test? If so, would we ever let her out in a car alone? Even if we wouldn't, she would have the legal right to drive. Would she ever take the car for a spin at a time we didn't know she had access to the car keys? We were talking about 'Miss Independent' here. Duh! We weren't stupid. However, we *were* perplexed. Should we refuse to allow her to take the test, or should we just see if she passed it and then cross that bridge when we came to it? Then all of a sudden, Windy gave up the idea, all on her own. I had taken her out for a practice drive, and she hit the brake too hard, and it scared her.

"Mom, I don't think I want to drive anymore. I could kill myself. Anyway, I have a lot of drivers, and I have a way to get anywhere I want to go. Is that okay?"

"Honey, that's great with me. For now we'll just say you have decided to wait. If you ever change your mind and you want to try again, just tell me."

That was that. She did go to the school office and sign up for a parking pass for the Junior Parking Lot, as she was eligible for the privilege. She didn't tell us anything about it. (Younger drivers had to park across the road and walk a good distance to school. We knew that part and weren't too happy with the kids having to cross the highway with no red-light at the school entrance. We were always concerned someone could be hit crossing on foot. Evidently Windy didn't like that either. Mikey drove her to school now, and he parked in this far removed lot every morning.)

A few days after her decision not to drive, she came home as proud as could be as she waved her pass in the air. "Look Mike, if you're *real* nice to me, I'll put this in the window of "our car", and *you* can park close to school from now on. No more long walks across the four-lane from the parking lot to the school!" Mike was only a sophomore and tickled at his big sister's suggestion. Mostly, he was tickled at her obtaining the pass on her own. We discovered that obtaining a parking pass was mainly why she had wanted to learn to drive. She wanted to be considered as a young adult. She was growing up, and she wanted everyone close to her to know it. And she wanted that pass. She got both, and she didn't even have to drive to get them. Now we understood her motivation, and we sought to show her we understood her desire for recognition as someone that was no longer a child. What a *woman*!

When Mikey was a freshman, and Windy was a junior, she helped her little Bro out in another big way. She knew all the teachers and principals by this time. After all, she had been there as a student for two entire years. Mikey came home after the first few weeks of school, a bit discouraged that his schedule was not as he preferred, and he was told by a teacher that no one could change their schedule after a certain date. He had passed that set date. Windy overheard him telling their dad about it, and she said, "Don't worry, Mikey, I'll help you out. Your Principal is Mrs. Johnson. Right?"

Yes, Win, but don't say *anything* to her. It won't do any good, and you can't do anything about it now. You'll just get me in trouble."

Silly brother. He thought his word held some kind of hold over her intervening in his life. Not so.

The next day they called Mikey's name over the loudspeaker to come to the Principal's office. He got up and left his English class, wondering what he had done to be called to the office. He'd only been there a couple of weeks. He hadn't had time to get into any trouble! When he knocked on her door, he was asked to enter by Mrs. Johnson, the freshman class principal, who he saw sitting at her desk. And . . . by golly . . . there sat his sister across from her, smiling big. "Hi Mike. This is your new Principal. She is so nice, and she's going to help you switch a class. Just tell her about it. I tried, but I don't know what you need exactly." A flabbergasted Mikey told his Principal his dilemma, and she was gracious enough to hear him out, and then she proceeded to sign a change order for him on the spot.

The two of them walked out together, and he thanked his sister with a kiss on the cheek. She was protecting him until he got used to the huge high school. Her job was a big one, but she was up to the challenge. She had surprised her brother *and* the Principal by her honest appeal and gutsy gesture.

It was not the last time she would help him out though . . . she helped him get a great job while he was in school, only this time it was while he was in Law School! And the job was at the White House! A favor he will never forget!

Mikey was searching for a job as an intern in an office where he could pick up some great experience for his future in the law profession. He decided to send in a resume for a position as an intern in the White House. He had some friends who worked in D.C. and would rent him a room if he got a job. Kari, his wife, was an RN and working as a rep for an orthopedic replacement appliances company. They figured she could drive up, or he could drive down, every weekend, so they could be together as much as possible. It would be hard, but worth the experience. He sent his resume on and found out he got the job. He was elated. During his tenure he worked long, long hours in the Personnel Department.

After a *long* summer, Kari came up alone for the last time, to help him move out. Mikey went to a last gathering where President George W. Bush came in to shake the Interns' hands and to thank them for the great service they had done for their country. Mikey was the last person in line. The President thanked him for his help and then in a joking matter (George W. Bush's style—his sense of humor is keen!) said, "Great job, Mike. We had many, many applications for your job. But you were highly recommended by someone special . . . your sister emailed Blake an impressive recommendation. How does it feel to have your big sis help you get a job?" Then he smiled at him and shook his hand.

Wait. What? Windy had written a letter? Yep, she sure had. And she had learned how to erase all traces of her correspondence so her parents couldn't get the wrong impression and mess up the good thing she was trying to do. She took matters into her own hands and did a wonderful deed for a guy she loved and respected very much. Dave and Mikey have been so kind and loving to their sister all her life, and she lives to do nice and loving things back for them.

Sometimes we just don't know what she has in mind, or to what lengths that girl will go to, in order to assist her brothers.

Her inherited 'dare-devilness' (from her daddy) was very evident when she attended another high school age youth trip with CSPC. She and Mikey went on a retreat to a place called, of all things, *Windy Gap*. The group could not have been there more than an hour, just barely time enough to find their cabin, claim a bunk, unpack some gear and settle in, when Mikey was walking with some friends to the site of the infamous camp zip-line. In a hurry, for they hoped to beat the crowd to get their turn on the much talked about activity. One guy asked Mikey if he was fearful of getting on it.

At that moment another friend yelled out, "I hope you're okay with riding it because your sister is already on it. Look at her go!" There was Windy letting out a big thrilling scream as she sailed along high above their heads! Mikey said he couldn't believe it! After they came home they excitedly told us all about it. And, of course, he rode it, too! Good thing he had wanted to, or he would have been humiliated into getting on anyway. No way was his sister going to try it, and he wasn't! That wasn't gonna' happen! Especially with all their friends watching!

During Windy's senior year, her art teacher, Ms. Whetsel, called me one day out of the clear blue, to ask if she could enter Windy's recently completed self-portrait, done in water colors over pen and ink, in the local Special Arts Competition. She told me that she had already received Windy's permission. She thought it was a fine piece of art and felt it had a chance of winning the area contest. I was somewhat surprised. We knew she liked to paint, to create, and to make things: draw fashions, decorate her room, but we didn't know she might have award winning talent. I gave my permission, and I couldn't wait to see the painting. She had never mentioned a drawing or a contest to us. Typical. So typical of her.

A few weeks later we went with Windy to the local Art Show and Contest. Special Arts is an art show and judged art contest for those who have a disability, and it encourages those with disabilities to be creative and allows them to compete against other artists. When we came to her painting, we were all delighted. There was a blue ribbon, a first place prize on her beautiful self-portrait! It went on to win on a state level, and then a place of honor in a display in the nation's Capitol, in the Rotunda. Later it hung on a wall in the official headquarters of the Special Arts Department in Washington, D.C. because it had won national recognition in a nationwide competition. (This is where it hung when it was seen and recognized to be the creation of Windy by Rod Paige, the Secretary of Education, later in the story.)

Farragut High was a great place for our daughter to dream dreams and achieve goals: goals once not even thought of as a possibility for someone who had been born with a disability. Now she, and many, many others all across America, were showing the world that they could make a difference, too.

While in high school, all the parents of the teams, Varsity and Junior Varsity Girls and Boys, got together, and with the Sixth Player Club overseeing us, cleaned and painted the gym of Farragut High. It had been a rural farm school district that had turned into an up-and-coming suburban school. County funds didn't cover all the needs, so we parents had meetings and assessed things. The gym was run-down looking and needed some tender loving care. The attendance at all basketball games was very low. We parents were embarrassed by the way things looked for the visiting teams that came there. Plus, a spiffy home court would do wonders for team morale! We all voted to clean the place up.

Windy helped us clean and scrub the bathrooms (think mops, paper towels and even toothbrushes here!), and then we painted the walls and doors of the stalls to refresh the decor. We put up mirrors, new soap dispensers and even painted the paper towel holders in Farragut blue. We all pitched in to raise the money to buy the paint and supplies. Some of us moms stenciled basketballs (real size) on the hall walls and put the players' numbers on them so the boys and girls could see them as they came up from the locker rooms on their way to the court. It was time to begin a new tradition of slapping your own number on the wall before appearing out there to the crowd. Windy helped me pick out the stencil and then a friend cut out a template for us. David and all the dads painted, washed, cleaned, and generally fixed all the broken things that needed fixing.

The gym walls finally looked new and clean, but very plain and bland. There's a limit to just how good you can make a gigantic room look using the colors of blue, gray and white! Windy told me of a boy who was a great artist in art class. She had come up with a wonderful idea. She and I called him, and we contracted with him to paint a larger than life school mascot, Admiral Farragut, a famous Navy officer, on the gym wall, all with the Sixth Player Club Board members' approval. She was real proud of the part she played in that endeavor. (Go Admirals!)

Other parents took down old dilapidated, faded hanging banners, had new ones made, and hung them high up in the rafters. Others painted the school's colors of blue and gray on the railings surrounding the upper balconies. The strategy worked: the teams took more pride in their school, the visiting schools had a nicer place to visit, and the students, parents, and families felt a unity and the satisfaction of a job well done! A bonus was the crowded bleachers

. . . sometimes not an empty seat in the place!

Oh yeah, and the girls' and boys' teams were getting a reputation for putting on a fine show, well worth the price of a ticket. That helped a whole lot! I knew all this involvement with her friends would be greatly missed by Windy when she graduated in three more years. We had to make the most of the time she had left in school.

Please God let me not borrow trouble and just enjoy the time we have now. But, please help us in that old dark future out there. Light the way we should go when high school is over and her adult years are finally here. Thank you, Father, for listening to me—just a mom, who's trying her best, and probably looking way too far into the future to find the peace you mean for us to have today. I know You understand though. I find comfort in that.

During her time at Farragut, Windy attended all the dances and proms and had a great time at each one of them. David and I would drive her, and her friends or a date, and we would usually dress up and stay as chaperones. She was none too happy about this, and we gave her enough space to satisfy her. Mr. Ken Stansberry, head of the English Department, put on elaborate proms at the old Tennessee Theatre in downtown Knoxville. Windy and I loved to volunteer to help decorate for them. We had a ball, as a mother and daughter team, working with the other parents and students to make the place look like a fairy tale come to life. Same thing for our church banquets and Missions Conference Banquets. We work well together. It's a blessing when moms and daughters can say that and mean it.

Her high school years were fun for her, and fun for all of the rest of us. Too quickly the years seemed to fly by, and her school days were coming to an end.

Windy was getting ready to graduate from Farragut High, after attending for five years. (She had been told by the Knox County School System that she could attend an extra year, until she turned twenty-one, because she was a special education student. We told her she was red-shirted like the athletes she liked to watch at UT! That worked for her, and it gave her one more year to learn more and to enjoy high school life! A bonus was that she got to go to school one more year with Mikey!)

So many wonderful things took place during that extra year of high school. One was when she received a letter from *The Knoxville News Sentinel* informing her that she had won a place on their prestigious list of Awards to Outstanding Seniors for the entire area! Her picture was to be in the paper along with the reasons she was chosen.

Several teachers had entered her name, along with a synopsis of her life as a high school student and her character and volunteer work. They told of her receiving a certificate for one-hundred hours of volunteer work at the East Tennessee Children's Hospital. (She had worked as one of the toy-cart ladies and had taken toys around to the rooms to let children chose a toy to play with. The hospital had put her on the cover of their monthly journal along with a featured article.) The teachers also listed the many things she was involved in as a member of her community and school.

She was one of the area students chosen and had her picture and a small article written about her in the paper. She was awarded this honor at a special presentation at the Knox City/County Building, by the Knox County Superintendent of Schools, Alan Morgan. We were so proud! Dave and Mikey were even happier than David and me; they had spent many hours loving, teaching and praying for their sis! They were thrilled that people all over our area would now know how awesome a person she really was.

Another highlight of her senior year came about a month before graduation. Windy came home one day from school and asked me to help her write a paper about her high school experience. We were in a hurry to get to a baseball game, so I jotted down a few things she said she wanted to say. I asked her what it was for, and she said, "Oh, just for a class thing." Her way of saying, "Don't pry, please!" So I didn't. She was almost out of school, so how much trouble could she get into for writing a paper about her true feelings about the school she loved and the people in it?

It was hard to sum up the five years she had attended Farragut High in just a few words. When we returned home, Windy and I sat on her bed, and we asked God to give us the right words for the assignment. We were tired, and we needed clarity and brevity as she began writing. She and I jotted down some sentences in a couple of paragraphs, things she wanted to say. She vetoed some thoughts I felt were good. I gave in because it *was* her report, and our collaboration was done in short order. Rewriting the paper in her deliberate, painstaking handwriting took her the longest amount of time. She thanked me with a big hug for my help, then placed the paper in her notebook and zipped the notebook back into her backpack to take to school the next day. It was very late when we heard her getting ready for bed.

We thought nothing about it . . . until we got a call from a teacher the next day telling us that Windy had been one of the five speakers chosen out of her class of nearly five hundred to speak at gradation. I was flabbergasted! Hearing the surprise in my voice, her teacher told me how it all took place. The announcement was made over the loud speaker at school, "for those interested in giving one of the speeches at graduation, please come to the auditorium for tryouts, and to fill out a form."

Guess who showed up and turned in their name with all the confidence in the world? You guessed it, Windy Smith! She had been listening to the announcement all week and had decided that she was going to give it a shot. Why not, she figured? She had been there longer than anyone else, five years, not just four, and she loved her school and her friends and teachers, and every aspect of the student life she had experienced. She wanted to be able to say goodbye and thanks for the memories "in style" . . . in *her* style, and loud enough for *everyone* to hear. What better way was there than this? It was a perfect "shout-out" for her, to her school.

The teacher went on to say, that when her name was called out she confidently got up and made her way to the stage. (This was all related again to me later in person by three teachers, who witnessed the speech tryouts first hand.) They said Windy held her paper up in front of her, so that she could read the words she had written down. She smiled at those teachers and students there to choose the speakers, then she began to read aloud in her quiet, sweet voice. She spoke of her loyalty for her school, and of the fears she overcame as she attended a big, huge school in the first LRE class at Farragut. She told how the students had made her feel welcome, and how they had accepted her as one of them.

She read her lines and then came to the end—where she thanked them all for being her friend. They said, "Everyone in the small audience was so touched that they were all crying when she finished. They stood and clapped for her and thanked her. Immediately the teachers took her and interrupted two other classes in session, and had her read it to them. The reaction from the listeners was the same: her fellow classmates and peers were moved to tears as they heard her words. She had touched their hearts deeply. Unanimously the judges agreed that something had to be done—the graduating class *had* to hear her words to them. This was just too special to miss knowing about, but Windy's speech did not meet the actual criteria for a speaker at graduation: she wasn't the Valedictorian or Salutatorian, or the President of her 1996 class, yet they felt like her words needed to be heard by the entire graduating class. After all, the message was for every student in her class, and for the lower classes as well. It was a speech straight from her heart to theirs. They promptly voted to place Windy on the graduation program as "a Special Speaker" . . . just before the Valedictorian spoke. The students' reaction had been a resounding unanimous vote for her to speak at the ceremony.

When the school called to invite her to speak, we asked her if she was really okay speaking to such a large crowd. (I know, silly us! Of course she was!) Her immediate answer was an enthusiastic response, "Oh, sure! I would *love* to!" Never once did she waiver in the days ahead. This would set a pattern for her public life to come.

We all anxiously anticipated the celebration. The entire family came to our house for dinner before driving over to the University of Tennessee campus. When we got to UT, we all streamed into the bleacher seats. We opened our programs and with pride read her name as a speaker. It *truly* was special! All four grandparents sat in those stadium seats so proud of their granddaughter. Their little darling had sure grown up to surprise them in mighty ways. God's power was so evident to us all that night!

She walked in with her classmates, the music already messing with our emotions, and as they took their seats, she walked up the steps in her navy cap and gown to take a seat on the stage. (I couldn't help but remember the steps she learned to walk up alone on those bus rides to Daniel Arthur years earlier.) When her turn came, she approached the podium with a purpose and singleness of mind. She was there to share her heart and gratefulness. There was absolutely no hesitation. The arena became silent as all eyes were focused on her.

She spoke that night to her classmates of her fear as a freshman at a new large, school. She told that she had transferred from a small, private Christian school, and was a member of the very first class at Farragut High for Special Ed kids. She thanked them for being so nice to her, and to her friends in the LRE class, and for treating her as an equal, and for giving her a chance to have a great time in high school. She related the story of the freshman boy who made fun of her at the beginning of her senior year and called her a name several times, the terrible "R" word. She explained that it had all turned out good though because, "about thirty-six of my best friends, members of the football and basketball teams, had a little meeting with him after school one day to help him learn how not to make fun of others." She said that they just talked to him and explained to him that he needed to be nicer to people, and then she said, "He got real nice to me after that." She had everyone laughing at that. She smiled out at her audience like an old pro and waited for the laughter to subside before she continued.

Then she proceeded to tell them all thanks for dancing with her at all the dances and proms. She thanked them for voting for her for the Admiral's Homecoming Queen's Court. She thanked them for helping her with her schoolwork as peer-teachers, and for helping her make her dreams come true while she was at FHS. Then she encouraged her peers to go out into the world and make their own dreams a reality. She finished by saying, "May God bless you all!" as she looked out, teary-eyed, at her peers.

The senior class jumped to their feet, and the audience followed suit to give her a standing ovation that lasted several minutes. She threw them a kiss, and the crowd went wild. Her graduation ceremony was held at Thompson-Bowling Arena at the University of Tennessee, in front of over three thousand people. It was the largest group of people she had ever spoken in front of, but surprisingly enough, and unbeknownst to us all, it would pale in comparison to the next huge audience she would be invited to speak to. It was certainly a great warming-up exercise! It was a wonderful night. (Whatever Farragut High was expecting and anticipating when they began accepting kids in the first LRE class we're sure it *wasn't this*!)

Thank you, Heavenly Father, for answered prayer for our daughter. She has had such a wonderful school experience! So far beyond our wildest dreams for her to reach her full potential. We had no idea how far that potential would develop and take her! Now show us where to go from here. Life after Graduation? Is there much out there for her? Show us your plans, please! This is just another path in our lives that looks dark right now, but we know You will reveal the next steps in due time. Help us in our waiting. That darned old waiting!

So many kids came up to us after graduation and told us that they would never forget her and how just knowing her had changed their lives for the better! They lined up to be able to say a few words to us about their sweet friend. It was awesome! Many pictures were taken of her with friends and family. One special picture taken that night was of Windy, and her friend, Emily Garman, in their caps and gowns, smiling their beautiful smiles as new graduates. It was the picture picked to be shown on the Jumbo Screen in Times Square for the DS Buddy Walk Celebration in New York City, a year later! (Her brothers had sent the picture in as a surprise for their sister.)

The National Down Syndrome Society's Awareness and Acceptance Campaign Press Release stated:

New York, NY-September 8, 1997

Windy Smith of Knoxville, TN, will appear in lights on Broadway as part of a national awareness campaign to demonstrate that people with Down syndrome can be successfully included in community activities, education, and employment. Ms. Smith's photograph was selected in the National Down Syndrome Society's nationwide search for images that illustrate the theme "Friendship Knows No Boundaries." Approximately 100 photographs will be arranged in a video PSA to be shown on the larger-than-life *NBC Astrovision by Panasonic* video board in Times Square.

We hadn't expected this! No, we hadn't expected this at all!

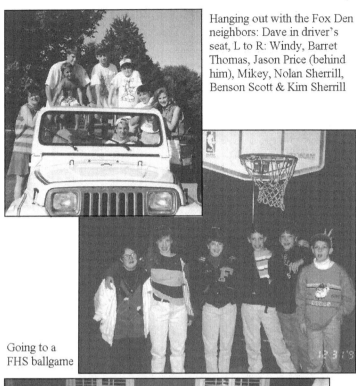

Hanging out with the Fox Den neighbors: Dave in driver's seat, L to R: Windy, Barret Thomas, Jason Price (behind him), Mikey, Nolan Sherrill, Benson Scott & Kim Sherrill

Going to a FHS ballgame

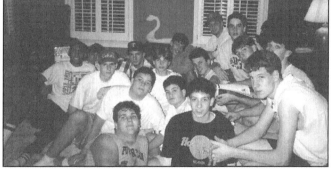

A bunch of Farragut friends (and other brothers!)

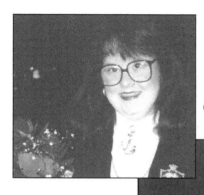

On FHS Homecoming Court

At the prom with friend (and future sister-in-law) Kari Hill

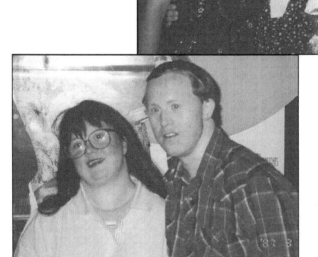

At the movies with actor Chris Burke

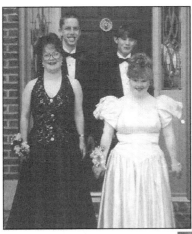

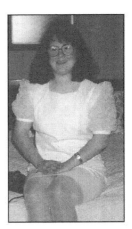

Ready to give a graduation speech, 1996

Prom night with friend, Susan Nichols, and their dates

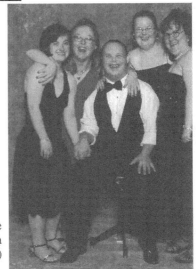

Matt Boyer surrounded by the girls (Heather, Pamela, Belinda and Windy)

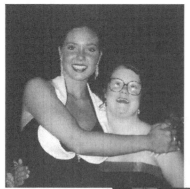

With dear friend Haley Holman

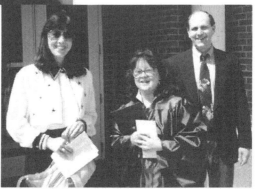

Graduated!

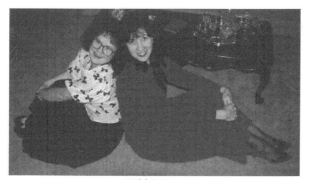

With Mom

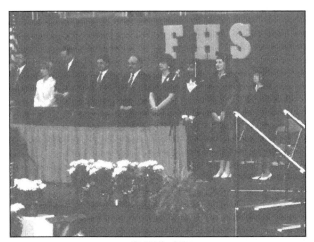

Speech time

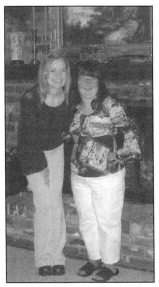

With cousin, Joni

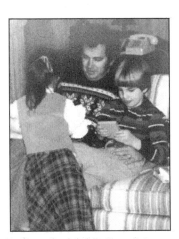

Uncle Jack with Windy and Dave

Chapter Seventeen
Life after Graduation

After graduation Windy and I went through a bit of a tough time. She was home with me all day. Mikey was still in school with some of her old buddies. She felt like she was missing out on the great active life she was accustomed to, and I no longer was free during the weekdays. I think we both were feeling a bit puzzled during this time. Was this how it would be? The two of us waiting for everyone else to get home from their wonderful, exciting lives while we sat at home? Wasn't gonna' happen. We weren't staying home! We hit the road after the first two weeks. We went out with friends on day trips. We went to visit with my parents and with David's parents, and we started looking into possible jobs for her. I hoped she would be an aide in a preschool. I kept talking it up.

She had taken several childcare courses, had even passed a CPR course, and was adored by "her students" in a daycare she had been involved with on FHS campus. Alex was the name of a little boy who had attended the class and wanted only "his Windy" to take care of him every day. He cried if she wasn't at school. (No wonder her nephews adore her now! She's a fun person to be with! Alex knew that!)

One night when we were talking over job opportunities, David asked her if she would like to work in a daycare. Her answer; "No way, Dad, Alex won't be there anymore. He's the reason I liked it so much. Would *you* want to go take care of little kids all day long?"

He looked away from her and looked straight at me, and said, "Forget working at a daycare, Vicki, she needs to find something else she'd *like* to do." "Okay," was all I said out loud, "But now what?" were the words I was thinking. I had hoped we had found her true bent, a career for her. Not so. I was stumped. When all else fails, pray about it. No, I have that backwards . . . pray first . . . so we did. Then we waited. And, we waited.

Windy especially missed her friendships. Her friendships in school had crossed over any boundaries high school kids self-impose on themselves. She had what was called "preppy" friends, friends that had special needs, friends that were the sports playing "Jocks", and anyone else in between. She even befriended those kids who seemed to lack close friendships. We had noticed she learned their names and spoke to them on a regular basis. She blurred the imaginary lines, and even erased them as she purposefully stepped on those "lines" with her small feet. She cared for all the kids. She was sincere. The kids knew this. We knew this. (Windy and her brothers have always been friendly and nice to *all* people). Kids, and parents of the kids, were always telling us this fact. We just didn't know to what extent, or how widespread and lasting Windy's influence had been on her peers—until after she left school.

She and I stopped by the school one day, almost a year after she had graduated, to drop something off for her brother, Mikey. She was reflective as we checked in at the main office. She looked around the office and spotted some familiar faces. Before I knew it, she headed for the door marked PRIVATE, and put her hand out to knock on the door. We heard a buzzer ring, and she turned the doorknob and entered to hug the women who worked there. Everyone was elated to see her. They even called out to others working out of sight in the back offices. Then after talking to them, she bounced out the door and walked right over to the open lunchroom area, where she hugged the cooks and staff on duty. Then, she effortlessly table-hopped from friend to acquaintance, giving out hugs and asking about their lives and siblings.

What a girl! I stood and watched her in action. I realized that I was probably holding her back. But I didn't know what to do to rectify the situation. She was in her element at this moment. I could see just how much she truly cared for other people, and literally blossomed as she came in contact with others. She could not have been more animated, and the feedback could not have been more receptive if she had been running for Mayor of Farragut! Heck, for Governor, even! (Some years later she would know several Governors personally, and she would win enough votes to be a Delegate when her name appeared on a Blount County ballot as a Delegate for Presidential hopeful, Mike Huckabee! Her 'meet and greet' before my eyes was a precursor for her future life as an adult.)

I always knew our daughter to be an exceptional personality, but seeing her at her old school reaffirmed for me that she had grown into a lovely lady in her own right. I couldn't wait to tell David all about our happy visit later that evening at dinner and "paint" the whole scene for him. He was going to love it.

Later, as we walked outside to the car, I happened to notice a girl, walking alone, dressed all in black Gothic-style clothing, who was picking up her pace to get closer to us. As she got closer I could see her short, jet black hair, pierced nose. Around her neck she wore a black, spiked, dog collar necklace. I wondered why she was approaching us on the sidewalk.

Before I could try to guess the girl hurriedly came up to Windy, and I heard her say in a low voice, "Hi, Windy!" She said it friendly, but reservedly. "Hey!" Windy said back to her in a very friendly voice. "Good to see you! How are you?" They smiled at each other as friends do. As we walked on, Windy looked sideways at me and said, "She's a friend, Mom," before I could make any comment. She said it in a protective way, hoping I wouldn't say anything negative about a friend who chose to dress differently than either one of us would have chosen. "I can see that, Honey, I'm *glad* she is! And you know what else? *Everybody* seems glad to see you. Everybody still remembers you, Windy! That's so special!"

"Yeah, it *is* special!" she said. We got in the car and remained silent on the short drive back home. She had her memories to contemplate, and I had mine. Public high school had been awesome for her. I was grateful! She had gone to public school for five years and had enjoyed the people, her studies, the extra curriculum activities, and yet never smoked, drank alcohol, tried drugs, fought with someone, nor had she even said *one* curse word. She had invited and led people to the flagpole to pray for their school and for our country every year, sometimes standing right beside her "little" brother. As CAK Alumni, they were comfortable praying anywhere. She had heard and seen all these things but she had remained true to herself, and to her Lord. In our book she was already a success in life—even if she never did another thing!

In the meantime, she continued to be the water girl (unofficially) for FHS's Varsity Basketball team. Mikey was on the team and the guys, his teammates, were so kind to her. They had always treated her like Mikey had treated her. (He and Dave had set that precedent from the start. It was obvious even years later!) She was kind to his teammates, too. She was at most of their practices, and at all of their games, and was a huge fan! She was vocal during the games and hollered out all their names as they went to the line to shoot the extra points.

Those big ol' basketball players treated her like a sister. It touched our hearts. We spent many, many happy hours in that tennis shoe-squeaking gym. (Thanks Brent Watts, Rudy Smith, Brandon

Clark, Andy Eagle, Brian Stickley, Landon Shewmake, Chris Garman, Scott Marshal, and Bryan Paylor.)

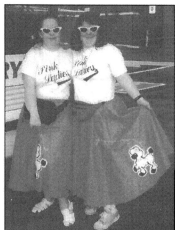

Windy with good buddy, Belinda Noonan

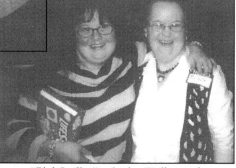

"Pink Ladies" enjoying Dollywood

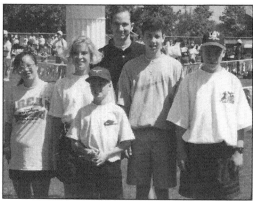

Windy with the Roberson kids

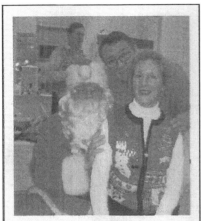

Dr. Larry & Mrs. Linda Rogers with Santa

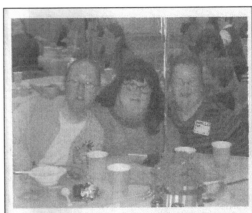

Pamela Balint, Windy Smith and Belinda Noonan were rocking away to the music of "Elvis"

With cousins
Molli and Emmalee Llar

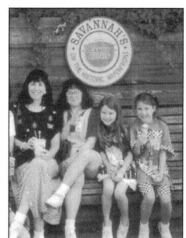

With cousins
Sarah and Lenzi Ilar

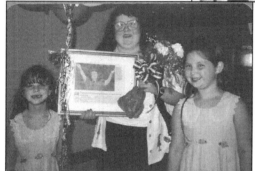

With friend Emily Goode

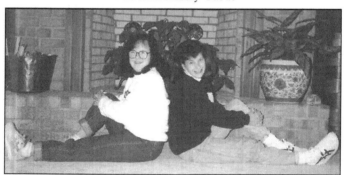

Chapter Eighteen
Nine to Five: On the Job

Windy and I were working at David's office, about a year after her graduation, when a patient stopped in. His name was Harry Call. (He was a CEO of a chain of clothing stores called Goody's. The president was Bobby Goodfriend, and the Corporate Headquarters was located in West Knoxville, not too far from our home.) David happened to ask Harry if there were any jobs Windy might do at the corporate office, maybe like delivering the mail? Harry knew of Windy, and had even heard her speak at graduation. He was very receptive to the idea, and said he would talk it over with Bobby and get back with us. A man of his word, he called back in a week and asked if Windy could come in for an interview. We were excited about the possibility of a real honest to goodness job for her!

Windy dressed up in a cute dress with matching sandals and bracelets on the day of her interview. She stood before me so I could get the full view and asked, "How do I look Mom? Like a career woman?" Then she laughed heartily. So did I, as I told her how great she looked. She was ready for the next phase of life . . . the workforce. Was I ready to let her spread her wings? For sure, but apprehensive as well. How would the other people in the workplace react to her? Would they all treat her with dignity and respect or would she be alone and lonely much of her day? We had to give it a try.

A job of her own would give her the self-worth she had been missing since she had been out of high school. She had sort of lost her identity without her own sphere of friends totally separate from her family's sphere of influence.

We walked into the large, glass entrance hall with white marble tile, went up to the receptionist's desk, and Windy asked where Mr. Call's office was. She wasn't shy about this aspect of her first day out in the work world. She *wanted* a job in this place. They went to New York and ordered stylish clothes there, didn't they? They had sample sales, too, she had heard. It was right up her alley, and she knew it.

The receptionist directed us to the elevator where we went up to Harry's second floor office. Soon we were both seated before him as he sat at a large desk in a well-appointed room. I couldn't help but think *this was a real interview for a real job*! Windy sat in the club chair, legs crossed, arms resting on the arm rests.

He asked her some pertinent questions, and she answered him with honesty. Then all of a sudden, he swung his swivel office desk-chair around and looked straight at me and said, "Vicki, for heaven's sakes, stop being so nervous. She's got the job here. I just want to see what she would really enjoy doing." He's a definite type "A", and they don't like to see someone else fidget! I had crossed my legs and was bouncing one foot, fast and furiously. I got still and sat back in my seat. His tone had made me smile and relax. He smiled back, and I let them talk. After he explained the job requirements to her and what she would be expected to do, she said she would like to start working there. She also liked the salary he offered her for a part-time job. I could tell she had really convinced him that she was ready for this job.

He stood up after a little conversation with her, shook her hand, and welcomed her to Goody's. She was on Cloud 9! She couldn't wait to tell her brothers and Dad about her new job. She was going to be in a department that distributed mail to all the departments and offices. Because she read so well, she was to hand-out mail to the respective parties. She would push a mail-cart all over the gigantic, multi-leveled building. It would be good for her to visit with all the people who worked there, and she would get great exercise because it involved walking several miles each day down those long corridors. She would probably lose weight. Or, so I thought.

Come to find out, she gained weight by celebrating with every department, for every birthday and baby shower. (Trust me, there were so many employees, that it was pretty much a sure bet there would be a celebration somewhere, on any given day.) We found out later that everyone there fell in love with her friendly manner. She could even walk into Bobby Goodfriend's or Harry's private offices to say a quick "Hi" if they weren't busy. They seemed to enjoy her little visits and would tell us about them when we ran into them at a restaurant, or out and about in town.

Windy worked at the Corporate office for six years. She liked the people. She enjoyed her freedom from mom. She was known all over that place. (David and I realized part of her purpose there was spreading good cheer. People would tell us how awesome it was to talk to her, and to see her smiling face, and how it made their day go better for having seen her!) She was treated with kindness and dignity at Goody's. Everywhere we went, we would run into someone who knew her from work. She loved that. She loved it when people yelled, "Hello" to her in a store parking lot, or stopped by to speak to her in a restaurant, or spoke to her at a movie theatre or at a concert. (This still happens years later!)

Most of the time she enjoyed work, but on an occasion she'd run into a situation. It *was* a situation the day her boss, Diane, called to ask me to come in for a talk. I told her I would come early to pick up Windy. There was a problem, I just didn't know yet what had happened.

Come to find out there *was* a problem all right, and Windy had been the one to find it to be a "big" problem. Her boss had asked her to open up some boxes that required some exertion with her hands and fingernails, to which Windy had replied, "I really can't do that sort of thing, I might break a nail." Those words hadn't gone over well with her superior.

Thus the reason I found myself sitting across from the boss and explaining, "Well, she didn't get it from me, as you can plainly see," I said as I held up my short, unpolished fingernails for her to inspect. "But, I do believe I know where she's coming from. She used to bite her nails. Did for years. Then one time she was asked to run in an opening ceremony for the AAU Junior Olympics with Gold Medal Olympic winner, the late Florence Griffith (Flo Jo) Joiner.

Flo Jo, and heavy-weight boxing champion of the world, Evander Holyfield ("Cute, with big muscles, and really nice!" were Windy's words to describe Evander.) were backstage with Windy, talking to her before the event. Windy asked if she could look at Flo Jo's nails. After telling her they looked fabulous, Windy said, "I wish I would grow my nails like that!" Flo Jo took Windy's hands in hers, and looked at her nails. (Besides being one of the fastest woman runners in the world, Flo Jo was also known for her beautiful, extremely long, colorfully painted fingernails.) She said, "Windy, honey, you shouldn't bite your nails. You let those nails grow and take care of them. I'll bet Mom will take you to get a manicure if you'll let them grow, okay?" Windy was in awe of Flo Jo. She would do as she said; I saw the look in her eyes as she looked into Flo Jo's.

I continued telling Windy's boss the "nail story." "Windy quit nail-biting from that moment. Really. She was determined to grow the longest, prettiest nails, and she has succeeded, and I *do* take her to get manicures. She is proud of her nails now. I do understand she needs to do what her boss asks her to do, but I also know why she feels she cannot risk the chance of breaking a nail. To her it would be defeating. Is there possibly a good compromise? Maybe she could open smaller packages and do some make-up work in another area?" Diane stared at me from across her desk. Here comes the part when she'll say, "We'll have to let her go," I said to myself, even braced for it.

Surprisingly, instead, she began to tell me about a boy who was born with a mental disability, who she had known when she was a child. Maybe she really wanted this job to work for Windy's sake, as well as for her own. She didn't let her go because of the nail incident. I was grateful. It had all definitely been a "nail-biting experience" for me. Probably for her boss, too!

For all the angst that interview gave me, that quote "I might break a nail!" has really given us something to laugh about through the years. Anytime any of us in our family really doesn't want to do something someone has asked us to do, we will say Windy's now infamous words. No doubt, Flo Jo would have loved it!

Something else big happened while we were in that particular desert time of our lives. That place on the timeline of our lives is somewhere after high school, and before God's big plan for her life was revealed to us. Right in that waiting period when God seemed to be so quiet, Windy made a big decision all on her own.

We had told her she could decide where she would attend church. Her high school peers had gone on to schools or jobs, and for the first time she felt left out of the loop. She felt the effects of lost friendships deeply. She had heard of a relatively new class that had been started. First Baptist Concord's Sonshine Class gave her a place she felt she could belong to comfortably. I know why she was drawn to it. She had loved the youth group at our church, but a new and growing class of young adults with special needs had been started at Concord First Baptist. She asked us if she could go to their Sunday School. A woman named Lois Walker had been instrumental in starting the class and keeping Windy up on all the things they were doing. The leaders were Steve Peak, Dr. Larry and Linda Rodgers, Norma Cuthell, Tim Blair, Becky Wyatt and Missy Fierley. (They have all gone the extra mile, for years now, to see to it that the people in the class have a higher quality of life. Norma and her husband, Robby, and their family have had several sleepovers at their house, just to host some fun time, and the girls have always had a ball.)

David and I told her it would be fine, although it would make us miss our own Sunday School class at church, but we could drop her off and still have time (barely) to go (fly) to our church's first Service, about six miles down the road. David hates to walk in late anywhere, especially to church! He didn't think we should try it. I pleaded her case saying that if she could drive, she would switch churches. It was only right that we take her and let her try it out. Windy and I assured him that it would work. If she didn't think the class was for her, she promised she'd go back to church with us. David already knew what she would decide to do. He knew she was going to enjoy her freedom from her parents, and enjoy being included in the many fun events.

For the next eight Sundays we dropped her off, drove to our church, went back to pick her up after her church's Sunday School and before their second service. We visited with friends, or bought a paper and read it in the car while we waited. It was a bit of a time sacrifice for us, but we were thrilled that she was happy worshipping there. We were always early to pick her up—and always late to our church service. Couldn't be helped.

She made many new friends. Pat, Rhonda, DeDe, Beth, Joseph, Michael F., Lisle, and Jenny B. were just some of the names we began to hear about at home. They really seemed to enjoy being together.

One particularly beautiful, sunny Sunday morning, David and I sat in the car waiting near the front door for our daughter to come out. She was always prompt. However, this Sunday she was late coming out, several minutes late, and of all things, her hair, which I had just washed and rolled that morning, was hanging wet and limp to her shoulders. I remember she spoke in an overly peppy voice, as she hopped in the backseat, "Hey, Mom! Hey, Dad! Sorry I'm a little late. Let's go!"

"Windy," I turned to face her as she put her seat belt on, "why is your hair wet? What happened? I just fixed it for you this morning?"

"Oh . . . about that!" she said, as she reached up with both hands to pat her damp hair. "I got baptized today. Brother Doug baptized me before church started." She looked steadily at me for a minute, and then at her dad. She knew full well beforehand, how this might go down with her parents. Her eyes were shinning from a glow within. She looked so grown up. All I could think of was why hadn't she told us? Wonder what everyone thought when her own parents didn't even show up for the baptismal service? *We're always there for our kids. This hurt bad!*

"Honey, you were baptized when you were twelve years-old, by Dr. Don Hoke in Fort Loudon Lake!" I said, none too calmly.

She kept a steady voice when she replied back, "But Mom, I was a child then. I'm an adult now, and it was something I *needed* to do."

David looked at me and nodded his head in agreement with her. I started crying. The shock was too much. I would have been there if she had asked me to. I would have been there for her. I've *always* been there for her. "Why didn't you tell us, Windy? *Why?*" I asked between sobs.

She answered me, now crying herself, "Because this was between me and God, Mom. Between *me* and *God!*"

I cried harder because I had to face the fact that she was right . . . it *was* between *her* and *God*. I was crushed that I hadn't been there for *her*. She had decided ahead of time not to ask us . . . so we hadn't been there at all. My heart was aching, but I had to release her, let God have her completely. He had given her to us, and now she longed to belong to Him. She always had, but because she had been born with Down syndrome, it had required more involvement and more control on my part as her parent. I know now, looking back, that it was for her sake, as well as mine, that things happened the way they did. Our Heavenly Father wanted me to learn something from this. I learned that I was not really in control or responsible for my daughter's destiny, and that God had His hand upon her life in a very unique way. Just like He does for each one of us. (Her disability was no hurdle for Him as He laid out plans for special jobs for her to do in life, one that would include helping thousands of others with disabilities—but none of us knew that on that Sunday.)

After we got home I had to recommit my trust in the Lord in this new stage of our lives. God was up to something. but it wasn't to be revealed just yet. Windy was preparing her heart for the life she wanted to lead out there in the world. She was certainly going to be ready.

Church attendance was a part of this equation. We had always attended church as a family, together. It had been a blessing to worship together, although church had been hard for us in one area. We never really had a support group or a class we felt Windy belonged in after she got to a certain age. David and I had each other, thank the good Lord, but there was no one I felt like I could go to and talk with when we went through tough times dealing with issues that came up when raising a child with a disability. Now ministries are aware of the parents and caregivers as a people group that could use some support and help. They really need the prayers and understanding, as they care for and minister to someone with a disability.

I had helped to start a Sunday School class for children with special needs at First Baptist, in Jefferson City and also at First Baptist Church in Clinton, years before, but there were not enough children to keep either of the classes open for too long. Since then Windy had attended the regular classes, youth groups, and youth choirs. (She loves to sing and even took voice lessons in high school and always knew every word, of every song.) All these things were in the past now. This new class sounded good.

As word spread about the Sonshine class, the group grew. It was rewarding to see the people flock to the class. We parents finally found a church that sought to minister to our kids, as well as, to us. Some of the parents were attending church services for the first time in years. There was such a need, and it was being fulfilled!

Our routines on Sundays were hectic, but worth the effort. David had been right . . . she loved her new church.

Chapter Nineteen
The Remarkable Missive

Speaking of Flo Jo again, Windy came away from her meeting with that famous lady with some sage advice that she passed along to someone else, who was to become a friend . . . George W. Bush. He found her advice very helpful, we were later told by his friends, Andy Card and Don Evans. Before running out onto the field at UT's Neyland Stadium before thousands gathered in the stands, Flo Jo had told Windy, "Be sure and smile," and "Just ignore the crowd and keep on running!" Great words of wisdom. Little did any of us know how those eight words would encourage a man running for President of the United States of America some years later. It's a good story all on its own.

The year Windy turned twenty-four, the whole family flew to the Hill Country of Texas to visit David's brother, J.W. and his wife, Dawn. J. W. has a 'rep' as a sort of 'call of the wild' outdoorsy man. He is one of those rare people that tall tales have been told about. Several authors have written about him in their books. He, himself, has told some amazing stories. (And, now we know he was actually being *modest* in his accounts.) He is even bigger than life *after* you meet him in person, than when you had only heard about him. For over thirty-five years he has co-owned a fishing and hunting business that guides people all over the world. (He has taken many well-known people as clients on some of those trips, including the singer/songwriter, Johnny Cash. He once gave Windy a picture of the two of them.) He has a colorful past when he "ran with some of the big boys" of Texas, including Rusty Rose of the Rangers, and many other famous, and many not so famous, personalities.

He then met and married Dawn who "settled him down so we could all enjoy his fun personality." It's always a treat to hear his "wild animal" stories. (Both sides of our families had lived in Texas for a while. My parents had always spoken fondly of the days during WWII when they lived in Seguin, Texas. David's grandparents had lived near San Antonio for a few years during the 1950s, before heading back to Tennessee. We like visiting there.)

On this wonderful family gathering we were all outside on their wide, covered veranda enjoying the lovely breeze blowing over us, making it bearable to remain outdoors on a warm evening. J.W. was telling us about his son, Steve, and his son's wife, Linda's, move to Washington state. All of us, but Windy, that is. She had slipped back inside to the air conditioned den to cool off and to check out her favorite television programs.

Midway through one of J.W.'s tales, she opened the French doors and announced to us she was voting for George Bush for President. (*What? She had been watching the news instead of her favorite shows? What was up?*) In my "Mother Knows Best" voice I told her *he* wasn't running again, that he could not run for a third term. She replied, in a somewhat exasperated tone of voice, that she was talking about "George, Jr., Mom!" I must confess that I didn't have the slightest clue who this *Junior* was. J.W. interjected that he was the Governor of Texas, but they had not heard that he was running in the next presidential election, which was many months away.

It was to become an almost prophetic statement made by Windy. No one else had heard he might run for President either! She said she liked what he said to the people in his state when she heard him giving a speech, and she thought he would make a great President. Shocked as we were, Governor George W. Bush *did* announce some months later that he was going to be running for President of the United States in the year 2000. She was interested in this presidential race, and she had her candidate.

In her enthusiasm and excitement, Windy immediately wrote Governor Bush telling him of her support. She came walking into our kitchen one day with a check and a long, hand-written letter she had composed herself. (We double checked the amount, and it was for twenty-five dollars.) She had really spent some time and energy on this. She was serious. David and I read her letter and helped her with the spelling and tweaked it as we edited it, with her input. She had the quote in there from Flo Jo, "Just ignore the crowd and keep on running." She loved that quote. It had helped her. She wanted to help him. We decided we had better get out of her way and let her do what she felt led to do. The problem was where to send it. We didn't know what address to tell her to put on it.

Turns out, we shouldn't have wasted a moment of concern over it because she took matters in her own hands. The following day she walked it over to Dick Powell's office. David had known Dick as a patient for years, but Windy and I barely knew him. We didn't know much about his family at the time. (Dick had told David about a commercial lot for sale, and we had purchased lots side by side, which had resulted in us building offices next-door to each other, built by friends of Dick's, Allan (Baldy) Houston, and Matthew Sturgill.) That's as far as Windy's knowledge of the Powell family went, up to that point in time.

She had boldly asked Dick Powell if he could send her letter off for her. Dick and she had become pretty good buddies in the last few months because she would walk over to his office to say "Hello" to him and his son, Russ, who works with him. Jan, and the rest of his staff, knew when she got bored with us at the office and would allow her to come in for a brief hello. She began teasing Dick that he knew everything, and Dick teased her back declaring that she was right! He had probably told her that, and started "that rumor", in the first place! This time she was going to test him on that.

We thought it was more than a bit odd that she would ask *him* to find an address for her letter, but in retrospect it was a Divine revelation after all. It so happened that, unbeknownst to *any* of us, he had a daughter-in-law, Dina, who had just gotten a new job working for the Republican National Committee. We had never met or heard him speak of Dina Powell. David had seen his sons and daughter at the office when they were younger, but he hadn't kept up with them since they had grown up and moved away. *We* barely knew what the RNC, or the DNC was at that time.

Windy wanting Dick involved in her letter surprised Dick, as much as the rest of us. I think he was amazed that she would bring it to him, just when his son, Rick, called to tell of his wife's new job. He knew Windy could not have known any of these facts. We still remember the perplexing look on his face when he walked back over with Windy to ask us *how* she happened to come to him for help. We could honestly say it had been her idea, and hers alone. He just stood there shaking his head. I don't think he knew quite what *to* say. He then turned to Windy, and he said he would try his best to get her letter to the right people. (He has told us that would always remain an important moment in his life.)

She was excited over his reply, and she was hoping to get back a small note and maybe, just maybe, she would get a picture of Governor Bush. (She is really into pictures. She downloads them on her phone. She posts them on bulletin boards, makes elaborate collages, and puts them in albums.)

For eight months, literally, almost daily during the work-week, she came to the office directly from her job at Goody's, and went through the stack of mail, looking for a reply. Then she asked Dick if he had heard anything, and she kept praying for Governor Bush and his wife and family. She had just about given up hope of ever receiving an answer back. Finally, instead of a message by post, out of the clear blue she got a phone call at our office, from a member of the Republican National Convention Committee.

(We now call her letter the "Remarkable Missive"! The one that catapulted her into the position of being able to help millions of people who have a disability.) We couldn't believe it when Darlene Gartman, David's receptionist, and our long-time friend, told Windy someone on the phone wished to speak with her and "her parents" and to, "Pick up on line one!" Windy picked up the phone in the kitchen, with me standing with my ear next to hers, so I wouldn't miss a word, and David listened-in on a phone in one of his exam rooms. After Windy said her initial hello, we listened together as the lady on the other end began to explain the reason for the call.

She said, "Governor Bush *had* received her letter." Windy grinned at this and nodded her head in a "Yes", and she gave a "thumbs up" motion to me! She continued on, "He had read it and been encouraged by it, all while he was in the middle of the political race. He loved the letter and passed it on to his close friend, Don Evans, who had passed it on to the head of the RNC, Ed Gillespie and Andy Card, another friend and advisor!" (We didn't recognize these names at the time, but Windy was to get to know them soon.) She continued, "They had all read Windy's letter, and when it was read aloud to a roomful of people, including Governor Bush, they had been so touched by it. Her open and candid words and heartfelt encouragement had made them shed a tear or two, and they wanted her to read her letter aloud at the Convention in August, in Philadelphia. Would she consider doing that?"

In surprise and shock, David asked the person on the line to please hold while we explained the situation to Windy, before she gave an answer. *We had assumed Windy might get a form letter and a photo back, if anything at all. Now they were asking her to speak? This was wild!* We really had no idea how big a thing this was.

David hurriedly came in to talk to Windy, face to face. We had her hold the phone away from her mouth, so the lady couldn't hear our conversation as we explained to her, who the person represented on the phone, and what they were asking her to do. We explained to the best of our knowledge, and believe me, it was very limited knowledge on our part . . . we didn't recognize any of the names, but George Bush's.

We privately asked Windy if she would, could, wanted, to speak in front of so many people about her letter, and she quickly replied, "Sure! Why not? All that crowd won't bother me. I spoke at my graduation in front of a lot of people, and I liked it!" We both explained that there would be *many* more people at this event than there had been at graduation, and that there would be more cameras and reporters than any of us had ever seen in one place.

We asked again, "Are you certain you will be all right speaking at something this big and with so many looking at you, listening to you?" She looked us right in the eyes and solemnly and quietly, yet confidently answered, "I'm sure!" She held the phone back up to her ear and spoke without any hesitation, "Sure, I'd love to do it!" to coin another Windy phrase. They were elated with her affirmative answer, and said they would soon be back in touch with the details.

I have to admit I was very, *very* torn. I was excited for her, very excited, and yet, fearful for her safety with the exposure to the world out there. I had spent a good part of my lifetime, and her *entire* lifetime, shielding her, protecting her. This was bigger than I could control. With much prayer, I began to realize that God was again asking me to trust Him as He led us down a path I had not imagined nor planned for her. I was afraid, so afraid that I trembled when I thought of her being in front of all those cameras. Why was God asking her to do something like this *now,* after I had worked so hard to make her life safe and normal as possible? We were finally in a place in our lives where everyone knew her and loved her and accepted her as an equal. Society, at least where we lived our lives every day, was accepting and kind to her. Would this be something that would put her out there with strangers, who might not be as kind and nice to her? I would love to say that I knew God's will immediately and embraced the idea like Windy had, and that I had the courage instantly to face her future in an arena that I had not ever imagined for her.

These kinds of decisions for our children are so much harder for a parent of a child born with a disability. We fight for years for their rights in education and place in society, and then when we are faced with something we did not coordinate or anticipate, well, honestly it's very difficult for us to relinquish control. God put us in charge of this child with special needs in the first place. We have to be their protector and provider, and to guide them in life. I felt He had put me in situations throughout her life, and *now* He wanted me to let her *go,* and let her go in front of the *entire* world? It was almost more than my emotions could take.

John Wood, who was now the head pastor at our home church, and Doug Sager, the pastor of the church Windy was attending, spoke with us as we sought God's wisdom. They imparted deep insight to us, and helped us to understand that this was between Windy and God now. If she chose to do what she felt He wanted her to do, we needed to allow her to go do it. Dr. Sager and Pastor Wood prayed with us and with Windy. (They prayed with her more than once. She had other people, who were important prayer warriors in her life at the time: Pastor Vern and Nancy Holstead, and David and Linda Ackerson.)

Windy saw this invitation as having the opportunity to help get a man elected that she knew to be a morale man—and a man that had qualities she thought a leader should have, especially a leader of the United States of America. She has always loved the fact that everyone, who is registered to vote can cast a vote. She truly wanted to help people. It *was* her decision, she was now an adult with a job to do. I had been raised to go vote and to keep my choice of candidates to myself or within my immediate family. My grandparents and parents had been registered Democrats *and* Republicans, David's too, and sometimes in the same household! We had learned to keep our voting private. Now there would be no more privacy, it would be everybody's business. At least for *this* election.

The day before we were to leave for the RNC, Windy and I turned the car radio on as we drove to work, and we tuned in to hear one of our favorite ministers, Chuck Swindoll, who was speaking on Jonah. He told how we must push past our fears and follow God. Windy looked straight ahead, but nodded her head and said, in a low voice, "Yes!", and she smiled a tiny smile. God was still using Jonah to help people, even in the year 2000. We were driving on Kingston Pike, but the signs were leading us to Philadelphia and beyond. Way beyond!

>I wish I could wisely say that following the Lord gets easier with time, and yet, I cannot. I trust Him fully, I do, but I do not *fully* trust myself. I know I sometimes vacillate between my will and His. I prayed and read the Bible for confirmation. I listened on the radio, and on CDs, to some pastors that David and I are always blessed by.

The GOP committee called back and gave us directions, flight numbers, and a date in August, 2000 to be in Philadelphia, Pennsylvania.

We packed, and asked our families and church pastors to continue to pray. Finally it was the day to go to the airport. On the way we stopped at our local *Chick-fil-A* to get a quick bite to eat. Windy and I ordered a kid's meal. We found a table and went to sit down with our tray of food. We said Grace and began to divide up our meals. Windy smiled, and said, "Look, Mom, God's talking to you again!" as she pointed to our kids' meal. On the bag, in living color, was a Bible story. It was the story of Jonah! I am not kidding! I nodded my head, yes, in acknowledgement to her. I got it.

Okay God, thanks for another sign. I really do get it. Forgive my unbelief, and from this moment on I will embrace everything on this trip that you have for us to experience. I'm out of my comfort zone again, but I WILL try really hard not to fear!

We were flying back home from a trip a few months before, and had a layover in the Nashville airport. Windy was looking at a magazine in the magazine rack when she looked up to see Senator Alexander standing close by. They said, "Hello" to each other, and then he recognized her as she shook his hand. (Who can forget Windy?) He looked tired, as he had been out on the road working to get the nomination of his party, for the chance to run for the Presidency. Support for George W. was coming on strong . . . the contest was almost over. Windy told Lamar, Goodbye, and we went to catch our plane.

Windy tugged on my sleeve and said, "Mom, I feel really sorry."

"For what, Baby?" I was clueless.

"Well, you know, for pulling for Governor Bush. I do want him to win, but I'm sorry I can't vote for Lamar, too."

That was so sweet, and so typical of her, to feel for the man who had been the governor of our state, someone she remembered as being friendly and kind to her and to her family. David had tried to help her with her sadness. She seemed consoled for a while, but we were to learn it was not a closed subject for her.

Several weeks later someone told us that Lamar and Honey Alexander were to be at Farragut High School for a political function. From the moment she heard about their upcoming visit, Windy asked me to take her by on the day he was to be there.

"We'll see," is all I could promise her. But, I did wind up taking the time to drive her over to her old school.

As we pulled into the parking lot, she spotted them speaking to some people on the sidewalk. She got out, closed her car door, looked their way, and walked over to stand in the line to say the something she had come to say. I hung back but I stayed close enough to hear her. I was very curious. I knew she might not tell me on the drive home, and I wanted to know why she had been so determined to seek him out.

When she got up to him, she shook his hand, and said, "I'm so glad to see you. You are a good man. I have something else to tell you, I'm sorry." That was all. He had other people in line to speak to him by then, and he probably had no clue, as to why she would apologize to him. Then again, maybe he did. She hadn't campaigned for him, and yet she wanted to let him know, face to face, that she meant no personal harm to him. She had just tried to do the right thing for the country at the time. I don't know if anyone else knew what she had said and done. I do know she smiled a smile of relief and almost skipped to the car. She had done the right thing, and her heart was no longer burdened. I looked over at her as we drove out past the school's work-out gym at the back of the building, and onto Campbell Station Road. Then I told her how proud I was of her.

Now I knew how she had worried over hurting someone's feelings . . . even if he had been a Governor. She had known him in the past. He was from her home state. Yet she had supported someone else for the job. Our daughter is a woman of character. She had had the guts to act upon her concern because she felt like she had let someone down. Even if they probably didn't know. She knew. She has taught us invaluable life lessons on how to live our own lives. This was a huge **WINDY'S LIFE LESSON**.

Now her conscience was clear and she was ready to go to Philly! We had an unbelievable time there. It was our first trip to that city, and we loved visiting. Our plane ride from Knoxville was exciting. Mikey flew with Windy and me. He was going to be our escort until David could fly up the night before her speech. When we walked out into the airport, we spotted a man holding a big sign with Windy's name on it—just like Windy had been told to look for. The man introduced himself as Mike, and said that he would be our driver for the next four days. (As we got to know him, we were so impressed with his manners and kindness to Windy.) He took us to our hotel—in a beautiful, large old building. Mike led us to the front desk, and he was given two keys for the room held in Windy's name. Then he took us to the room, with our luggage, and said he would be back to pick us up that evening.

He was giving us time to settle in. He suggested we go back downstairs to watch the activity in the lobby, that it might be fun for Windy to do a little people-watching, and that he would pick the three of us up at a designated time to take us to the place where the Convention was being held: in the Arena that the Philadelphia '76ers pro basketball team called home court. Mikey was very excited over this aspect of the visit. His love for the game of basketball was legendary back home in his old alma mater, Farragut High School. (He used to fall asleep reading about the famous LSU, and professional basketball player, Pete Maravich. He couldn't wait to see the arena, and to see where the movie character, Rocky, played by Sylvester Stalone, had run up the steep steps as he was training for the fight of his life.)

I couldn't wait either, because from a mother's perspective, a mother of a child with a disability, we were in the same city depicted in that movie, with our own "event of a lifetime" about to take place. I could almost hear the trumpets in the theme song from the movie as we headed down in the elevator.

She was ready to speak to millions because she had first learned to *listen* to God. She was faithful in prayer and in her daily life, and we believe He was honoring her faithfulness and allowing her to speak on behalf of all the people in America, and on behalf of all those who had a disability, in every country of the world, to prove their lives mattered too! She was also a Champion, and not afraid— just like Rocky. Good thing, because she was about to enter a "huge ring".

We found the people of the city of Philadelphia to be friendly as we wandered through the Market in the downtown area across from the hotel. (We heard they had had a major cleanup, spiff-up campaign that took several months before this Convention came to town. The results showed!) We finally got to eat our first original

Philly steak sandwiches. We ate one every day while we were there. They were scrumptious.

Seeing the cracked Liberty Bell later, on a quick sightseeing side-trip, was very moving, and it reminded us of why we were all there in the first place, because we had the freedom to vote the way we saw fit. We were also just as adamant for those who chose to vote the opposite way because America, after all, stands for liberty and justice for *all*. We were awed by the sheer magnitude of what Windy had been asked to do—she was the first person with an intellectual disability *ever* to speak at a GOP convention, and they had put her at such a key spot in the program. *She* was to be a *keynote speaker*!

Headed back down to the hotel lobby, the three of us looked out at the incredible sights before us when the doors of the elevator opened. There were people everywhere. Some were carrying in luggage and laptops. Many were on the phone, and some were busy speaking with each other. Reporters were all around the lobby, trailed by their camera crews holding onto large cables as they ran around the room in pursuit of someone to interview before their deadline, at the various media places they worked for. It was then that we realized that we were staying in the same hotel where many familiar faces from the nightly news were also staying. Political leaders, Stateswomen and Statesmen from across the nation were filing by. It was like being in a movie. Concerned over all the commotion around us, I began to wonder if Windy was beginning to feel overwhelmed. Just as I was leaning over to ask how she was, she elbowed her brother, who was raptly watching everything and everyone right along with her, and said, rather loudly, "Isn't this great fun, Mikey?" I looked at her face. She was smiling big. That answered *that*!

Time seemed to fly by and soon it was time to go back up to the room and get ready for our first night out. Mikey stayed to enjoy the "people watching" and we girls went to heat up the hot curlers and lay out our clothes for the night. Windy loves to shop for new clothes, and she had a wonderful time picking out the outfits we took with us. The only trouble was, we didn't know what one was to wear to something like we were going to. The ladies who worked at Steinmart, where we ended up, were really sweet to Windy as we tried on many items. (They didn't know the magnitude of the task she was headed to do in Philadelphia, and I wonder, if we had told them the story, if they would have believed us anyway. It was pretty unbelievable to *us*!) They had wonderful suggestions as we went through the usual trying on, and weeding out, until we came up with the best outfits. It was important to Windy to look her best.

Many clothes were tried on and vetoed by the both of us. Finally, near the end of both of our patience and stamina, success came. She picked out a cute little bright red suit consisting of a jacket and a skirt. It fit her to a 'T' and would look so nice with her new black glasses, which she hadn't worn yet by the way. She loved her old red ones. She would not part with them, nor could we talk her into wearing them, even for short periods. She always said she was "saving" them, just to keep us off her back. Remember 'pick and chose the battles', we kept telling ourselves, as all good parents tend to do, so as not to be disagreeable about *everything* coming and going. When the time was right, or when the old glasses broke (which usually had to occur before she would try a new pair of glasses), she would have to wear them and adjust to the change. Always she ended up liking the new ones better, but NOT until *she* was ready. Okay?

Her words as a little bitty girl still bring us laughs when her Dad changed her glasses prescription for the first time, and we had picked out a darling little pair of pink glasses. Windy consented to try them on, and to walk in them across our rough, hilly front yard, where she promptly tripped and fell. She stood up, and yanked those glasses off, tossed them into the dirt, and said rather sharply, "I can't see! Do you want me to get killed?" With that being said she stomped to the front door, noisily opened and shut it behind her, leaving us out in the yard with the offending spectacles. It took several days of coaxing and bribes by Dave and us before she would try them on again.

Finally, after leaving them on *and* sitting still in one place (no more of that walking about on rough terrain with 'new eyes'), she realized the improvement in her vision and left them on, only taking them off at night, where she placed them ever so gently, on her bedside table. It is always so with a prescription and eyeglass change. (Hey, maybe the *only* change she has not embraced with gusto!) We persisted on her wearing them, but allowed her to adjust at her own rate. After all it was her eyes and her life, and we were gently reminded of this fact by her, and we respected that.

This time we were confident that at the proper time for Windy to wear the new glasses to look stylish on national television, she would do it. She was older now, wiser. That being settled, we now we had another little problem: shoes. We had to find a pair of black high heels, not too high, so she could walk without tripping, up on that stage, and they had to look grown up, not childish, yet in her small shoe size. That would take another miracle, just a tiny one though (well, two tiny ones), and not life changing! Just life challenging. We were used to that.

(Jama, Mikey's mother-in-law, made Windy a beautiful, colorful scrapbook of all the pictures of her trips to Philly and D.C., and it is still amazing for us to look through it and see all the famous people Windy has met and talked with. Only God could have orchestrated all of this in her life. She has been such a blessing to so many people, and she has been blessed by so many people. Finding these words, in Proverbs 11:25, confirmed to me, David, and our sons this very thing, *"Whoever brings blessing will be enriched, and one who waters will himself be watered."* Another one of **WINDY'S LIFE LESSONS** for everyone reading this. Go out and bless others!

Nighttime came, and we three—Windy, Mikey, and I—went down to the foyer of our hotel where we were to meet our driver, Mike.

Recognizable faces were everywhere. We rode down in the elevator with several Senators and Governors. At the hotel entrance, we stood with well-known people as we waited for Mike to pull his car to the door. Mike got there, got out, and opened the door for Windy to get in the back seat. I got in on the other side. Mikey took the passenger seat up front, and we were off.

Mike told us some interesting facts of history of the city as we made our way to the Stadium where the Convention was being held. When we came to the check-in point, we stopped to give the police guard our names, and he checked us off the list, and we drove slowly forward until another group of police asked us to stop and for Mike to open the hood and trunk of the car. Police bomb-detecting dogs smelled under and around the entire car, and under the hood, and in the trunk. When everything was double-checked, we were allowed to move forward.

We pulled up to another check point where we disembarked, and Windy and I placed our purses on the table to be checked while we walked one-at-a-time through the metal detector gate. When we got the okay to proceed, we gathered our purses and papers, and walked down the sidewalk to the front doors of the Stadium. (This was pre-9-11, and we had never been through such a thorough inspection. After 9-11 it was even more intense. We have now accompanied Windy to many places where guards have been armed with visible machine guns, or heavy weaponry on a few occasions. We never imagined this in her future, either!) We were aware of potential danger in a large event with so many important people present from our government, and we were grateful for the enormous presence of security everywhere we looked: on foot, on horseback, on motorcycle, and in patrol cars. It was very reassuring.

About this time I was so busy taking note of all the security, that I bumped into the man standing in front of us, and I hurriedly apologized to him. I heard a friendly answer, "That's all right!" coming from the person I had just bumped. I was surprised when I looked over at Mikey. "Mom," he whispered, "Look *up*! Don't look down. That was Newt Gingrich you just ran into. There go the newscasters from NBC News. Look up, and you will see people you'll recognize. For instance, that's Fred Thompson from Tennessee right behind us, and just behind him is that TV star Windy likes to watch, and his wife." I took a good look around and decided that was wonderful advice from my son. I held onto Windy's arm and asked her how *she* was doing, and she said, "Great!" She was. No intimidation for this little lady. She behaved as though she rubbed shoulders with people like this every day. The wonderful thing is, that for her that was the truth, every person there was on a level playing ground to Windy. No one is ever better or more famous, nor deserved more special treatment than anyone else she knows or interacts with.

We walked into the large arena. We had never attended a political convention, of *any* size, much less on this grand a scale. The Republican and Democrat conventions in the United States are, to politicians, and those interested in the politics of our nation, something like the Super Bowl, except it's celebrated and played out every four years instead of yearly. And here *we* were. It's as if we had never been to a single football game in our lives, and now we were on the fifty yard-line, at the biggest pro football game of the year, with the most famous players suited up for the game of their lives. (Please forgive us, all you who are politicians, or citizens who are very politically savvy, but it is the comparison we feel best describes the scene for us, the common voters, who had faithfully gone to the polls to vote, but had never been to anything of this magnitude.) We had seen these functions only on TV, and then mostly just snippets.

Honestly, we had previously found it a bit boring to hear all the speeches, definitely not riveting enough to keep us glued to the television screen for several consecutive nights. We stand corrected! In real life, it was truly amazing! The atmosphere was charged with electricity one could feel, an intensity so exhilarating. The masses of people, the extraordinary display of patriotic colors everywhere your eyes wandered, the passionate words of the speakers on the massive stage, mingled with the loud continuous conversations on the expansive floor. We found it arresting and highly contagious! It was almost impossible to be in attendance and not clap or whistle or stomp your feet as people stood on the mammoth stage and addressed the ever-talking, ever-moving, teeming crowd on the multi-leveled floors of the coliseum. The show was on stage in front of us, as well as on the floor, all around us. Those of us in the stands were meeting and greeting and talking state and national topics of interest . . . exercising freedom of speech in a big way.

Soon Mike was walking us to the escalators. Up we went to our seats, we assumed. At the top floor, we followed him to where we were to be in a skybox, he told us. Well, okay, now I wouldn't have to worry about Windy being able to see everything. It was going to be a bird's eye view for her. We looked in a small room, next to the door we were to go in, when Windy patted me on the arm, "Look Mom, Larry King is getting his makeup on for his show!" she said under her breath, so he couldn't hear her. Believe me, we were close enough for him to hear! At just this time, a tall, lean distinguished gentleman in his early fifties, and his attractive wife, began walking towards us. With hand extended, he introduced himself to Windy first, and then to me, and then to Mikey. He told us his name was Don Evans, and he introduced us to his wife, Susie. He then got down on one knee in order to be on eye-level with Windy, as he took both her hands in his larger ones—all this, amidst the moving crowd, that he seemed oblivious to. Susie leaned in to look into Windy's eyes, and to hear what her husband was saying. Mikey and I also moved closer, so we wouldn't miss a word of what was spoken between them.

Don told Windy how honored he was that she had consented to speak to the nation. He told her how pleased he was to meet her in person, and how much he admired her commitment to come and speak up for his friend, George W. Bush. He said they were old buddies and they had both been in the room when Windy's letter had been read aloud for the first time to about twelve or so people. When the person reading her letter came to the end, he said, "There wasn't a dry eye in the room". He continued, "Windy, your letter made all of us cry, and it touched our hearts. I think it will touch the nation's heart when you read it to them. Susie and I will be praying for you. We have a daughter, who was born with a mental disability, and she can't do the things that God has blessed you to do. I love you honey, and Susie and I are proud of you!"

With that said, Don hugged Windy, and she hugged him back. Then Susie hugged her. Don stood back up to shake my hand and said, "Thank you!" with his eyes brimming with tears. I choked back tears as I said, "Thank You!", with the deepest appreciation I could muster. He squeezed my hand in both of his, and then he and Susie turned to go on down the hallway. What a tender memorable moment that was, and one that none of us will ever forget. We later discovered he was one of the people instrumental in having Windy come to speak. (Andy Card and Ed Gillespie were two other men who had cast their votes for her to speak, we found out that night when she met them.)

(Don later became the Secretary of Commerce in George W.'s Presidential Cabinet, and he also became a friend to Windy. She would see him again in the years to come at the White House where he showed her around his office, and to her delight, he showed her a picture of him and George W. in their basketball uniforms when they were in high school together. I believe she giggled.)

There were so many moments and sights that we will never forget from that Philadelphia trip. One great moment was when we saw hundreds of police motorcycles lined up as they circled the building we were in, with an officer standing at attention beside each cycle. They were there on duty to protect all the former Presidents of the United States of America, and the current President, who were all present at one time, in one place, in that very building where we were. We were to be in the very same room with them, within the hour! The officers' stateliness and complete command of their job, and of the situation, was stunning.

Entering the large private skybox was a once in a lifetime experience. We followed Windy, as she followed the people assigned to get her to the right place. We had no idea we would be in a skybox. The head of the RNC, Ed Gillespie, and his wife stopped by to say hello and to visit with everyone in the room each night. Don and Susie came by for several visits. We got to meet Dina Habib Powell and her husband, Rick, who were there along with Dina's father-in-law, Dick, and his wife, Docia.

For the first hour we were really overwhelmed by the parade of people who came into that skybox. Politicians, movie and TV stars, singers and entertainers paraded in and out to talk and eat from a buffet table over at the side of the room. All were familiar to the Smiths (us) only because we had seen them all on the TV screen back home. The more we looked at the sea of people before us, the more Windy and I began to feel the enormity of it all. She and I went to "our" private bathroom to catch our breath. We had found a bathroom to the side of the big room, that hardly anyone ever used. Maybe no one else knew it was there in a back corner. The two of us escaped for a few moments every night to pray, reapply lipstick, and find the strength "to go out there and face the crowd." This was big. We knew it would be, but did we know it would be THIS big? Not really.

That first night we said a prayer and asked for His strength to see us through. We went back out, with shoulders erect, heads up (My mama had taught me some good advice, "Never let them see you sweat." I had passed it on to Windy. Now we were going to test this family maxim to the nth degree, in this environment!), and we walked to the edge of the room that looks out over all the goings-on on the floor below. All the fifty states and the U.S. territories were represented. All the delegates seemed to be speaking at once. The jumbo screens surrounded each wall, with every known news agency there to report to the world the process of America's Democracy in action. Politically it was like being in Williamsburg in the 1700's, only on steroids! Our founding fathers would never have believed how this dream of theirs—this republic thing—had grown so BIG!

I slide onto a sofa, next to the wall, and closed my eyes to the crowd, below and all around us. *"God this is so overwhelming! Did we hear You right in all this? It's so scary to think that in two days our Windy will be up on that stage speaking. Please God, please reaffirm to me real fast if this is really Your will for her life. Forgive my wavering confidence and for asking for a sign. If You would please give me a sign, any indication, that You want her here, we will follow You in all we do. Forgive me for even asking, but I'm scared for her.*

Truly, before I could say, "Amen," I heard a masculine voice from a few feet away, above my bowed head, say with glee in his voice, "Windy! What in the world are *you* doing here?" I opened my eyes in astonishment to see Dean Rice hugging Windy. Dean had gone to school with Windy and her brothers at CAK. He had played soccer with her brother, Dave. It was in Dean's parent's yard, on Fort Loudon Lake, that Windy and Mikey were baptized. This was **not** a chance meeting. None of us had any idea that Dean was working in D.C. We hadn't seen him in years. Our appearance there surprised him as much as his appearance had surprised us.

I quickly told him that Windy was to speak on the next to the last night of the Convention. He was amazed and delighted and told her how proud he was of her, a former classmate! I told him *he* was an answer to my most recent, (*very* recent), prayer, and I knew God had sent him at just that moment to reaffirm to me, her mother, that she was to stay and do what she had come to do. He told her he was so glad she was speaking, and that if God had brought her this far, He was not going to let anything get in the way of her Divine duty—

not even her own mom's nerves! He patted me on the back and said it was all going to be fine. I believed him. His presence was a reaffirmation that we were where God wanted her to be. Dean told us that he was in D.C. working at the Faith Based Initiative Office. I asked him to pray for Windy, and for all of us, and he did, quickly and quietly, and he promised to pray all that week. He told Windy that his entire office would be holding her up in prayer.

Oh, Boy! I felt like a burden had been lifted. With God's help we *would* persevere. (Back home we had several people praying. Besides our family and Windy's friends, she had others praying: Dr. David and Linda Ackerson, Pastor Doug Sager and his wife, Faye, and their secretary, Melinda Burnett, and Pastor John Wood. Darlene Gartman, Norma Cuthell, Susan Iglehart, and Paulette Neely were praying for her at our office. We could feel their prayers. Years before, other ladies worked with us, and prayed for her, as she grew up, and we are so grateful for their friendships: Betty Foster, Jan Nash and Felicia Gaddy and Debbie Bunch. Now in these later years other special friends and prayer warriors that we have had the pleasure of working with are: Amy Mynatt, Dru Ellis, and Abby Lance. They have all done so many nice things for her. There is no such thing as too many people to pray for you or to love you. Windy has coveted their prayers. So have we.)

The second day of the convention, Mikey, Windy and I met our driver in the lobby of the hotel, and he took us to the Center to practice Windy's talk and to let her get familiar with the stage and microphones, while the stadium was mostly empty. Our car always had to be stopped and the bomb-detector canine made an investigative inspection, I.D.'s were double checked, and lists were looked at to be sure we were going where we said we were going. After arriving at the stadium, we three were led down a long hall to a door that was labeled *Speech Writers*. We knocked, and a pleasant, middle-aged lady answered the door. She introduced herself to

Windy, and then to us. She told Windy she was there to help her make her talk the very best it could be. She was a former special education teacher and a speech therapist, she told her. She came with high credentials and experience.

She had Windy stand before a podium in the front of the room. She had Windy's letter on an overhead projector behind Windy's head, and she had a copy for her to hold and read. (We couldn't say this teacher didn't come prepared.) She asked her to begin reading aloud. Windy began to read, but very slowly and deliberately, and in a *really* quiet voice. It was most painful to listen to her speak. Mikey and I squirmed in our metal chairs seated before her. We knew her, we knew she was terribly uncomfortable having to perform on-call. The woman asked me if she always read that slowly, if that was her normal speed. I replied that she could read faster, but that she was not too comfortable in this setting. I also told her that she did read slowly, but this was really slower than her natural reading aloud speed.

The former teacher, under much stress and honestly quite exasperated after two or three reads, said Windy would never get finished with her talk at this rate. She also said my daughter had only so much time blocked off for this televised event, and she was way over the minutes they had given her. I agreed, "We will have to cut out some of her letter and condense it down to the main points."

I got up and looked for a pen in my heavy, over-stuffed purse, ready for anything any of us might possibly need on a trip. Finding one, I walked up to stand beside Windy. I asked to see the paper in her hand, and I had her look at it with me as I began cutting and editing the content. I asked her if she felt uncomfortable saying aloud certain words or sentences. She was definite in her honest answers back to me. Mikey gave his suggestions, and he asked Windy about several key points. He had taken mental notes of where she seemed to hesitate too long over a word or stumble over one. (Now I'm not implying we know everything there is to know about special education, but we *do* know our Windy. Our family has adapted and adjusted many things so Windy can learn. It's just second nature to us now, and we don't even stop to think about it, we just start right in throwing out ideas to her that she might comprehend and adjust to easier. We know what she usually can, and cannot do, and what she usually will, and will not do.)

Mikey and I started instructing and guiding her to help her feel at ease and confident with her talk. To begin with, I took a look at the spacing and size of the print on the written pages on the podium before her. "If you don't mind, this needs to be changed, please. One big problem slowing her down is that she is having trouble reading this fine print. It needs to be larger print, preferable all capital letters, and double spaced, so she can look up at the audience, and the words don't all run together when she glances back down." We looked out into the room behind us surprised to find that the back of the room was now full of strangers, people on the Committee responsible for asking her to speak.

They had quietly entered the door in the back of the room to listen to the girl who had written *the* letter. So engrossed at out task before us, Mike and I had been in our own little world and hadn't seen the standing audience. She had though. I realized I shouldn't have been surprised. They were probably a bit nervous too. They had asked someone, who had a disability, to speak at a major event for the country and on live TV. It was a big first, and maybe a risk. They didn't know her or know what the outcome would be. It was a gutsy move by all involved.

All of a sudden someone who had been in the back stepped up, grabbed the papers from me, and said they would be right back with the corrected pages. Then, Mikey walked up and pulled the microphone down to place it closer to her mouth. A man walked up and asked me if we felt comfortable helping Windy. They had been observing the three of us and felt sure that we had a handle on the situation. They were considerate, and did not want to wear Windy out or have her become frighten or upset. They didn't want her to feel pushed or uncomfortable. I think her quiet voice had made them rethink this "special speaker spot" on the program schedule. It might not work out like they had envisioned.

Mikey and I looked at each other and smiled. This is what we had both been hoping for the last hour—a chance to help her. I turned and faced those in the room and said, "I have been adjusting things for twenty-six years so Windy could learn to do things. We appreciate any help or suggestions you have for her, but because we know her, know the ways she learns quicker, we probably are the people who could help her more than anyone else in this situation."

From that moment on *we* were in charge of helping her, and the woman they had brought in to help her was there if we needed her help. She quickly affirmed that Windy was responding better to her mom and brother, than to a stranger. She was there for Windy and wanted what was best for her. She stuck close to us in case she could help.

The papers were brought back with corrections made, and we began to cut and paste where needed. More corrections were made, and finally we had a copy we three felt good about. Windy was much more confident. Mikey and I stopped fidgeting. The talk was sounding like a real interesting presentation, even to us. People walked in and out of the room continually. Windy now ignored the distractions and kept plugging away at her task at hand. Mikey and I would turn to look at them occasionally. The revolving audience came in, listened a minute, smiled, nodded in confirmation to each other, and walked back out. They were beginning to hear a young woman put her touch to her talk, and they evidently liked what they heard.

After about an hour, someone came in and asked Windy if she was ready to try out the actual stage. It was freed-up for the time being they told her, explaining that it was a rare moment that no politician or entertainer was scheduled for practice on the stage with the mics and lights for the next hour. She looked up at them and said, "Sure! I think I'm ready!" She gathered up the pages of her talk. She was more than ready to be out of that smaller, stuffy room. We could tell she hadn't bargained for all this preparatory stuff!

Off we went, following half a dozen people up the wide stairs to the gigantic stage set up on the main floor. The walk up was fun for her. She stopped and met many people walking the hallways. The people with us introduced her, and us, to many people she had seen only on television. She met and had her picture made in the hallway on the way up with several people, and later on, with many more including: "The Rock" Dwayne Johnson, Tennessee Senator and Mrs. Bill Frist, Allen Simpson, Wyoming Governor Jim Geringer and his wife, Fred Thompson, Bo Derek, and J.C. Watts, to name a few. They even took her to look in the locker room of the 76ers. She really liked seeing where the team got ready to play ball, and where they went to rest up during halftime. She said she would like to be there when they played a real game. She loved the team colors and liked the jerseys and tennis shoes. Mikey didn't mind getting the chance to go in with her one bit! After her fun and relaxing tour, we followed her to the main stage area.

She didn't hesitate when they asked her to walk up the big steps, stage right. She looked so small up there with all those "big" people walking around on the stage before us. (By big I mean that in two ways: first "big" as in everyone up there was much taller in stature than she was. Windy is only four feet and ten inches tall. Secondly, I mean "big" in the political, news network personalities, and entertainment arenas.)

Only a few people in that room knew who Windy was, or why she was standing up there at the microphone. Mikey and I took a seat in two of the thousands of empty seats, a few rows back, so we could see her face, and so she could see ours. Mics were lowered and tested. Someone asked Windy to start reading her letter aloud. She was obedient, but still reading in a *very* slow, quiet voice. People were straining to hear her and to understand her words. Mikey whispered and asked me if it were possible for her words to be shown above her head as she read the letter out loud, so her audience could follow her words with more clarity. (There were already jumbo screens in place on the walls behind her.) "Ask them, Mom!" *Great idea, brother!* I looked back and could see people positioned in different sections shaking their heads, "No," telling the sound system people that they could not hear her. So, I stood up at my seat and asked those on stage with her if it was a possibility to have her words visible for the audience.

The women and men on the stage with her put their heads together in a quick discussion. Then they turned to Mikey and me and said it was a great idea, and they would have it by the next day's final practice run. Windy was asked several times to start over and to speak up as the sound system was retested and readjusted. Each time she began over, she spoke in her small sweet voice as she pronounced each word slowly and deliberately. We knew she was really trying hard to do just as they asked, but we also knew she was feeling a tremendous amount of pressure.

I was wondering if she was getting cold feet over the whole thing. Maybe it was just her reaction to all the attention, and to all the pressure to read as if this were the real thing. She wouldn't do that. Windy was not into faking anything.

I suddenly realized that was it! She felt like it was faking to read aloud, with feeling, when it was just a practice run. We had seen her do the same thing when she went over her gymnastic routines in preparation for her participation in the 1987 International Special Olympics at Notre Dame. She had gone over her floor and ribbon routine probably hundreds of times, but had never performed like she did, with pomp and enthusiasm, when she competed as an American against people from seventy-four other countries.

It was as if God had specifically reminded me of that moment as she stood up on the winners box and bent her head forward so they could place her medals over her head, and then she stood back flashing a huge smile to all of us watching her. Practice was, and had always been for her, just that—practice. If her heart was still in this, and Mikey and I would have to be sure for her sake that she still wanted to do this, then we had no doubt that she would do her best at the right moment. Windy always gives her best to what she believes is right and just. Would we have really "walked" if she had decided not to do this? Are you kidding? We would have gone home in a second. We felt being asked to speak was a great honor, but Windy's well-being was way more important to us. Now we had to discover if her heart was still in all this.

> *Please, Lord, help us to find out her heart in this. We don't want to make her too uncomfortable and scared, neither do we want her to feel like she has to give her talk now because we have come this far.*

We had to make sure she understood we were with her no matter what she decided to do now. No matter what that decision entailed. We took a needed lunch break. Being so close to Reading Terminal Market, we walked over to get some sunshine and exercise, and to order a Philly steak and cheese. A break from work always makes everything look brighter when you return!

Revived again, we three took a deep breath for the first time that morning. Mikey looked right into his sister's eyes, from where he sat across the table from her, and asked her if she was still okay giving her talk. "You gotta tell me, Win. Level with me here. Are you okay with all this?"

"Yes, I am Mikey!" she said with a little disgust, implying "why would you question my commitment?"

"OK, just checking. I want you to feel good about this. You don't have to do it if you have changed your mind. Mom and Dad won't be mad at you. I won't be mad at you. It's okay. Just tell us, and we'll have a good visit up here, and then we'll go home. No big deal."

I supportively chimed in with the words, "The reason your brother is asking you is because you are speaking really, really quiet honey, and it may be hard for people to hear you. Can you speak a little louder? You want people to be able to hear you, don't you? Think how Hillary Duff would just speak out loud for her TV show character, Lizzie McGuire?" I tried to encourage her by using her favorite star of the moment. Hilary was all over the Disney channel at that time, and Windy really liked her.

She rolled her eyes and put one elbow on the table, and put her opposite hand to her forehead, and said, "I *will* Mom. When it's *time*. I want to do this thing."

"Great, that's all we're asking," I told her. We knew her well. She meant what she said. No mincing of words for this woman. Come game time, she would make it happen. This was only practice, and she was saving most of her emotions and ability for the big night.

The trouble was, those in charge did not know Windy, or her personality, and so Mikey and I both saw the glances between the support people when we three went back after lunch to practice again. They were probably more than a *bit* skeptical. This was the first time someone with an intellectual disability had spoken before such a huge, televised live audience. I felt like I needed to say something to them that was reassuringly positive.

After our discussion with Windy, Mikey and I felt confident that she would be able to handle this, that she still wanted the opportunity to speak. I stood beside her as we were getting ready to leave for the day, putting my hand out to steady her as she walked down the steep stage steps. I then turned and faced the people who had been there with her all day, encouraging her and instructing her on where she would stand and where she would walk in. Everyone had been very kind to her and most respectful. They hadn't talked down to her, or discussed things with us. They had directed all conversation to her, as was only right—they had treated her as an equal. Mikey and I were very touched by that. They had worked long hours and given so much, they needed to hear something positive.

"Don't worry," I said, "if she says she'll speak up when her time comes, then she will. She knows this is only practice, and she reserves her biggest and best for the real thing." I smiled. They smiled back. Windy smiled. She's pleased with her mom's assessment. We saw how they watched for Windy's reaction to what I had just said. They took note of her smile, and of her nod in agreement. All of a sudden, we saw them all look more relieved than they had looked all day.

Please, God, give Windy strength and discernment to speak up at the exact time she needs to. And please, send Guardian angels to watch over her. I can't be standing beside her up there when she goes on. I don't even think I could if they asked me to. But You are with her, with her every step and word, because Your Word promises that. Thank you so much for her willingness to do this. Thank you for Windy. What a courageous woman she is! What a strong woman of faith! What an example of how we should stand before You . . . quietly trusting You for everything. Amen.

The Remarkable Missive

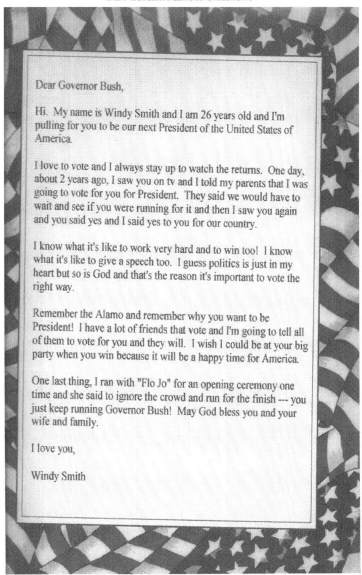

Dear Governor Bush,

Hi. My name is Windy Smith and I am 26 years old and I'm pulling for you to be our next President of the United States of America.

I love to vote and I always stay up to watch the returns. One day, about 2 years ago, I saw you on tv and I told my parents that I was going to vote for you for President. They said we would have to wait and see if you were running for it and then I saw you again and you said yes and I said yes to you for our country.

I know what it's like to work very hard and to win too! I know what it's like to give a speech too. I guess politics is just in my heart but so is God and that's the reason it's important to vote the right way.

Remember the Alamo and remember why you want to be President! I have a lot of friends that vote and I'm going to tell all of them to vote for you and they will. I wish I could be at your big party when you win because it will be a happy time for America.

One last thing, I ran with "Flo Jo" for an opening ceremony one time and she said to ignore the crowd and run for the finish --- you just keep running Governor Bush! May God bless you and your wife and family.

I love you,

Windy Smith

A TX Governor's Reply Back

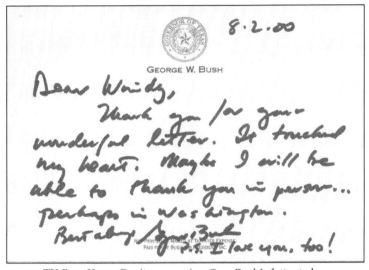

TX Rep. Henry Bonita presenting Gov. Bush's letter to her

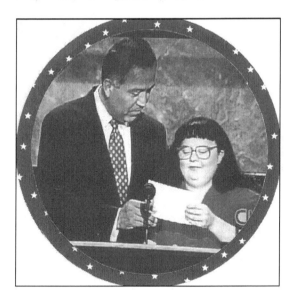

Windy is the tiny speck on stage

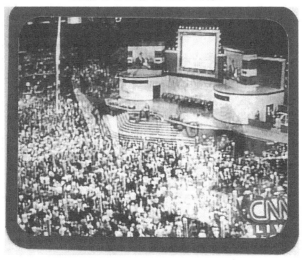

Attendees at the RNC

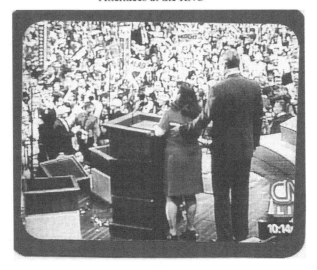

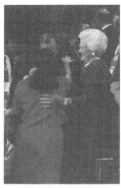

Windy and President
G. H. W. Bush

Meeting the TX Governor

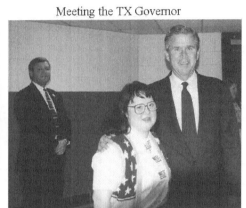

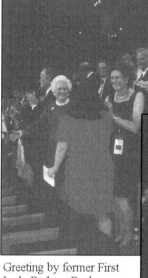

Greeting by former First
Lady Barbara Bush

Our seats with the
Bush family

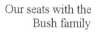

A letter back from Gov. Bush

GEORGE W. BUSH

July 7, 2000

Miss Windy Smith

Dear Windy,

Thank you for your thoughtful letter and your contribution to my campaign. Laura and I are honored to have your support.

As a silver medalist gymnast, you understand the unique challenges and sacrifices of competition. So your advice about focusing on the finish means a lot to me. I will remember it in the coming months. And I will remember my new friend from Tennessee.

You're right about our states' close ties. Tennessee gave Texas some legendary heroes like Davy Crockett and Sam Houston. And all Texas ever gave Tennessee was the Houston Oilers. Not exactly an even trade.

I can tell from your words that you not only have a good heart, but also good sense. You know what really matters most in life: faith, family and friends.

Laura and I are grateful to have you on our team.

Sincerely,

George W. Bush

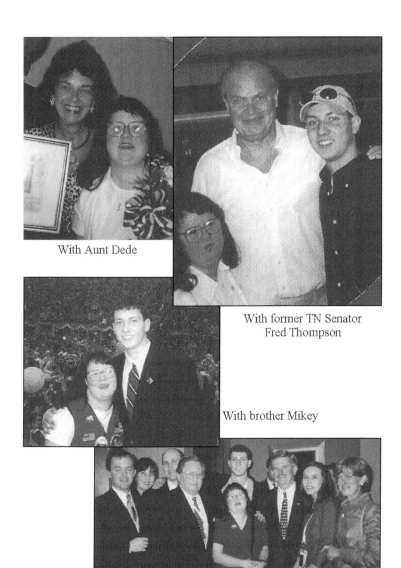

With Aunt Dede

With former TN Senator Fred Thompson

With brother Mikey

Ed Gillespie and his wife, and Dina, Rick, and Dick Powell

Chapter Twenty
The Speech of a Life Time

The BIG night finally came for our family. It was the night before the nomination of George W. Bush for the Republican candidate for the President of the United States of America. Windy was to speak just before the nomination and introduction of Dick Cheney. Her dad flew in and was ready to escort us. His flight had gotten in very late, and we had already gone on to bed. Forgetting about telling him the minor detail of our room number, we slept peacefully away. He arrived in the hotel lobby with no info of our whereabouts, and the staff, rightfully so, gave out no information to someone claiming to be looking for his daughter's room at 2:00 in the morning. Someone that knew about Windy, and had a room close to ours, happened to be walking by the front desk at just that moment! He overheard David's plight, and out of kindness walked him to our door. A grateful David, shook his hand and thanked him. Then he knocked quietly on our door. (Grateful, because the man had saved him from a fitful night's sleep in a chair in the lobby!)

We girls started getting ready early in the afternoon for the night ahead of us. We did our hair and nails and makeup. It always takes me awhile to fix both of us up. When Windy was finally ready, she walked out of the bathroom, and Mikey and her dad whistled and told her how beautiful she looked. She grinned. She had on that cute red suit we had bought. I had pinned a sparkling red, white, and blue pin on one lapel. It was a pin a lady had given her to wear, a gift from a new friend back home. (A kind stranger had insisted she take it as a gift when Windy had admired it!) Black heels, in a children's size three, had been hard to find, and we were thrilled when at long last Target had the perfect style and the perfect fit. She had on the *new*, stylish black glasses. Her outfit was complete. She looked darling!

We hopped on the elevator and said hello to Bob and Elizabeth Dole, who were already in there, on their way to the ground floor. Windy smiled at them, and they were kind enough to allow us to take her picture with them when we all got to the lobby. We went to the front door of the hotel where people were lined up to get into the cars to take them to the event. We got into our car, and Mike, our volunteer driver, shut Windy's door and went around to the driver's side and got in. We already had the feeling that this night was going to be vastly different from any night we had ever experienced in our lifetime. We looked at Windy, and she was taking it all in stride. She was absolutely savoring every detail of the evening.

When we arrived at the skybox, Dick Powell told her how beautiful she looked and that he was so proud of her. She beamed a big smile and hugged him. (He and his wife were there as guests of their daughter-in-law's. Windy thought it was pretty cool that he was there. She has always loved Dick from the moment she met him. They had a rapport. He always teased her about her always wearing the color pink.)

Two young women came by to take Windy backstage for 'make-up' they said. She loved the fact that they were going to redo her look for television just like she had seen the newscasters there that week getting their make-up to be camera ready. She had seen most of the leading reporters from all the major networks as we walked around on the news media level, on the two previous nights. Before she took off, I told her again how nice her new smaller black glasses looked on her, very stylish, I assured her with a warm smile. She heard me, but made no outward indication that she had. I knew very well she had heard my compliment. Unbeknownst to her (*or so I thought*) I had hidden her older red frames with the older style big lenses in my purse. Just in case her new ones fell off and broke or something, she would have a back-up pair.

We all kissed her and wished her well. I hugged her one last time, and whispered in her ear that we would be praying the *whole* time for her. "Thanks, Mom, I love you!" she said. Then she bravely walked off down the big hall, never looking back. True grit if we had ever seen it! A few minutes later someone came to escort us to seats on the floor level, so we could see and hear Windy better when it was her turn to go on.

"This is it Daddy! From the day we heard the words, 'She will probably never talk or walk,' . . . to this? Isn't God good?" I said in his left ear.

"Oh yeah!" he said, as he swallowed back big tears. It was the climax of all those years of love and sacrifice, and tears of deep pain, and of joy unspeakable. We, as her parents, couldn't have been more proud of her if she had been the person running for President. There was such an air of "unrealness" to all of it.

Then suddenly, reality brought me back to earth. I was tapped on the shoulder by a volunteer floor runner. "Mrs. Smith, Windy is feeling a little dizzy, and we need her old eyeglasses. She said you had them in your purse. I'm sorry, but we need them in a big hurry, please!" I obediently opened my purse and felt for the old red glasses. I grabbed them and held them out to her. She took them from me, said a thank you, and quickly walked away.

Well, Windy, you won that contest. You got your old glasses back, AND I couldn't say one word! You go girl. Now knock a home run with this thing you've come to do, and we get to go home!

We sat listening to the speakers, and I was astonished that it was sometimes hard to hear because so many conversations were going on down on the floor, all around the entire building, at any given time. Well, okay, if this is how it is at one of these things, so be it. If Windy did mess up, or mispronounce a word, who would hear her? At least there was some consolation in that fact. It seemed sort of rude to me that people talked and politicked right over the speakers on stage, but we had never attended a Convention before, and from the looks and sounds of it from our main floor vantage point, it was standard behavior. So maybe that was an advantage, not a negative?

Finally! The big moment was here. Windy's name was announced on the main stage, and she was being escorted out onto the stage from behind a large curtain, by Texas Representative Henry Bonita. The music, "Windy," written by the musical group, The Association, *her* song, was being played loudly and lively, by the live orchestra as they presented her to the Floor. No one had told us that would be her "stepping out" music. She held to his proffered arm and walked out with aplomb and confidence. She looked as if she had walked out before thousands every night, and this was just another night. (Docia, Dick's wife, said afterwards to us, "that she looked as poised and confident as Nancy Reagan walking onto that huge stage!") And, she *did,* yet with dignity and humility!

Poised and smiling at Rep. Bonita and then at the audience, she stood waiting while Henry Bonita gave an introduction of her and her letter written to the then Governor of Texas. He then said, "Every week Governor Bush receives thousands of letters from supporters all across America. But one letter in particular, that came eight months ago from a young lady with Down syndrome, from Knoxville, Tennessee, stood out. Please welcome Miss Windy Smith to share some of her letter with us tonight."

To my surprise *and* fear, the room that had vibrated *every* night with a thousand voices, all at once became *totally* and *utterly* quiet. My mother's fear was so palpable that I was afraid everyone around us could see me begin to shake in my seat. David sat transfixed on our daughter up there on that huge stage before us. I must have been shaking only on the inside, I guess, because he didn't even glance my way. I grabbed his arm and held on tight, much like I do every time we take off on a plane ride together. This was going to be the ride of our lives. I felt his bicep tense up under my grip as an acknowledgement that he was right there with me in this. He *always* has been, bless him!

All of a sudden it was show time. Windy stood alone at the podium, cleared her throat and raised her small right hand to pat her throat, for a brief second. (We knew it to be a slight sign of fear and hesitation, the very first we had seen. We held our breath, as if we were trying to give her our own breath to use—willing her our strength. And then in a split second, we prayed again for God to fill her with **His** strength. And also . . . for Him to get the glory. Not her. Not us. Him.) We watched as she nodded slightly, crooking her head and dipping her chin, affirming her readiness to do this thing she had come to do. She looked down at the letter in front of her.

She hit the ground running. She began to speak to the thousands present, and to about thirty-eight million people watching on the televised newscasts. She read her letter, the one she wrote to George W. Bush months ago. She had written it for his eyes only, but she was willing to share it with all of America in order to help make the world a better place. She had referenced the Alamo as a link to the strong friendship and allies Tennesseans had been to Texans in the past. She had been to San Antonio, visited the Alamo. She wished for Governor Bush to know she was a person from Tennessee, who would stand up for him and for the country.

We looked around us and *all* of the crowd, on the floor, in the balconies and sky boxes were watching her in stunning rapt attention. They were evidently so touched by her sweet voice and heart-felt words, that many, many people had tears coursing down their cheeks unchecked. It was such a rare moment: her pure heart was so evident, probably *very* rare for any kind of political rally, especially for a Convention of this magnitude, to see such a pure heart: no agenda on the mind, wanting only what was best for others, and totaling forgetting self. People didn't know any other way to react, except to cry at her presentation.

I had DC Talk's song, "*I Took a Dive,*" playing the whole time in the background of my mind. She was definitely taking a dive, and so were we.

When Windy read her last word, she looked out at the people, and then so like her spontaneous nature, she said into the mic, "I love you all!" Then she threw a kiss to the crowd with both hands, and threw her arms up, palms facing the crowd before her, with a big beautiful smile on her face. She had never rehearsed that action or told us she was going to do it. Her smile let us know that she knew she had done a great job. Sure enough, she did what she had come to do when it came down to the wire.

When she finished, she was given a standing ovation, for several long minutes camera flashes were going off to capture the moment. Her attitude was infectious, the entire stadium rose quickly to their feet in a long, loud, standing ovation. (Several newspaper writers and news commentators said her ovation rivaled the Vice-Presidential nominee's, given after her talk that night!) People were crying unashamedly, as they clapped and clapped for the pretty, little dark-haired lady.

David and I will never, *ever*, forget the feeling we had that night for as long as we live. It was the most amazing thing that had ever happened to us. We learned afterwards that we had *both* felt it in *exactly* the same way. It was miraculous. It was really just as if time actually stood completely still, and the past and the present were combined into one time zone! We felt like God was holding Windy, and us, gathered up to Him. The only sound we could hear (strange as it sounds, because of the deafening noise, it was to us as if there was complete silence and out of that silence was an almost audible voice saying, *This is why you needed to follow Me in faith at Windy's birth. . . . because your daughter was meant to do great and wonderful things for others, and only time could reveal these things.*)

Be still and know that I am God, had never been more potent in our lives than at that moment! She had walked and talked and lived a faithful and productive life—despite a disability—to show the world that people with disabilities are really more like them, than not. They have hopes and dreams and opinions, and are just as vital to our society as anyone else. As I stated in the introduction, they teach us more about ourselves. The way we treat them and love them and care for them enriches us and teaches us patience, perseverance and character. She showed the world that it *was* possible to triumphantly overcome obstacles and great odds.

Henry Bonita walked back up to hug Windy and stand beside her. The noise from the floor was still quite deafening and showed no sign of ceasing. Henry put up a hand to hush the crowd. Finally, quiet prevailed again as everyone strained to hear, interested in what he had to say. He then said to her, "Windy, I have a surprise for you." (No one had said anything to her or us about this. We were as curious as everyone else.) "The Governor personally read your letter, and he gave me a handwritten note that he asked me to pass along to you." She politely said, "Thank you" and stood still while he began to read it aloud to her.

>Dear Windy,
>Thank you for your wonderful letter. It touched my heart. Maybe I will be able to thank you in person . . . perhaps in Washington.

Best always,
George W. Bush
P.S. I love you, too!

Wow! The crowd went wild for a second time, and Windy stood before them smiling and looking happy. Rep. Bonita handed her the note, and they walked off the stage together.

After Windy left the stage, they announced the candidate for Vice President, Dick Cheney, and he was about to come out to give his speech. We sat up straighter in our seats. All of a sudden, someone tapped me on the shoulder, and asked, "Mrs. Smith would you and Dr. Smith and Michael like to go over and sit with the Bush Family? Windy has already joined them and is waiting for you there." *Really? Well, if you insist!* I was thinking with merriment. "Sure, we'd love to!" we said quickly, and matter of factly, as if we received invitations of this caliber *all* the time. We got up and followed her up the aisle, out the doors, to where Windy was now seated.

Wonders never cease, we soon learned. She was sitting right next to Barbara Bush and the former President George Herbert Walker Bush, and *all* of their family: Jeb, Marvin, Neil, sister Dora Koch and their spouses and children. J.C. Watts walked up and shook everyone's hand and sat down with us! (We are still not prepared for the surprises we get when we follow Windy around, even today!) We shook hands as Windy introduced us as her parents and brother, and then she ignored us completely, as she and Mrs. Bush whispered and laughed over shared funny stories and accounts of the day. I felt like she was acting much like the Queen of England would have behaved in a similar situation. And I mean *Windy* as the Queen, for she had acknowledged our presence with a consolatory nod of her head in our direction, and then had dismissed us for more entertaining company.

We stole a few glances at Windy while she was listening to Dick Chaney give his acceptance speech. She sat stately and upright, with her hands folded in her lap, feet crossed at the ankles, listening with rapt attention to the man on the stage. My goodness! She had become such a grownup. We were very proud!

No nerves showing, no regrets. Looking ahead to the future with hope and determination. That's Windy, and that's another **WINDY LIFE LESSON** for all of us!

In the end, it was all about a young adult born with a disability who was given a chance to have her voice heard in America, on a grand scale, for the very first time. She was a pioneer for those who needed to be represented as full-fledged citizens!

Windy wanted to call her brother Dave, first thing after she left the building with us. She smiled as he answered on the other end. She said, "Well, what did you think, Dave? Did I do okay?" We heard her laugh her little low giggle. Dave was shouting out all kinds of accolades to his little sis. He was so proud, and frankly, in awe of her. All his life, except for the sixteen little months he was an only child, he had loved her, prayed for her, stood up for her to their peers, protected her. Now he, too, was realizing, more than ever, that she was her own person. They sent love and kisses over the phone to each other, and then she called her grandparents. The Smiths were just as proud of her as the rest of us. Papaw and Nannie had watched her speak on television from their home, and Nannie told her they couldn't wait to give her a big hug and that she had been praying the whole entire time for her.

She then dialed up Gaymom and Poppie, who were as ecstatic as everyone else. They laughed with glee, and said they had prayed for her *and* for all of us. Dianne's entire family had crowded into their den over at their house. Windy's cousins all did a shout out to

Windy, as Poppie held the phone up in the air, on speaker phone. Windy smiled a wide smile. She could just see them in her mind's eye in that cozy room with the dark-green painted walls, the shelves loaded down with beautiful things Gaymom had collected through the years, and all the familiar faces of her family members.

We heard her say, with an excited tenderness, "Thanks for praying, I *knew* you were! That's why I could talk to everybody out there! I love you all! I'll see you soon!" Windy pressed the end key and handed the phone back to her dad. She could not hide the loving glow in her sparkling brown eyes that was a direct result of true love for her family, and knowing assuredly she was truly loved back!

After it was all over, we got back into the car and drove back to the hotel. When we got there, we got out of the car and our driver Mike came around to let Windy out. He opened the door for her, and she stepped out and hugged him and thanked him for his help. He instantly gave her a big bear hug back and said, "Windy, it is I who thanks *you*! You did a fantastic job tonight, and the entire country thanks you!"

We walk into the front door of the hotel, and even though it's really late, we went into the restaurant to eat a bite. We had promised Windy practically all day, we would eat, and we had only had time to nibble on a snack here or there. We walked through the room and noticed the CNN channel was on several televisions hanging on the walls. Windy was on the screen speaking in a news clip.

Soon everyone in the crowded restaurant began to look over at her, and then they rose to their feet and clapped for her! Regardless of their politics, they were touched by her ability to speak to such a large audience, as a Keynote speaker at a national political convention. She was humbled and felt so honored at their response, and she smiled shyly at the attention. We were so very touched ourselves. We knew again that we were in the company of someone who had done a great feat. She no longer belonged just to us, her family and friends, but to our country. She shouldered the responsibility with great dignity and grace. All her life we had spent protecting her and looking out for her, and on this night we had shared her with the world, and the world *is a better place because of it.*

We ordered and ate, but only barely, because people actually stood in line to speak with her and to get her autograph. She graciously spoke to each person and gave out tons of hugs and signatures. It was truly a night none of us would ever forget!

She finally got to sleep in the wee hours of the morning. I stayed awake until I heard her slow rhythmic breathing. It was as if I could not rest until I knew our girl was finally getting the rest she so desperately needed. Ah, rest and sleep, and right before I closed my eyes to fall asleep myself, Mikey, using his key to open our hotel room door, called out softly, "Dad. Mom." He couldn't wait to show us the headlines for the new day.

He had been down hanging out in the lobby where all the reporters and the very-late-to-bed crowd hung out. (To his delight, while eating a late dessert, he had gotten the chance to speak with Ben Stein, and have a picture taken with him.) Computers were not readily available at the time. We didn't all carry around laptops or have smart phones and thus, instant news. So it was still fascinating to us all that he could have the page headlines for tomorrow's paper, printed from the Internet, before the actual papers hit the stands.

There in our Knoxville paper dated Thursday, August 3, 2000, was a large color photograph of Windy, along with an article about their hometown girl. It told how she had spoken to an unusually quiet audience, "so quiet you could have heard a pin drop" as one reporter on national television had reported. (Very, *very* quiet, especially for a Political National Convention!) It told how she had captivated them with her presence, presentation and honesty. There she was with her arms lifted up to all the people with a beautiful smile on her beautiful face. The caption below the picture read, "*Windy Smith of Farragut, who addressed the delegates of the Republican National Convention on Wednesday night, blows a kiss to the audience after speaking. Smith wrote a letter to Bush explaining why she would vote for him and sent him twenty-five dollars. He later invited her to read the letter in Philadelphia.*"

"You're not going to believe this . . . She's in nearly every newspaper in the country this morning!" Mike exclaimed with fierce pride for his big sister. Our hearts were deeply touched at the obvious love he had for her. He looked over at his sleeping sister and shook his head in astonishment, saying in a whisper, "Isn't God good? And, isn't my sister *something*?"

Long ago we had worried *so* much about how having a sister with a disability would affect our other children. Well, here was an answer to that: our sons loved and cared for other people, and they had real concern for people with any disability. Dave and Mikey both had become men of character and responsibility. David and I were *just* as proud of the two of them as we were of Windy. We were so grateful for them, and way beyond tired. We were asleep before Mikey turned off the light.

Following is the article about her talk, written by Tom Humphrey from News Sentinel Bureau:
    Philadelphia

Windy Smith of Farragut sent George W. Bush 25 dollars and wrote him a letter, saying she liked him even better than that "nice" Lamar Alexander, who knew her name.

Bush "loved the letter," a spokeswoman said, and surprised Smith, who has Down syndrome, by inviting her to read the letter to the Republican National Convention. The daughter of Dr. and Mrs. David Smith, Windy is a 1996 graduate of Farragut High School and once served as a Poster child for The Association of Retarded Citizens (Now known as The Arc, one of the first to do away with the "R" word!). Smith, who read portions of her letter Wednesday to the packed auditorium, concluded by wishing Bush good luck. "May God bless you and your wife and family," she said.

Smith then waved to the crowd as the audience gave a standing ovation.

Rep. Henry Bonita, R-Texas, presented Smith with a handwritten note from Bush thanking her for her letter.

She started out her letter to him by saying:

Dear Governor Bush,

Hi. My name is Windy Smith, and I am 26 years old, and I'm pulling for you to be our next President of the United States of America. I love to vote and I always stay up to watch the returns.

One day about two years ago I saw you on T.V. and I told my parents that I was going to vote for you for President. They told me we would have to see if you were going to run for it, and then I saw you again and you said, 'yes' and I said 'yes' to you for our country. I know what it's like to work very hard and to win. [Referencing her Special Olympic competitions.] I know what it's like to give a speech too. [Referencing her high school graduation.] I guess politics [Meaning to her: Public service.] is just in my heart, but so is God, and that's the reason it's important to vote the right way.

Remember the Alamo [Meaning to her: The long, close relationship between Tennesseans and Texans She has friends from Mexico, too!] and remember why you want to be President. I have a lot of friends that vote, and I am going to tell all of them to vote for you, and they will. I wish I could be at your big party when you win because it will be a happy time for America.

One last thing, I ran with 'Flo Jo' for an opening ceremony one time, and she said to ignore the crowd and run for the finish. You just keep running Governor Bush! May God bless you and your wife and family.

I love you,
Windy Smith

Her postscript was something like:
P.S. I am sending you twenty-five dollars from my own paycheck for your campaign.

We have all of these letters and newspaper articles and many, many more put away in albums and boxes. *All* of the words "Down syndrome" have been rubbed out carefully and methodically with a black, permanent marker. Windy had gone through every article, read each one over, word by word, and had taken it upon herself to wipe out all evidence of the term she felt unnecessarily descriptive of her. It was premeditated, too . . . she had bought her own marker at the office supply store while I was shopping for David's office supplies. It was touching and *so* telling.

What a **WINDY LIFE LESSON**! Bottom line: Keep attempting to do great things, and ignore any disability others may try to label you with! *Way to go Windy! We learn invaluable lessons from you every day!*

We slept in for an hour or so longer than usual the day after Windy spoke. We probably could have slept another couple of hours, but "duty called." We took our time doing our hair and makeup again, so the guys went down to breakfast before us. It wasn't too long until we followed them down to the cafe, and it began to dawn anew just how big of a deal her talk had been. People from all over this nation would stop us and ask to have their picture made with Windy, and they wanted to hug her and shake her hand. Moms and dads told her, and us, about their daughter, or son, who had also had Down syndrome or some other disability. People came up and told her stories of their brother or sister or niece or nephew who had a disability. Teachers and educators came streaming by all day, wherever we went, and asked for a picture of Windy to put up in their school or classrooms to encourage their students—all of their students in the regular classes or in the Special Ed classes.

It was the same on the streets of Philly, in the Market Place where we attempted to eat lunch (We didn't care if we missed a meal, the stories of the people were so incredible we wanted to hear them all!) and at the exhibit where we went to see the historic display of the American Revolutionary flags, and the fashionable attire on display that was worn by some of the earlier First Ladies. (Windy especially liked those.)

Each person had a touching story to relate about their family, and as they spoke the love that radiated from them to Windy, and from Windy to them, was astonishing! It was energizing to all of us! Talk about a ministry! She listened and shed tears many times, really moved to tears, because of some of the things they told her. Some stories were joyful, some were sad. She has so much compassion for others. She feels so deeply, and can visualize the children and people as they told her about them. Her hugs and sweet, heartfelt comments sent each person off with a lighter, brighter heart!

Many, many people asked her about Governor Bush. "Was he *really* a nice man? Was he as kind in person as they had heard he was? Was his faith real?" These questions were asked of Windy, and of us *hundreds* of times. We read the pulse of the nation during that Presidential election year, *everyone* was curious to know if the man behind the name was a sincerely good man. Would he do what he said he would do? Our country needed a sincerely good man to lead us.

Windy always answered, "He is a really *nice* man. So are his wife and family. He will be a *great* President!"

"OK, Windy, we're trusting you in this, so we're going to vote for him for President!" were the very words we heard time and again.

"Oh, Great!" she would reply with enthusiasm and gratitude.

We were amazed at everyone's passion to find someone who could become our next President. They looked to Windy to give them the insight they needed before making up their minds on a candidate. People felt the need to state the fact that they were Democrats or Republicans, or Independents. Some even said they had never voted before in a national election, but they promised her they would now. She was enjoying speaking to them all so much, but I saw her getting tired before she voiced it to me. I saw her shift her weight from foot to foot, and I realized her new shoes were hurting her feet like mine were. We had to go upstairs and kick off our shoes and rest for a while.

We began to steer her out the door so we could let her recoup before another big night, the night the vote was taken from all of the states represented for a candidate for the next Presidential race in the year 2000. She was a virtual stranger to them, yet since she had revealed her thoughts and heart to them in her talk, they felt as if they knew her, could trust her word. It was so gratifying and uplifting to witness the multitude of people asking someone who had been born with a disability to help give *them* more clarity and knowledge on a subject they felt she knew more about than they did.

She did know more at the time. She had been with many of his family members, his closest friends and top advisors for several days now. They had been with her many times backstage or to a private group gathering. Knowing about the people closest to someone can give you a clearer understanding of the person in question. She already had a good indication of who the man behind the name really was. She gladly shared what she knew without any embellishment. The rest of us were all more than curious.

Talking to people all day was taking its toll on her stamina. David and Mikey had also seen signs that she was getting exhausted. Protectively they stepped up and flanked her left and right side, and began to escort her towards a doorway. David took her left elbow to direct her out when a young man, in his twenties, came up quickly to stand before her, and he said, "Windy I am very proud of you for standing up for what you believe and for trying to help our country." As he spoke, he presented her with a patriotic necklace with little flags that lit up. She smiled, and thanked him.

Then he looked directly at her dad, then at her brother, and then at me, and said, somewhat nervously, "I don't know Governor Bush, and I don't know the people backing him, but I hope that they are really sincere. I hope they don't just use her and forget about her after all this is over. That's when we'll know if they are really good people, if they don't forget Windy months from now! I want to think he cares about what happens to her, and if he does—then I'm going to vote for him!" With that said, he turned away quickly and was gone. It was a bit startling but we had heard the same sentiment more than once that day, the part about people hoping they weren't just using Windy to get a tear-jerk reaction from people. They wanted to know they truly cared about her.

On the last night of the convention, the biggest night for all for National Conventions, the nominee for the Presidency speaks to the Party who elected him or her, and to the whole world as it watches on television. We were almost headed out the door of our hotel room, ready to go to the Comcast First Union Center for this big night, when David's cell phone rang, and we heard him say, "Oh, I'm sure she would be honored. Tell me when and where you want us to bring her." He had all of our attention now. Windy stood by her dad and looked at him quizzically. She knew the phone call was concerning her. He held up his pointer finger, indicating he would tell us in a second. We were completely silent, but anxiously awaiting his explanation. After a brief conversation he hung up and turned to look at Windy.

"Windy, how would you like to meet George W. Bush tonight? He has asked if you would join him on stage tonight after he speaks."

"Really, Dad? I would *love* to meet him. Sure I'll go. I don't mind going back up on stage! She turned to me, and before I could ask any questions, she stated, "Mom, I'll be fine! *Don*'t panic!"

She turned to her brother and said, "Mikey, you go with me as my bodyguard. I want you with me tonight." She turned to look in the mirror hanging on the wall behind her, for a last quick glance to check on her appearance, then grabbed her pocketbook, slipped the shoulder strap over her arm and turned to leave. We three obediently followed her out the door. This was beginning to be a habit . . . following her to places we'd never been before. We could tell, she liked it lots! (Flashbacks of her leading us on those hiking trails in the Smokies came rushing back to my mind. This girl had been training for this moment for years! And we thought *we* had taken her hiking to teach *her* something!)

We found out later that the GOP had received an overwhelmingly large, positive response and feedback about the young woman who spoke about her support for George W. They informed the man running for President of this. After hearing it, George W. had requested to meet this amazing woman. She had been a fan of his . . . and now he had become a fan of Windy's!

We soon arrived at our destination, after security check points had been done. Dina greeted us cheerfully, but briefly, telling us she needed to whisk Windy off to "makeup". Did our daughter love that she was going to get made up for television again? That's a big affirmative! Before she went, Windy hugged us bye, and softly said, "Don't worry about me, just pray for me, please!"

"Oh, Windy! We will be praying the *whole* time! We love you!" Words a mom couldn't have meant more. I loved her so much, and I was in awe of her strong faith and bravery in pressure situations—the likes of which she had never seen before! We let her go knowing she was in good hands, in God's hands, first and foremost, and then, in her "little" brother's. Windy had turned to Dina and requested, in a very determined tone I might add, that she hoped her brother Mike could go with her. (*Wow, authoritative and decisive. Had we overdone the independent training? Nope! Win was using it at the right time, and in the right place. She wanted the support and company of her sibling. She made a proper plea, and it was affirmed immediately.*)

Off the two of them went, somewhere in the recesses of the backstage, and David and I were left to be as surprised as the rest of the crowd as to when, and how, Windy would be back on stage on this important night of the Convention. They took a camera with them, and the pictures are amazing! Windy is in a picture with so many people she met backstage. There is Windy—in a white shirt with embroidered American flags running down the front tab, wearing a red, white and blue cotton knit sweater vest over it and a skirt—smiling away with many well-known people in the political and entertainment circles.

The two of us were led to fantastic seats on the ground floor again, and we sat back and took a look around us. The air was electric with excitement. The majority of people were dressed in red, white and blue apparel, milling around everywhere, stopping to talk with old friends, or making new ones right on the spot. It seemed as if no one was staying in their seats as they switched places and walked the aisles continually. Political leaders, Statesmen, and Stateswomen, thousands of average Americans that cared about their country, and news reporters from around the world were mingling together. Some were there to make some news, some were there to report the events and news, yet most were there to watch, weigh the evidence of what they had come to see and hear, and report back to their respective states so everyone could make educated decisions on who, and what, to vote for in the coming elections.

The lengthy votes from the states were finally counted, and announced. Each state had a representative who was chosen to stand up, microphone poised, to present the distinct accolades of their state before giving the final vote count. The results were blasted over the gigantic speakers hanging all over the stadium: Texas Governor George W. Bush had received the most votes for the nomination to be the Republicans choice to run for the Presidency in 2000 from the delegates. (Talk about shouting it from the roof tops! This was from the rafters too!) A roar from the crowd grew louder until it seemed *every* person in the room was shouting, "George W.! George W.! George W.!" in unison. The noise was deafening. All present were now up on their feet, clapping with glee, and stomping their feet. It was a sight to see!

After several *long* minutes of this, we began hearing faint strains of music being played by the orchestra. Then, the noise from the crowd turned up several notches. (Didn't think that was a possibility, but we were proved wrong!) George W. Bush was officially introduced to the thousands present, and to the approximately 40 million viewers via televised newscasts. He stood smiling and looked truly grateful for the accolades.

It took a long time, but quiet again reigned, and he began to speak of his hopes and dreams for America, and for his goal to become the 43rd President of the United States of America. He really seemed sincere and focused.

After he spoke, he asked his wife, Laura Bush, and his two daughters, Jenna and Barbara, to join him on stage. Then Dick Cheney, and his wife, Lynn, joined them. The applause was stunningly vibrant and louder each time the group on stage grew. Then his parents, Former President George H.W. Bush and Barbara Bush, joined him, and another wave of applause began. Next, George W.'s brothers and sisters, and sisters-in-law, and brothers-in-law, accompanied by their children, came on stage to surround him. Dick Cheney's two daughters joined their dad and mom. More shouts and whistles and clapping emitted. All the speakers from all the nights of the Convention came out: Condoleezza Rice, Elaine Chow, Henry Bonita, 'The Rock' and many others walked out to join in the celebration.

And *then*, David and I zeroed in on Windy, with Mikey right by her side. We watched as if it were all taking place in a movie. Suddenly we saw our kids being ushered to the front, and right next to President-Elect George W. Bush! We saw him bend down, amidst all that confusion and noise, and look into Windy's eyes and hug her. She hugged him back for all she was worth. She had finally gotten to meet him in person, and the entire world got to witness their introduction to each other. Another huge roar came from the audience as the newscasters described the scene live on the air. By this time confetti, the most we ever hope to see at one time, began to drop from the ceiling, and it was also blasted by blowers from the front of the room. Tons of tiny, tiny red, white and blue colored papers floated down to rest on everyone and everything. What a sight!

Then the singer and entertainer, Chaka Khan, walked out to center stage, just in front of George W. and Laura (and our kids!), and began to sing her well known hit song, *"Through The Fire."* We had certainly been through the fire, and now the smoke was clearing, and we were beginning to have a better understanding of why Windy had been born to us with Down syndrome. She had big things to do as God directed her life, and in the process encouraged us all in our own lives. As Chaka Khan belted out her song in her perfectly pitched voice, David searched to see our children.

Always the gentleman, and always looking out for Windy's good, he located them, and he began to put his right hand out to indicate to Windy to keep it down, to be cool, and keep the celebrating to a decent level. I just lost it at that gesture. "Honey, Honey!" I yelled at my husband. Had to yell, it was impossible for him to hear my words, even at that. It was hard for me to *see* him standing right beside me, because of all the confetti floating in the air. Windy couldn't possible see us out in the crowd. *It's okay, Daddy. She's fine. She won't go wild with the dancing or try to show off. She knows this isn't the time or the place. It isn't her show. She knows that. And I know she knows that.* And sure enough, she was ever the lady. Daddy could relax.

It was so sweet, his love and protection of her. He was trying to avert a possible catastrophe, or embarrassment. Heaven knows, she had been such a big ham in the past, and she knew how to cut up at celebrations. Please note, that girl can dance! She has won several dancing contests in the past. This celebration time, however, she remained calm and dignified. (She's no dummy, it was being televised!) There amidst all this was our youngest, now grown up son, Michael, and his big sister, Windy. He was smiling and swaying to the music along with everybody else. Windy was standing and smiling a big ol' grin with George W. standing next to her with his right arm around her shoulders! And that's just the way they looked in the papers the next day. This time I think her picture *did* make it in nearly every newspaper across the country.

We have a framed copy in David's office from one of the nationally known papers *and* from our local News-Sentinel, dated August 4, 2000. Each time we look at it it's a reminder of God's goodness and grace.

After the ceremonies were over, we didn't get much sleep for a fourth night in a row. People came up to Windy, until late that night, just like the night before. She really loved meeting and talking and having her picture made with them. Eventually, we all fell into bed and slept for a few hours. Our flight home was late the next afternoon, so we could see a little bit of the beautiful city of Philadelphia, before we had to leave. We took Windy to see the Liberty Bell, and we rode in a cab to do some sightseeing. She looked out and pointed out things for us to look at. The kids got to see the famous "Rocky" movie statue, although it was behind a high fence at the time, and you couldn't get real close to it. Windy made Mikey pose like the statue, with it in the background. Both of them laughed over her request. (Big sister demand, was more like it!) They still laugh over that picture. They still laugh when we all look over all the pictures of that trip that Jama, Kari's mom, made for Windy, in a beautiful large scrapbook created as a memento of those days. It's cram-packed.)

The trip home was also very memorable—kinda' like it must be to travel with a "Rock star". In the airport at Philly, Windy was a head turner: she was recognized, watched, followed, and stopped for pictures and autographs. She was so kind and sweet to each person. They were very kind and respectful to her. Then we boarded the plane, and the pilot announced her presence on the flight, and the entire plane clapped for her! We were quite surprised and elated with everyone's response to her. No matter what each person's political affiliation was, they were all supportive of *her*. How awesome is that?

When we landed in Pittsburgh it was the same thing all over again. Educators, Special Ed and regular classroom teachers, recognized her and came up to talk to her by the droves. Many were parents, siblings, or friends of someone with a disability. Wherever she went they patiently waited in line. All joyfully spoke with our daughter, Dave and Mikey's sister, and took a little piece of joy and hope back home with them. It was all a blessing for them . . . and for us!

Our daughter was inspired by her teachers—Windy's ability to read and write has now inspired many teachers. Years after her school days, Windy wrote a note to the Tennessee Commissioner of Education, Lana Seivers, the mother of Matt, a friend of hers, who had attended Daniel Arthur with her, and she mentioned her teacher from Daniel Arthur "Miss Bertie . . . how she would not give up on me, and so . . . I learned to read." Windy has been an inspiration to teachers everywhere for a long time, not just after her speaking at the RNC Convention in 2000.

Her opportunity to speak before millions did catapult her into the view of hundreds of educators, who took hope for their current students. Teachers attending the Convention took her picture to share with their classrooms around the country. Some wrote to tell her about what it had meant to them, how it had encouraged them to see her speak before the nation. Some sent her pictures of their classrooms. Others stopped her in person to tell her what they were planning on doing, what she had inspired them to do when they got back home. Still others, on the streets of Philly, D.C., and in the airports, recognized her, stopped her to speak to her, and have their picture made with her. All for their schools back home!

I also emailed Lana a personal note. Lana emailed back and told me about her love for Windy, "because she would *always* remember how sweet she was to her son, Matthew, when they attended school together." She reminded me again of how Windy would walk down the school hallway a few paces, and then encourage Matthew to walk to her. He had been one of the students she encouraged to do his best way back in the 1980s.

Lana asked Windy, in 2006, if she would be in a television spot to help recruit Special-Ed teachers for the state of Tennessee. She and Miss Bertie appeared with Lana on TV, and all three had a line or two to say. It was a great encouraging message, and when it was completed Windy sent it to First Lady Laura Bush to encourage her. Windy wanted Laura to know she was still out there doing her part for the education system. Miss Laura wrote back a gracious note of acknowledgement and thanked Windy, and all of them, for their recruiting efforts to enlist great teachers, a theme close to Miss Laura's heart as a former educator.

Our daughter has always been associated with people from both of our country's two main political parties. Windy's sincerity and faith in her friends has overridden any political affiliation. Lana knew this and she knew her heart. She had seen her in action. Another life lesson for us all . . . live your life in love and faith . . . and others will know your *heart,* and there will be no boundaries on who you will be able to encourage. If anyone can coax someone to reach across the "aisle" to agree on a topic—with the express purpose of helping others—it's Windy. Yep, Windy is your girl.

We finally boarded a small plane to take us back to Knoxville, and the late night flight was more than half empty. Just when we felt like things were settling back down to "normal", the pilot came on over the loud speaker and acknowledged Windy's presence on the plane and thanked her for "a job well done in Philly!" Everyone clapped for her gallant effort.

After about twenty minutes the *pilot* came walking down the aisle and reached out his hand to shake Windy's hand. She stood up, holding onto the high back of the seat in front of her, to greet him. He had seen her on television and had been touched by her talk. He told her he was voting for Bush, and that *she* was the reason. He told her it was an honor to meet her, and he was proud that she was a fellow Tennessean! She was impressed that a pilot would know her name and would come to talk just to her. She thanked him and smiled up at him. He saluted her and then turned to walk back to the cockpit.

"Wasn't that special, Windy?" David exclaimed to her, "The pilot of this airplane came back just to talk to YOU!"

"Oh, yeah, Dad, that was *so* nice of him. But, I've got a question . . . should he get out of his seatbelt? He needs to fly this plane and keep us all safe. I want to get home!"

We all busted out laughing! A couple behind us was from Blount County, a Mr. and Mrs. Johnson, and Mr. Johnson laughed right out loud, and then said, "I'm with you, Windy!"

Mikey loved it. He was really belly laughing across the aisle from us. *Windy, Windy. What joy you bring into our lives!* Then all grew quiet. Only the hum of the plane's engines could be heard. She sat in her seat next to me, by the window, and closed her eyes. I was afraid she was scared of flying, or maybe getting sick after this exhausting trip.

"Sweetheart, are you all right?" I whispered.

"I'm great, Mom. I'm just talking to God," she said as she kept her eyes closed. She reached her left hand out to find my right arm resting on the armrest between us, and patted me lovingly. I started to cry, very quietly, so I, too, shut my eyes in prayer.

> *Wow, Heavenly Father! You are amazingly wonderful! I thank you for this surprising trip You had planned for us, and I thank you for our Windy, for the joy she has brought us, as well as the tears we have shed at times in her life. It's in those tears that I have learned to depend on You . . . and You alone. I can honestly say I haven't always liked the journey, but I do love the destination. Thank you for being with us at her birth, and here with us now, and forever. Amen.*

When we landed at our smaller, but very attractive airport in Knoxville (we have a model of a Smoky Mountain stream running down the middle of the long beautiful entrance hall, complete with statutes of our native black bears), we were glad to be back! We got up to gather our carry-on bags, and said goodbye to those we had met on this flight. We had talked back and forth to each other throughout the trip, since it was not a very full plane. Most of us had attended the Convention. People again thanked Windy for speaking at the Convention and told her to "watch those polls in November" as they filed out. She told them she definitely would be watching. Then she got to the door of the plane, and the flight attendant, pilot, and co-pilot stood at attention as she passed. We thanked them, and we were *very* touched by the respect they showed our daughter. With a grateful and happy heart, we followed her down the steps into the dark night—*especially* dark and quiet in contrast to the hustle and bustle and bright lights we had been around for the last week.

We walked up the stairs into the airport and into the waiting area, and we were so surprised to see many of our family members waiting for Windy. (This was before 9-11 when people were still allowed to come and greet you as you got off the plane.) They held large posters saying, 'WELCOME HOME WINDY!" Her big brother, Dave, was the first person to come running up to her, hugged her tightly, and told her how proud he was of her. He handed her a big bouquet of fresh red, white and blue flowers wrapped in a ribbon of the same colors. Then he held onto her shoulders and held her back at an arm's length, as his lighter brown eyes looked down into her darker brown eyes, "Windy, honey, you did a great job! *I* couldn't have done it. I couldn't have spoken to a crowd of that size. You never cease to amaze me, Sis!" She was delighted in his pride in her and for her warm reception from "The Fam".

Then Kari gave Windy a big kiss and a bear-hug, before making a beeline for her future husband, Mikey. Gaymom and Poppie were there to give their big hugs and joyful accolades. So were Nanny Juanita, and her Aunt Dede, with a framed picture of Windy from the front page of The *Knoxville News Sentinel* to present to her as a gift. Her cousins Kristi, Jim, Danny, Dana, and Jackie, all presented her with a half dozen red, white and blue balloons. Many of her younger cousins were there: Molli, Emmalee, Linzi, Sarah and Blake. This was the kind of celebration Windy adored, all the people she loved in one grouping. She had come home to people who loved her.

We all filed into our local Waffle House to eat and visit. They wanted to hear all the stories, and we four related everything we could remember. It was loud and fun. Everyone was talking at once, but we all got quiet when Windy began to answer any specific questions. We all wanted her 'take' on the whole thing, her perception of everything. All her responses and her understanding was remarkable. She was full of humorous comments as she told all that had taken place. What a lovely way to end a whirlwind trip. When it was time to go, we hugged and kissed each other goodbye. We all went our separate ways. David, Windy, and I got in our car to drive home. Windy totally relaxed, fell asleep in the car on the way home.

Sleep peacefully, you deserve some much needed rest. May God continue to bless you. And Lord, please keep us all on the right path as we follow You. Forgive us the doubts and fears we have at times. We do love you Lord, we just don't always show it. Thanks for loving us anyway!

Those words, "Maybe I'll get to see you in Washington!" were to echo in our minds in the upcoming election returns of the 2000 Presidential election. Bush has won . . . No, Gore has won . . . And so it went . . . back and forth for 36 days. Windy stayed up to watch the returns until David sent us all to bed saying it was going to be awhile before we learned the final outcome. He was right, it was going to be a while before it was all figured, votes counted . . . and recounted . . . Windy would ask every day, "Is Governor Bush the President yet?"

Finally the counting was done, and George W. Bush was declared the 43rd President of the United States of America.

At the suggestion of Dick Powell, we put that handwritten note from Governor Bush to Windy in a lock deposit box. It may be worth something someday as future Americans look back on American History in the year 2000. It was almost prophetic in the very wording. (She would later offer the note to be "on loan" to The George W. Bush Presidential Center at Southern Methodist University in Dallas in 2012.)

With Elizabeth Browning, Dina Powell, and Knoxville TV newscaster, Ted Hall

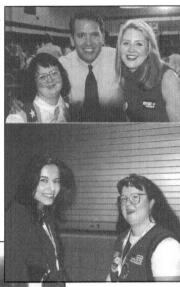

Waiting in the East Room

With Madeleine Will

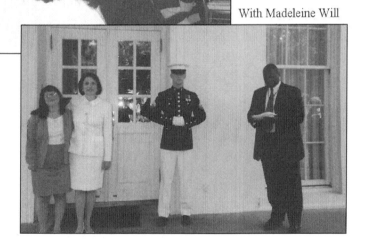

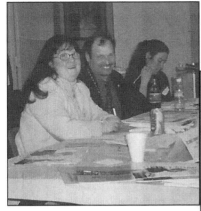

With buddy, Michael Rogers

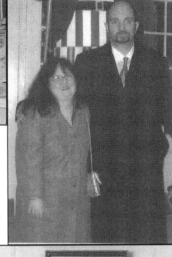

Attending a Christmas Party

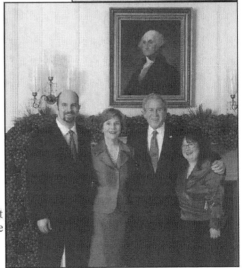

With big brother Dave at the White House

Chapter Twenty-One
Box Seats Next to the First Lady

The events following our introduction to Michele Tennery, who worked as a Senior Associate in the Office of Public Affairs, are really amusing, comical really. She had sought us out and introduced herself when we were standing in the Presidential greeting room, in the White House, on the night of President Bush's first address to Congress in January, 2001. Miss Laura had asked Windy to be seated beside her at her husband's speech!

Michele had been told we were coming, and she knew to look for us. We were milling about the room, meeting the others who were to be seated in the First Lady's Box for the evening. Windy was having a wonderful time meeting all the people and making small talk with everyone. She looked so cute, all dressed up in a black skirt and jacket, with a pink blouse underneath. She was so polite, and so lady-like, as she sipped her water, in a glass someone had served her on a silver tray, while she walked around looking at the historic wallpapered-walls and at the lovely china, that had graced past Presidents' tables, displayed behind the various, glass cabinet doors.

Suddenly my daughter turned to me and said, "Mom, I hate to tell you this, but I have to go to the 'you know what'." Now I'm wondering what to do in a situation like this. It was almost time for us to load into the cars and vans parked in front of the entrance, near the room we were standing in. Time was not on our side here. Plus, I saw no bathroom, nor anyone to ask where the nearest one was. I knew we could not go looking for one on our own. Awkward. (Thoughts of the movie's main character,

Forest, in *Forest Gump,* and his untimely announcement that he had to go to the bathroom as he was being introduced to the President quickly came to mind. Oh, my! It was going to be a *long* night, and it had just begun. We had to find a bathroom fast.)

Who do you ask and where do you go? Windy didn't know what to do, and I certainly didn't know either. The room was filled with the other guests, who were to be seated in the First Lady's box in the Galley of the Capitol, for the speech later that evening. I looked around the room for David. He and our sons were speaking with the mayor of D.C.. Couldn't disturb them. Okay. The servers, who had earlier been everywhere, were no longer in the three rooms we were free to walk about in.

That's when Michelle walked back into the room from the hallway beyond, and I gladly motioned to her. We told her of our dilemma, and she was so gracious and asked us to follow her. We walked behind her as she leaded the way through a door and out into the hall. She explained that the stairs to our left lead to the personal quarters of the President and his family. Windy and I turned to look and nearly ran into each other. (Windy has a way of stopping on a dime, and I swear, one of these days as I'm trying to avoid running into her, I'll turn and flip, head over heels, and fly right over her head. Thankfully this wasn't the time.) We recovered quite nicely I believe, and continued down the hall. Michele turned to see our antics and laughed with us. (So much for looking totally in control and dignified. Our secret was out. Windy and I *are* funny. *Really* funny sometimes. This was definitely an "I love Lucy moment" as Windy coins my funny, and sometimes embarrassing moments.)

Michele pointed to a bathroom door on the right, and we went in. We were so excited. It's just a bathroom to some people, but to us . . . it was a special bathroom because it was in the WHITE HOUSE! I washed my hands and dried them off on the lovely paper napkin with the Presidential seal on it. They all had a seal on them, I noticed, stacked so nicely on the counter for anyone to use. It was so stately looking, I had a hard time just tossing it into the wastebasket. The gold embossed emblem looked so regal, even on a throw-away, paper hand towel. Knowing how my mother, who was always teaching us what she considered the essential niceties of social graces, would enjoy seeing one for herself, I turned to Windy and said, "Let's take one to keep, and one to take to Gaymom, shall we?" "Sure, okay," she says, as she shook her head at me, as if to say, "Mom you are crazy, it's a napkin for gosh sakes, but take it if you must, and let's get on with the reason we are here!"

I wondered how I would explain the napkins in my purse when they searched us as we entered the Capitol. Is it a crime to take a paper napkin provided for the drying of your hands IF you are not planning to get a drop of water on it, and instead you are planning to put it in a scrapbook? (Don't you know I'm kidding here? I knew they wouldn't really ask about the napkin.) But as soon as we came out, I confessed to the waiting Michelle, and she laughed and told us that we were welcome to take the napkins home with us. (Later we learned that many women present that night had a napkin with the seal on it, stuffed in their own handbags. It has become quite a thing to do, this taking a paper napkin home as a memento, so much so that the White House Staff has considered doing away with them and replacing them with regular old paper towels. That would be a real shame I think.)

Windy and I still smile any time we look through her scrapbook of those days and see that seal on the remnant of paper. Next time, I'm going to suggest they pass out an official napkin to all the visitors, straight out, sort of as a token souvenir of the important evening. At least it will keep everyone from having to declare their purse contents in personal confessions!

We left the boys back at the White House. They had been invited to stay behind and watch the televised speech with some of the men in the Secret Service. Before it began they were treated to a brief private tour of one of the weapon and ammunition rooms, and had their playtime with the First Pet, a black Scotty dog. Fun and unique memories they will never forget.

When we arrived at our destination, Windy and I were led to our seats in the First Lady's Gallery, where Windy was seated, it turned out to be at the right hand of Laura Bush . . . when Mrs. Bush came in to be seated at the appointed time. Lynn Cheney, the Vice President's wife, came in, was applauded by the crowd, and then took her seat behind Laura's empty chair. Then the people that were invited to sit in the box seats began to fill up the remaining seats. The mayor of Philadelphia, John Street, sat down on the other side of the empty seat, between him and Windy. He turned and nodded hello to her, and she smiled back at him, and said, "Hi."

Windy and I watched the seats also fill up down below on the floor. The House Representatives and the Senators filed in. Then came the Joint Chiefs of Staff and the Generals. The previous First Lady, Hillary Clinton, came in and looked up at the Gallery where she had been seated for the last eight years. She now had a seat on the floor as a Senator. Windy saw and recognized her. I could see my daughter smile sweetly at the people down below, but ever so slightly. It was a very solemn occasion. At last, the First Lady was led into the Gallery, and she came to stand beside Windy. We spied David as he walked in with the Secret Service, and they methodically sat down on each one of the steps in the aisle. (We knew he'd be fine on the steps. He used to sit on the aisle seat of the bleachers at some point at all the basketball games we went to so he could talk and visit with people during the games. He was used to, and comfortable with, a seat on the steps!)

Miss Laura warmly greeted the Mayor, as she stepped up to walk in front of him to find her seat, and then she turned to Mrs. Cheney, whose seat was directly behind hers, and spoke a greeting to all the others in her Box. She then turned to Windy, and said the words, "Hello, Windy!", and she smiled, first at Windy, and then at me, Windy's mom, who had the honor of being placed to my daughter's right. Her strikingly direct gaze was magnified by the beautiful aqua-blue color of her eyes. (Windy once said she knew why George W. fell in love with his wife . . . it was her beautiful eyes when she looked back at him! I'll bet she's right about that!)

Laura stood straight and poised, and seemed at ease, as the entire room applauded for the Nation's new First Lady. The applause went on for several minutes, and then "Miss Laura," as Windy calls her, leaned in to Windy and me and asked in a voice meant only for us . . . so down to earth, and still smiling . . . "Do I remain standing?" Windy looked quizzically at me, and I was horrified that I didn't know the protocol to help advise her. For a split second I wished I had looked up the protocol, to be her personal advisor and protector, but like everyone else, we were 'winging it.' (Americans are not like other countries with their Monarchs. We are not as 'stick to the rules' driven, so I guess there are many things one has to learn as they go! This was one of those moments.) Nothing our First Lady could have done, whether she remained standing for a longer period, or whether she sat down immediately, would have been improper. She is such a real lady, and she didn't want to appear as someone trying to seek the limelight.

(She probably wished to sit down and turn the focus to her husband, the new President. She is a gracious person and wanted to stand only as long as people wanted her to stand, so they could pay homage to the position and honor that being the First Lady of our country warrants.) My heart went out to her. I apologetically confessed to her that I did not know. I shook my head in a 'I don't know' reaction as I lifted my shoulders ever so slightly. I think I said, "We'll do what you do." And, we did. (My one big chance to shine, and I failed miserably! I did learn a lesson in humility though. I will never forget the moment. If she ever asks me to help her out again, or, if any First Lady ever needs some advice, I will be ready to help.)

Miss Laura stands just a few seconds longer, and then decides to sit down, to take the focus off herself, and the rest of us followed suit. She had displayed leadership qualities all on her own! I was so touched by her honesty. She was just like the rest of us, a real person who needed some time to learn the ropes. And, she wasn't ashamed to admit when she did need some help. Windy and I knew at that instant she was going to be a wonderful First Lady. (And did she ever prove herself in the aftermath of 9-11, and in the many events that took place during her husband's eight years in office. She was steady as a rock. She was a wonderful First Lady, and the country still respects and adores her.)

President Bush spoke from his heart that night as he told everyone the direction he hoped to lead the country in for the next four years, and during his speech he looked up at the Gallery several times. Windy sat perfectly still listening to his every word. She clapped and stood many times, along with the crowd. After the speech, and after we had all filed out into the hallway, Windy and I met back up with David. She was so cute walking in her little high heels. "Did you see him? Did you see the President look up at me and smile?" she elatedly asked her dad and me, as we flanked her on either side, walking a slight step behind her.

"Honey," I said, in an all-knowing, motherly fashion, "He was looking up at Miss Laura, his wife." I had to be truthful with her, I thought. No use in her going back home and telling something based on an assumption. Neither did I want her having false hope.

"Yeah . . . he did," she said slowly, . . . "but he looked up *at me* one time and smiled." We could tell she was playing the moment over in her head, and then she slowly nodded a yes to herself, as if to assure herself that it must have been as she called it.

"Well, I think he and Miss Laura are just so close, like me and your dad, and he was probably looking at her because he loves her, and he wanted to get Laura's approval."

She thought about that a second and then replied, "Yes, he did that too, but he looked at me one time and smiled *just* at me!"

"Okay, sweetheart, if you say so. He might have looked at you, too. It was just such an honor for you to be asked to be here. I will never forget this, will you?"

"No, Mom! *Never!*"

Then we realized that we were not being led to an exit near where we left our coats, as we had expected, but were being led into another large reception room. One of the nuns, who had been in the

First Lady's Box with Windy, saw us looking quizzically, and she came over and told us we were all going to get a chance to shake hands with the President and First Lady. Also with the Vice President, and his wife! It was a surprise to us, for sure. No one had mentioned this added honor. Sure enough, in what seemed like a short wait, in walked the President and Laura, and the Vice President, Dick Cheney and Lynn. Everyone stood all around the room waiting for a chance to speak with them.

There was no formal receiving line. It was more like a large party held in someone's home, not what we expected at all. In just a few minutes George W., full of life, as he always was when we got to observe him up close . . . was going to walk up to us, very soon. When he saw Windy, he immediately came striding across the room, leaned down to hug her, and looked right into her eyes, as he said in his loudest, friendliest voice, " Windy! Girl, did you see me look up at you and smile one time?"

Windy hugged him back with enthusiasm. Nodding her head in happy affirmation, as she said quickly, and proudly, "I sure *did*! You did a great job tonight! I was praying for you!"

"I know you were. I could feel everyone's prayers for me tonight!" He stood upright to look directly at all of us. Then he thanked her for coming and thanked us for bringing her. We assured him that it was *our* honor to have our daughter invited and for us to have the opportunity to come with her. A great honor!

She stood up and turned her head ever so slightly to glance at my face, as to be sure her mom had heard his words to her. Being a Lady, *always a Lady*, she never gave me away to those present. I was humbled though. Big time. The Leader of the Free World had befriended our daughter. What did *I* know? I didn't know him. She really knew him already: his electric, fun personality, and even his genuine smile. (If everyone in the U.S. could have met the man face to face, I don't think there would be one person that didn't like the man. I'm not talking differences in politics, just personality here. He was fun to talk with.) She already knew if he was smiling a smile meant for a special friend, or not.

Our daughter turned to direct her hand in our direction, and said, "I want you to meet my mom and dad, David and Vicki Smith." The President greeted us with a "Hi, Mom and Dad. It's a pleasure to meet Windy's parents. Laura and I are very fond of this young woman." Again her manners were impeccable. Again she was in charge of the moment. She was beaming with pride. (I hoped some of it was pride in her parents!) We shook hands and were impressed with his personality. He *was* bigger than life! (Windy's descriptive words to us once.) He was personable and caring. He was enthusiastic and bright. He never forgot a name. Like never. (It was reported to us that he knew, and spoke often to all the staff at the White House, no matter how insignificant and small a job they appeared to have. No job was insignificant to him. He was friendly to everyone and would even ask about their family members and friends, by their names, too!)

He really seemed sincere and kind. We were beginning to understood why Windy thought so much of him now. He was a real man, with real integrity. He was also a brother in Christ, even though he was the President of the United States of America. She felt compelled to pray for him and his family every day. Now that's tr*u*e friendship.

Windy also got the opportunity to speak with, and hug, Miss Laura, and thank her for asking her to sit by her at the President's First Address to Congress. Laura was a former teacher and obviously, intuitively, knew that Windy's great education and wonderful lively personality, were a direct result of many great teachers, loving parents, and a supportive family. Windy was living proof of the importance of inclusion, no matter the ability, the disability, race or age of the student.

All too soon, the reception was drawing to a close, as the President and Miss Laura continued around the room, making a point to speak, if only for a few minutes, with every person in attendance. Soon they had circled back to the door they had come in, and were escorted out. After about five minutes, the door was opened and people began to file out. The three of us went to fetch our coats in the cloak room where we had checked them. Windy purposely walked to place herself between us as we stepped out into the hallway, and took one of our hands, in both of her small precious ones. "Thanks, Mom and Dad, for bringing me here tonight."

"Oh, Windy, thanks for bringing *us!*" we both exclaimed at the same time.

We hugged her, and then put on our coats and walked hand in hand out the door and into the night. The three musketeers. Again.

"Windy, he *did* look up at *you,* and you knew it didn't you, honey?" I asked her, still amazed.

"Yes, I did!" she answered affirmatively, but very sweetly, as she smiled up at me with those enchanting, sparkling brown eyes.

"Well, thanks for not telling on me. I didn't think it was possible. I'll never doubt you again, baby!" I said with great feeling. I meant it!

She laughed her distinctive, cute little giggle. (Her 'Kappie laugh,' that's what we call it. My aunt Kappie (Kathryn Stansberry) had been an English teacher at Oak Ridge High School, in Oak

Ridge, Tennessee, for over thirty-five years. She never married, and never had any children of her own, yet she considered all the students she taught as 'her kids' . . . she had hundreds of kids! When Windy came along, she got to enjoy being around a baby. She used to hold little Windy in her lap, and they would both giggle at each other. She would be thrilled to know that she is still remembered today whenever her great-niece laughs!)

Forging ahead and taking full control of the night out, Windy said, "Let's go to Old Ebbitt Grill. I'm starving!" So that's just what we did. We called our boys to meet us at the restaurant. They were still at the White House and within a short walk to our destination. They were all for it. Why not enjoy the nightlife while we were in D.C.? That was Windy's philosophy, and we were game. We followed her into a cab for the short ride, and then out onto the street and into the large revolving door. She was in the door section before us, and she confidently walked into the foyer, went up to the hostess station, and asked for a table for five.

She ordered for us after we were seated. (She was relishing this role reversal. She was in charge, and it not only didn't intimidate her, she took charge with great flourish!) She ordered two appetizers of Maryland Crab Cakes and five iced teas with lemon (Alas, no sweet tea this far North!). She couldn't have chosen better! But really, after all these years, what did we expect? Windy was learning her way around Washington, D.C., and if we wanted to learn along with her, we had to be "on our toes and follow her lead!" People stopped by our table to say hello and to tell her they saw her in the First Lady's Box. She thanked them and told them it was an honor, *and* a lot of fun!

Windy, Windy, You *are* a lot of fun! What's next? We are on a great adventure with God, and this girl, and that's a fact! No doubt about it!

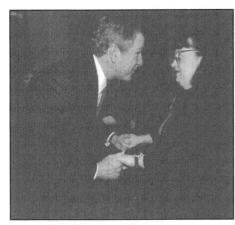

President Bush asking Windy, "Did you see me looking at you one time?"

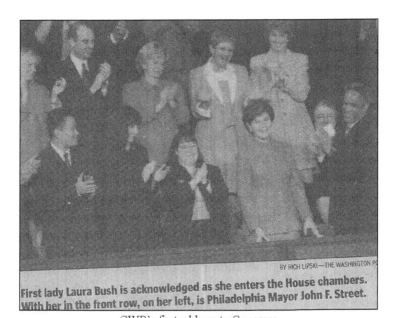

First lady Laura Bush is acknowledged as she enters the House chambers. With her in the front row, on her left, is Philadelphia Mayor John F. Street.

GWB's first address to Congress
Windy next to the First Lady

THE WHITE HOUSE
WASHINGTON

August 4, 2006

The Honorable Windy J. Smith

Dear Windy:

It was great having you and your family to the Oval Office last week. I am fortunate to have good friends like you. Thank you for coming and for the wonderful gifts.

Laura and I send our best wishes.

Sincerely,

George W. Bush

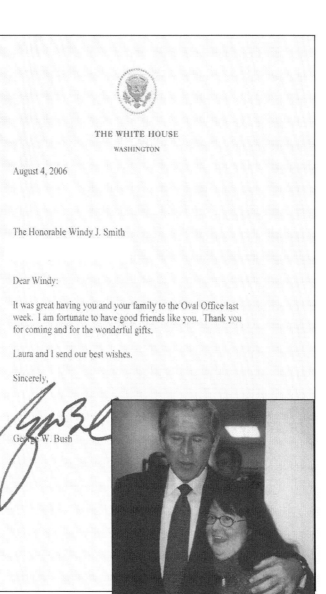

A personal visit at the airport

Chapter Twenty-Two
Presidential Appointment

Open your mouth for the mute, for the rights of all who are destitute. Open your mouth, judge righteously, defend the rights of the poor and needy.   Proverbs 31:8-9

The following is how Windy began her work in Washington D.C. Please let me preface by saying: **Everyone** played an important role in the big Committee name change. I don't mean to imply Windy Smith changed the Committee's name single-handedly . . . I am telling about the important part she and others had in the changing of it, though. It's really a great story of one spunky young lady, and how she got the ball rolling with the first push! She was only a part of the whole successful process. Thank heavens for Committee members, ex officio members, tireless working Staff members, and others who work together for the good of this country and the citizens! Thank you for putting people *first*—and putting aside politics. Hip! Hip! Hooray! To all of you!

We returned home to Knoxville and to normal life after she had attended the President's First Address to Congress. Windy kept busy at work, but we think she missed the hustle and bustle of D.C., which was now only memory—or so we thought.

A few months later she was appointed to a Presidential Committee—a federal level committee which happened in a unique way. When a search committee set out to find new members, her name kept popping up as a possibility—from all over the country, from people who had heard her speak at the RNC. Even the Secretary of Education knew about her and called her former high school to inquire if the Windy that spoke at the Convention was the same one whose self-portrait he had seen on the wall of the Special Arts Council in D.C.!

A funny story in itself, the high school secretary had called me out of the blue one day, four years after Windy had graduated from Farragut, to say, "Some secretary, a Mr. Rod Paige, called from Washington to ask questions about Windy". They didn't know who he was, but they told us he seemed very happy when they affirmed that she was indeed, the one and only . . . their Windy Smith! They were surprised to learn that he was *the* Secretary of Education, not just some unknown "secretary", when we recognized his name and told them his position in the government. They got a big laugh out of that one!

I called Secretary Paige back. His office then informed me that they had been doing a national search for the President, for new committee members for something called The President's Committee on Mental Retardation. They said they had been asking for names of self-advocates, people who had been born with a disability, who would like to serve. They said Windy Smith's name kept coming up *all* over America as someone who should be asked. They told me someone would be getting in touch with Windy soon, to talk about this possibility. I hung up the phone and just stood frozen for a moment.

> Who would have thought that our child, born with a disability, and in the first LRE class at Farragut, would be responsible for the school receiving a phone call about her, as a former student, from such an important man! And, who would have believed she would be taking us back and forth to Washington, D.C.? On federal business, no less! (What a humbling role as her parents David and I have had, and what a privilege we have had to serve our

country and help all those who have a disability, by assisting our beloved daughter, and accompanying her to the PCPID meetings.)

Windy received another important phone call—this time from Washington. Someone on the other end asked Windy if she would be interested in serving on President George W. Bush's Presidential Appointed Committee. (She smiled into the phone.) Then they said the name of the committee was The President's Committee on Mental Retardation (PCMR). (Her face *fell*.) The person on the other end said, "Ms. Smith, will you accept this Appointment?" At that moment Windy asked the person to "Hold, please," and she laid the phone down, and turned to David and me, and said, "Mom, Dad, I *want* to serve my country . . . but could they *please* change the name of the committee? I *hate* that name! My friends hate *those words*!"

"Windy, sweetheart, nobody can change the name! It's an honor to be asked to serve! It's a great honor. The name is what it is. Would you like to go to D.C. and be on this committee? You can do many things to help people! It'll be a wonderful thing!" We both were spouting out these statements to her quickly. We thought we were giving her helpful, wise advise.

She stood there for only a second more, then she said to us, "It *needs* to be changed. I'm going to pray hard about this!" Then she walked over to the phone, picked it up, and said sweetly, "I would love to be on the committee! Please tell President Bush, I'm ready to come to D.C. to help."

That's the last we heard of that request. (We thought!)

A week later she received a letter from President George W. Bush, thanking her for accepting the Appointment.

The PCMR called back and gave her the times to be at her first meeting. They also told us that one of us could go with her as her support person. Only one of us would receive a plane ticket along with Windy's ticket. We would have to buy one ticket. David and I decided we would both go—me to do her hair and makeup—him to chauffeur her around town. We kept smiling at each other the rest of the week, and kept saying, "Can you believe *this*? We're following Windy back to D.C.? And, we'll celebrate her *birthday* in Washington! How cool is that? Wish we had known *this* 28 years ago!"

On September 23, 2000, Windy was appointed to serve on the President's Committee for Mental Retardation. She was the only one, out of the nineteen members, with an intellectual disability at the time of her swearing in. By the time the committee was completed, she was one, of two, with a disability, out of twenty-one members. They met in Washington, D.C. four times a year. They helped shape the future by breaking down the barriers that existed for Americans with Disabilities in the workforce and in their everyday lives. She proposed a committee name change that was voted on and passed in Committee and signed by President George W. Bush in an Executive Order. She served as Co-Chair of the Public Awareness Sub-Committee, under the Chair Kim Porter-Hoppe. It all started with an unexpected happening.

It was an awesome, overwhelming and exhausting day, that first day Windy was sworn in to her position as a member of the President's Committee on Mental Retardation (PCMR). We had no idea the magnitude of these meetings.

When we got to the White House gate to go through security, we learned all about the routine we had to go through before we could be admitted into the Old Executive Building. (Renamed the Eisenhower Office Building, completed in 1888, located next to the West Wing. It houses a majority of offices for White House staff.) It has carved wood, elaborate stenciled ceilings and walls, beautiful marble wall-panels, eight-hundred-pound bronze sconces, and gold leaf-covered ornamentation throughout, with amazing handmade, multi-colored tile floors. There is a stained glass skylight over the double curved staircase. The stairs are made of granite, with cast iron handrails. It took seventeen years to build, and it contains 553 rooms on 5 floors. It has housed many private offices of past vice presidents, the Navy Department, the War Department and the State Department. The PCMR held their meetings here until they moved to the Health and Human Services building, close by.)

This was no *little* meeting in some *little* place on the outskirts of D.C. (We had believed that was what her meetings would be like before we attended the first one with her.) This was HUGE! (Later, on two other occasions, Windy and her brothers got to explore the old building with a guide, even getting to look out the attic windows to the White House grounds below. They enjoyed the unique perspective of the private grounds.)

I watched Windy to see her reaction to the security check and to the surroundings. No big deal, to her. She was all business. She followed the instructions to the letter and placed her purse on the table before her, and walked through the metal detectors, when the officers told her to walk, after they had checked her name off the list of approved guests for the day. She kindly waited while David and I went through the same procedure, then we all headed to the elevators for the room number she had been given. (Later she was issued an ID which she wore on a lanyard. She could come and go as needed.)

We got off and walked down the *big* hall (total corridor length 1.73 miles or 9,160 feet long!) to the doors of the meeting room. The room was *very* large and filled with light from the windows on the walls opposite the entrances. The walls were decorated with columns, and carved cherubs looked down on us from the corners of the room, and the ceilings were magnificently stenciled in beautiful colors. The huge tables were set up in a rectangular formation so everyone, when seated, would face each other, with a microphone at every seat. There were cardboard (painted to look like) brick boxes set up on the tables, representing a wall, all along the interior square, to represent the barriers people with disabilities encounter in everyday life. We learned later in the meeting that one of the main committee goals was to try to break through some of those barriers (such as in education, society's conception, and in the job market by advising the President on pressing issues that need to be addressed by our government about this segment of Americans).

There were chairs set up for the audience, lined up at the back of the room. (I'll swear, it looked like a setting for a television show, and I just hoped we were in the *wrong* room. How could Windy participate in something like this? I knew it would have been intimidating to sit at *that* group of tables, among *this* group of people. What could she bring to the table that hadn't already been said, thought or introduced before? How was Windy going to handle something like this? (We had wondered what a PCMR meeting would be like, but initially figured it was probably held in a small room, on the outskirts of town, with several people who had disabilities, and with mediators to help in the discussions. We still would have considered it an honor for her to serve on *any* scale.) That is all we had expected. Not in our wildest dreams had we imagined all of this. Wow, and more wow!

There was going to be a short swearing in of the new members by the Secretary of Health and Human Services, Tommy Thompson. There were so many important people in that room, gathered at one time: Don Evans, Secretary of Commerce, Elaine Chao, Secretary of

Labor, all the Committee members, who had served for the last several years. The Staff: Madeleine Will, Sally Atwater, Laverdia Roach, and the members of the Press present.

We walked around the tables and looked for her name. There it was: WINDY SMITH, KNOXVILLE, TENNESSEE. Windy smiled at the impressively large, white place card, with black printed letters, and put her purse in her chair as if to claim her spot with confidence to face what came next. Let me just say, the surroundings were not having a negative effect on *this* lady appointed to be there from Tennessee. Soon everyone that had been at the reception the night before was making a beeline for their own place cards, shaking hands and saying hello to one another. David and I slipped to the back of the room to find a seat. (We *had* no reserved seating.) Before I left her I told her where we were going to sit (in the seats open to the public), just in case she might need us. She said, "That's fine. I'll be busy up here for a while." She knew from the looks of things that this was going to be a time-consuming morning. She sat down and began to look over the agenda printed out for the next two days. We had been dismissed, it seemed.

Don Evans and Elaine Chao are two of the people who made a point to find Windy and tell her how pleased they were that she had accepted this Appointment. (Elaine even told her she looked so pretty, and how she loved her makeup and hair style.)

Soon everyone found a seat. Some stood at the back of the room because all that was left was standing room only. By now, several people stood at the front of the room where a podium and mic were set up. Madeleine Will introduced herself as the Chairperson. She then introduced her staff; Sally Atwater, Executive Director, Dr. George N. Bouthilet, Research Director, Laverdia T. Roach, Special Assistant to the Executive Director, Lena Stone, Program Specialist, and Sheila Whittaker, Budget Officer. I wondered how we could remember all the names. I wondered if Windy would ever get to talk to any of them at all. (Windy not only learned their names, she came to know them all as friends!)

Madeleine also introduced the ex officio members:

The Honorable Tommy G. Thompson, Secretary of the U.S. Department of Health and Human Services, (who would soon be swearing Windy, and the other new members in, in a Swearing-In Ceremony, and from then on Windy would have the title of "The Honorable" on her mail addressed to her. *All* a surprise to us, and all in God's plan!) represented by The Honorable Margaret Giannini, M.D.

The Honorable John Ashcroft, Attorney General, U.S. Department of Justice, represented by Mark Gross, Deputy Chief, Appellate Section Civil Rights Division

The Honorable Don Evans, Secretary, U.S. Department of Commerce, Represented by: Nique Fajors

The Honorable Roderick R. Paige, Ph.D., Secretary of the U.S. Department of Education, represented by Troy Justesen, Ed.D., Acting Assistant Secretary Special Education and Rehabilitative Services

The Honorable Tom Ridge, Secretary, U.S. Department of Homeland Security, represented by Daniel W. Sutherland, Officer for Civil Rights and Civil Liberties

The Honorable Norman Y. Mineta, Secretary of Transportation

The Honorable Alphonso Jackson, Acting Secretary of Housing and Urban Development, represented by William O. Russell,

Deputy Assistant Secretary, Office of Public and Indian Housing

The Honorable Elaine L. Chao, Secretary, U.S. Department of Labor (Who was the first Asian Pacific American woman/Taiwanese American, ever to be appointed to a President's Cabinet in American history. She would make a point to find Windy and talk to her about the Committee and about fun things like makeup and hair. She said she thought Windy looked so pretty, and they reminisced about getting their makeup done at the same time in Philadelphia! How kind of Sec. Chao was *that*? Windy *always* loved to talk to her, and she got several opportunities to do so.) Secretary Chao was represented by The Honorable W. Roy Grizzard, Jr., Ed. D.

The Honorable Jo Anne B. Barnhart, Commissioner, Social Security Administration, represented by The Honorable Martin H. Gerry, Deputy Commissioner, Disability and Income Security Programs

The Honorable Carl Dominguez, Chairperson, Equal Employment Opportunity Commission, represented by Mary Kay Mauren, Senior Attorney/Advisor

The Honorable David Eisner, Chief executive Officer, Corporation for National and Community Services, represented by Michele Tennery, Senior Associate, Public Affairs

The Honorable Lex Frieden, Chairman, National Council on Disability, represented by Milton Aponte, Esq., Council Member

This was the impressive list read aloud. Many of them were present in the room at the time. They had come to the first meeting to be introduced, and to meet the members, and to watch the swearing in of new members. David and I were completely astounded—all these important people here to insure equal and fair representation for people with disabilities. It was so wonderful to know that so many people cared about this segment of the population and that they willingly gave of their time to see that they received given their God-given rights to be included in all aspects of our laws. We were encouraged to see "behind the curtain", and to realize we were not alone in our quest for our daughter's best interests, and for the thousands of others with disabilities. All the names mentioned were dedicated to helping make these Americans' lives better.

We learned later that many of the Committee members and Staff had a child, a sibling, or a family member, who had been born with a disability. Their hearts were in this committee work all the way. It was so gratifying, and we were so humbled by it all.

This was a big honor for Windy to be asked to join them and to be a member of the same committee, but we wondered what her role might be in this environment. Would she ever have a chance to speak during any future meeting, with all these brilliant minds and ideas floating around the room? Would we even *want* her to say anything on any subject? How would they react to her comments? How would she know just when to comment? Would they overlook her? Would she get bored during the long hours the position required? She looked so little among the giants in the room, yet she sat attentively and smiled or nodded her head as each person was introduced. She was already familiar with some of them, and she evidently felt perfectly at ease.

David and I felt like flies on the wall, watching all this amazing governmental stuff take place. Truthfully, we felt we would have a challenging time just following the discussions that were surely going to take place. I started to feel sorry for Windy. Would she be so intimidated that she could not stand and say her name and state where she was from, when her turn came to stand up and walk to the podium, in the front and center of the room? I really wondered what Windy's job was going to be in Washington, D.C.?

God what are we doing here? Why have You allowed her to be on a committee like this? We trust You, Lord, but we just don't get it. Please help her now as she sits there, as she takes her place among all these people. Please give her wisdom. In Jesus' sweet Holy name. Amen

All the members were asked to come to the front of the room, one at a time, speak into the microphone, tell their name, where they were from, and say a brief introduction. We had no knowledge of the position Windy was taking, of the thing she was about to do. We watched for her turn to stand up and go forward.

I think it was Sally who kindly adjusted the microphone down some so Windy's voice could be heard, and then we heard her say in her beautiful soft, yet strong voice, "Hi, my name is Windy Smith, and I'm from Knoxville, Tennessee." (*Yes! She did it! She made it through the first hurdle, and in flying colors I might add! I was anxious for her to take her seat and for the meeting to officially begin.*)

And, then . . . we watched as she continued to stand before everyone, with no indication that she was going back to her seat. Everyone's eyes were upon her, and the room was quiet. (Should I *do* something? Do I subtly motion for her to come back, and point her to her chair? Is she suddenly frozen in fear? I had never seen her fold, but this could be *it*. I didn't know what was going on with her, and I didn't want to embarrass her *or* to make her look helpless. She had never been that! I didn't want her to give everyone in that room the wrong impression, especially on her very first day! What would they think?) All this took only a few seconds in real time, but it felt like an eternity to me. (Now I know that a Divine moment happened for our daughter to make a huge contribution for all people with disabilities in this country, and consequently, in the whole world.)

She deliberately looked around the entire room, at the strangers and familiar faces alike, and said, "Would you *please* change the name of this Committee?" (*No! Windy, don't ask now, honey, it's not the time or place. Why ask at all? We thought you had forgotten all about your question to us when they asked you to be on the President's Committee on Mental Retardation! Forgotten? Not hardly!*) She continued her plea, "I hate the name. My friends and I have to *live* with that name, (the "R" word). It needs to be changed, and we need your help to do it. Thank you for helping people like me." At this extremely rare admittance, the first time, really and truly, she had admitted to having a disability herself, tears were coursing down her cheeks. She politely thanked them, and then wiped her eyes with her hands as she lifted her eyeglasses up. Then she walked confidently to her assigned seat, pulled her heavy chair back, and sat down quietly. The meeting was called to order, and the roll call was taken.

She had gladly joined a team of people who were willing to serve their country by serving others. Only it was under a heading that Windy abhorred. We know now that she accepted her position to help change the name, and ultimately allow better words to be used to describe people born with a multitude of medical conditions that affect their cognitive abilities. She totally had a motive behind her acceptance!

Who's to say? Maybe the name would have never been changed if not for Windy's hope for a change! After her plea, we realize that difficult work took place behind the scenes; many committee members and staff worked tirelessly for hours upon hours to make it a reality. It definitely would have never taken place without their efforts, for sure. But, all good happenings must have a perpetrator who starts the ball rolling. Windy became the first 'ball roller.'

After she spoke we looked around the room at the people gathered, and we understood her true motive. Up to *this* day, Windy had *never, ever* admitted she was born with Down syndrome. Sure, she knew it. We had explained to her many times, in different situations, through the years. Why was she eligible to be in Special Olympics, and her brothers were not? Why could she not attend the same schools as her siblings, in those early school years? Why did she not get to stay in regular classrooms all day? We had talked at length many times with her about the reasons why, but we always ended each conversation with, "Remember, Windy, God made you just like He wanted you to be. You can do *anything in your life* with His help."

That day Windy had laid down her pride and bared her soul to all those strangers present at her first meeting in Washington, so that other people who had disabilities could live with a greater degree of dignity.

Her audience seemed somewhat surprised at her request. Believe *me*, there was no one more surprised than her dad and me. The weightiness of the moment had been almost more than either one of us could bear. She had said nothing to us. She had done this on her own. It had to be a God-given job that she had discerned was her duty. She had stood in a room of giants, taken her one long-shot at a goal most people would have said was unrealistic and unobtainable. Yet, she stood firm, firm as any soldier who has stood in the gap for what is good and right in this world. She knew that even though it looked like she was all alone, she had faith enough to know God was with her. She just had to have the courage to take the first step.

She had proven she had the courage all right, and she had come all the way to D.C. to do the job, even though it had cost her, her pride, her dignity, and broke her heart, as she had revealed to all present that she had a disability. We knew she had lived her entire life, for twenty-seven years, trying to refute the hurtful fact, and she strove daily to prove to all of us, and to the world, that it wasn't so. Yet, somehow, this precious girl, had been coached by her Creator to bare her soul, to sacrifice self, in order to help others—and in the process to make *all* of their lives better.

We were the only ones that day that knew the *depth* of her revelation. We were stunned. Windy was a hero to us already, but *this, this act* was the epitome of what makes a hero. Was it the right timing? Was it even necessary? We didn't think so . . . but our daughter *did,* and we were there to support her and, by golly, we would do the job we were there to do. Windy had grown up and become an awesome lady! My heart *ached* for her, but now it was simultaneously bursting with pride for her.

Windy's benign request was surprisingly tackled immediately by some members. The adamant feelings against such a proposal was surprising to our naive way of thinking. Comments something like these were made: "Those of us who have been on this Committee for many years have seen us waste years with this name change issue." "It's always voted down. Let's not start another year on this." "Let's take a vote to forget this nonsense and get on with more important things, like how to really break down those barriers in a society that holds these people with disabilities back!" Windy took the reaction she got as a challenge, and not the answers to bow in deference to.

It was obvious to all three of us that the Committee's name had been the subject of more than this meeting evidently, and the opposition began to take the floor. Madeleine took control of the room and, after hearing many of the reasons some thought it should remain the PCMR, she recognized someone, we can't recall who, that said, "Maybe it's time to change the name. Maybe after all these years you are the very group to do it. Perhaps Windy's idea is a good one?" Madeleine said they needed to think through this, since there was a strong difference of opinions, and vote to discuss the subject at length, and do some research, before taking a final vote on it. They agreed and went on to other business.

The decisions the Committee had made through the years had already made a huge, positive impact on public opinion. Now, the new committee, and all of their new discussions would begin. Windy sat there and shook her head in agreement with her fellow committee members, as they all began to see a pattern of familiar suggestions as each member got a chance to speak and make comments on what they hoped they could accomplish as a group during the next four years of their tenure. There *were* many subjects and common threads. Some goals were perceived as easily attainable, and some were very lofty goals, and seen as time consuming and less realistic. Some believed Windy's suggestion to be the latter: a waste of the Committee's time and efforts . . . a Committee name change had been attempted several times, and each time had been voted down.

Windy listened, and took notes. I saw her pick up a pen they had supplied, turned it to read it, and put it back on the table, giving it a small push away from her tabletop space. She then reached down to her leather handbag and pulled out a small pink pen with a pink feather plume attached—a feather-pen, if you will. I was displeased, not too businesslike, but she seemed nonplused. She had purposefully rejected the Committee's blue one with their logo on it.

I cheered her choice of pens later, when I found out her reasoning. I couldn't read the logo on the pen from my seat. She had quietly refused to write with a pen with the "R" word written on it. At first, I was hoping no one would notice her choice of pens. But, they did, and several people later said they loved it! Her propensity for color and flare had already torn down a few "barriers". If she wanted to use her own pen, so be it. They would find out soon enough how much she adored the color pink. Her outfit and boots were pink and she would wear it again at most all her meetings. (She wore the color pink in D.C. before the movie, *Legally Blonde* was released. The choice color for everyone in D.C. seemed to be black with black, and maybe a touch of white! Not Windy's color choice. She was a trend setter for sure!)

David and I looked at the notes she had taken for the two days of meetings, and they were so insightful. Included in them she had drawn a stick person on one page, then out from that was the word JOBS, then she had drawn a smiley face. There were other words written such as: SCHOOL and LAWS, and she had written out from those words, ACCEPTANCE and CHANGES. She had seen the words on the handout they had been given. She might not get a chance to talk much, but she sure was listening to everyone else, and she was a quick study. We already knew that about her. They were 'fixing to learn' it too!

After a lively discussion they were called to order, and it was agreed upon to take up the discussion of a possible name change at another time. The meeting continued on covering several more topics.

The lid had been temporarily set back on the "boiling pot" but it was just a matter of time. It was obvious that everyone in that room had a strong feeling one way or another about a potential name change, and here we were, the three of us, right in the *middle* of it all! Who knew?

After a couple of hours they adjourned for lunch. Windy got up to gather her purse and favorite pen. The three of us slowly walked out the door.

At the adjournment, people, about half the room, began to come up to Windy, and to us, to shake her hand, and our hands, and to pat her on the back in a congratulatory gesture. We were astonished at the reactions and comments—the Nays *and* the Yeas. "Please hang in there, Windy. You're right, the name of this Committee really needs to be changed! It's time!" One person with The Arc, came up and spoke with her. "Keep pushing for this! I'm the person who told how our organization changed our name. This committee *can* change their name, too!" (Windy didn't remember the association's name, but David and I did. Vividly. Our daughter had been a Poster Child for them in our state of Tennessee when she was a little girl.)

Many comments and discussions had ensued. Some of the members had rolled their eyes and said, "Oh, No! Not this subject again!" Others had agreed vocally that it was way past due to change it. Windy had listened quietly.

Someone in the audience representing The Arc had been recognized by the Chair, and he told about their own organization's quest, and subsequent name change, to The Arc, deleting the "R" word in their previous title. He had assured the committee that it *could* be done.

(I remembered being ever so glad to hear The Arc organization had changed their name, now that he mentioned it. The old name *was* truly awful sounding to *my* ears, too, and I didn't have to "live with that name" as

Windy had put it to us, not to the degree our daughter did. I had learned many things at Windy's first day of meetings, and I had been a witness to "more firsts"!)

Then Sally Atwater, Madeleine Will, George Bouthilet, Laverdia Roach, and Dr. Margaret Giannini circled us in the hall as we were exiting, introduced themselves to Windy, and began to encourage her to keep pushing for this change of committee name she had been bold enough to ask for. They told us that it had been tried for ten years now (*Ten* Years! Who knew? Not us. Not Windy), and each time the idea was introduced, it was voted down, but now they felt like it was the perfect time, this time. (It was obvious these people had been faithfully committed to a name change for a long time.) They also warned her and us of the impending opposition it would receive. "Some people don't ever want to see a change made, even if it's for the better. They'd rather leave well enough alone, when it's a matter of good enough!" we were told. Forewarned is more like it.

So much for thinking (with rose colored glasses on), we could all go to Washington, and see many good things happen as the committee went right to work, and in the process, make lots of new friends. We *would* make friends, but I guess a few "frenemies" along the way, too. You can *not* please everyone, all of the time. You have to act upon your convictions and try to make the world a better place because you are in it—and let the chips fall as they may.

"Oh, well, that's politics!" as Windy rightly describes it in the many talks she has given. She said as much to the Special Olympic Board of the Greater Atlanta, Georgia Area, at the Cherokee Town and Country Club, on February 27, 2004, when she was invited to speak as a Community Speaker at an honorary Board luncheon. (Jean and Jim Callier are her dear friends from Atlanta/Highlands, North Carolina who invited her to speak to the group.) She has also stated those words to various church groups across her home state, readily admitting her suggestion for a name change brought about "some trouble." As she said, "Pardon me for saying it, but it opened up a can of worms!" And how!)

(It was a great honor for us to meet Dr. Margaret Giannini, or Dr. G., as she was lovingly called in D.C., at Windy's first meeting, so many years after those classes. Dr. G. had been one of the main people responsible for initiating those first Infant Stimulation classes for DS babies across the nation. Windy was one of those kids who had benefited from those classes as she sat at her rightful place, with her nameplate in front of her at a huge table, among the many distinguished members and guests, as a full fledged member of the Presidential Committee. Who knew *the* Dr. G. would be present at this meeting? That point alone was *awesome*! We don't think this fantastic point was lost on Dr. G. when she met Windy, either!) When she came up to Windy to shake her hand and to introduce herself, she said, "Windy, I am so proud of you. Don't give up on this. The name does need to be changed, and *who* knows that better than *you*! We've tried for ten long years to do it. And here *you* come along and surprise all of us with your suggestion. It will be a fight, Windy. Some people never want to change things, even if it is for the better for all people with disabilities. Change seems difficult at times. You can show them why it needs to be done. It may take them some time to sink in. I think *you* just may be the person to finally get this done. Don't give up the fight!"

Windy didn't know her, but she immediately read her heart. She hugged her and said, "Oh, I won't! It needs to be changed!" They hugged again in agreement. Here was a woman who had made it her life's goal to educate these children born with Down syndrome, and a woman, born with Down syndrome, who was living proof of the woman's life-devotion! Not many people get to see their reward here on earth, or see it so obvious. We think Dr. G. left very happy that day because of our Windy. (We also know she had to be smiling at the irony . . . wrong word . . . at the *miracle*, that a graduate of one of her own programs she'd started to give the babies a great start in life—to have one of "her babies" be instrumental in bringing about a name change for a federal level committee! Thank you Dr. G., and all those who believed these kids *could* learn, and could be productive in society. It's true, they can be, and are!)

Someone in the group gathered around Windy said, "There are some other new members joining the group in a few weeks. We think you'll have some good support on this real soon, they have expressed their desire for a name change possibility, too!"

"Great!" our girl said.

She was all for support, but she'd fight it all alone if she had too. We had never seen her so driven, and focused on a cause. She'd never had a *larger* cause.

We walked down the hall and waited on the elevator to take us down to the main floor. The three of us were wondering about the impact of what had taken place that morning. Well, two of us were wondering. Windy was not. (Later that night she would tell us that she had prayed for a miracle about the name change, and the conversations she had just had with some of the people had been a confirmation to her that she was doing the right thing!)

We quickly went back over to our hotel to change into more comfortable shoes, so we could go walking and grab a bite of lunch. When we arrived in the lobby, Windy informed me that she needed a drink. (It's a well known fact that she carries a glass of water or iced tea around with her wherever she goes, and she had been through quite a dry spell on this particular day.) She and I popped into the restaurant to get her an iced tea to go. We walked back in the large lobby to look for David, who had told us he would wait at the elevator door for us. He was there all right, and so was Coach Stallings, giving him a rather loud talk on why it was so improper for us, as Windy's parents, to come up here to Washington and cause the committee to waste more precious time on the question of a name change for the committee. (He assumed incorrectly, that it had been our idea for Windy to ask for a name change. Who could blame him? He didn't know her at the time, and he thought we had planted this strange request in her mind. How could this sweet, seemingly quiet young woman have deep feelings on something like the name of a committee she was asked to serve on?)

Neither David, Windy, nor I have ever wondered since that day, what he might have sounded like at halftime in one of his talks to his team, especially to a team that was way behind in scoring, 'cause we know how it might have played out'. David was getting a halftime talk! The "talk" had taken him by surprise really, and he didn't deserve the reprimand. (We all three love Coach now, so *please* keep reading the book for the whole story!) David listened politely, and then he made it clear that Windy had acted of her own accord. He informed Coach that she held her *own* opinions on the name change. Gene Stallings was only trying to let us know that for years the Committee's work had been hindered repeatedly because the subject of a name change always came up and resulted in hours of discussions and yet, nothing ever changed. He wanted to ensure that these new sessions would be productive, and that the committee got something worthwhile done for the people with disabilities they were there to represent. A noble cause, a very noble cause, but presented poorly to a father who had escorted his daughter all the way to D.C., and didn't know *"squat"* about any of the history of the committee. All David knew was the history of our family with Windy, and the amazing courage that it had taken for his daughter to speak her mind to them.

Coach accused David of coming to the meeting with his own agenda! David kindly listened again, out of respect for the man, his age, and his position. Then, when he got a chance, he firmly told him, "My daughter asked your committee to help her. It is not *our* idea. We told her *not* to do this, not to ask for the name change. It is *her* idea, and she feels like it is the *right* thing to do, a job she believes she has been given to do, so I am going to help her with this. It may pass vote, and it may not, but at least I would have done my best to get *her* thoughts across to the committee. That's the *only* reason I'm here, as her *support*. You are incorrect in assuming *we* are pushing this thing! *She* is!"

That's the day we learned about agendas—evidently everyone comes to Washington with his/her own agenda. David and I hadn't, but we had to admit to each other that our daughter *had*! Good, Golly! She came here knowing all along that she was going to ask a very big question to complete strangers, and to some relatively new friends she recognized from the convention, and consequently, it didn't take us long to get involved in a big way! Windy was our beloved daughter, and her voice and opinion mattered. No doubt it counted *especially* because she had had to live with "that word" like none of us ever had, or ever will. It only made her request more powerful, more potent than any empty accusations. Windy had watched and heard it all. Her face looked pinched, and she bit her bottom lip, but remained calm and silent. I knew her looks . . . she was not going to let this idea go, because of what was happening—she was all the more ready to push on!

"Let's just pack up and go home! Who needs this conflict in their lives?" I asked the two of them when we were alone. (Silly comment, but I was thoroughly deflated.) We sat in silence for a moment, then I asked Windy to please *forget* the name change for a moment, and try to enjoy our first meal in Washington in peace. I was tired, I knew she must be, too. We had traveled a long way, and had prepared for *days* in advance. Then, there was the let down, the trouble we felt like we had fallen into.

The trip had cost us time and money. One of us had a free plane ride along with Windy's, but the other one had to purchase a ticket, and David and I had to pay for all of our meals, cab rides, tips, and any other expenses. We run our own business, he is the sole practitioner in the office, and when he is absent from the job there is no income coming in. It was something we were willing to do for our daughter, *and* our country, but this persecution (in the light of our sacrifices to get there) was not anticipated or expected. I was frustrated and wanted to get us all away from the line of fire.

But, because of the passion involved in the misconception that a name change wasn't her idea, Windy was all the more determined to push for a name change, and David was, all of a sudden, ready to help her take on her cause: to help her get her proper plea on the table before the entire committee at the second day of her scheduled meeting. He wanted to explain her feelings so they could understand the urgency we knew she felt. Here I was almost ready to retreat for the sake of peace . . . and these two "warriors" were ready for a good fight!

Forget a peaceful meal in the Capitol's city. David started plying her with questions. She was so willing to talk and tell him about how much she hated the words "mental retardation", and what it had been like to live under the consternation and connotation of the words. (This aversion to the term had been growing larger and larger over her entire lifetime, and now it was spilling out all over the place!) We finally gave up all pretense of dining, and we pushed our plates aside. David began writing on his napkin. (None of us had any paper.) He began to take notes on what she was trying to say to us . . . *and* most importantly, to all of *them*.

That night, back in our hotel room, David sat down on one of the beds and faced Windy, who sat on the other. "Okay, Windy. I heard what you said today. You want the committee's help in changing the name. I understand now *why* you do, but could you tell me *why* you asked your committee *today*, of *all* days?" We were trying to get the whole story from her. She returned his steady gaze. It was then that her side of the story was revealed. She told him that, "I have prayed and prayed about this. I was praying for a miracle, and God told me to ask them right from the first. Not to wait. I wasn't being rude to you and Mom. I know you told me at home to wait until later if I still wanted to ask . . . but I *had* to do it then. *Everybody* was there to hear me." She nodded her head to one side, her look that means "that's that." Then she looked over the top of her eyeglasses at her daddy, to see what he would say.

He replied to her confession in an apologetic manner, by saying, "Sweetheart, we apologize to you. Mom and I didn't know how strongly you felt about this thing. We are very proud of you for listening to God on this." (Now I was *all* in and ready to do anything to help! Her need became my own.) "If God tells you to do something, then you *have* to do it. We understand now." She smiled a smile of relief! We could see her whole being relax as she leaned to her right side, settling back up on the bed against the pillow shams, her feet hanging over, toes barely touching the ground.

"Do you want help in explaining to your Committee tomorrow just why you think they should take a vote to try to change the name?" David asked her.

"David!" I interrupted, "Do you think you *can* get permission to speak at a meeting? We're not members."

"I think I have to ask. How can we not try to help her with this? If she was brave enough to ask the entire committee, then I have to at least ask. He repeated his question to Windy, "Do you want me to ask if I can speak?"

"Oh, Dad! *Would* you? I need *help* here!" She sat straight up. She was getting fired up now—she had her parents' approval—and they were willing to back her up on this. He turned to me, and said, "Get me a pen and paper, Vic. Let's get something down so we'll know how to get her idea across to those on her Committee." For the next two hours he would ask her something, and then write fast and furiously. Windy leaned back on the pillows and almost went to sleep. I asked him to wrap it up—we had another long day ahead of us. It wasn't too much longer until he finished it, and then he read it aloud to us. Windy smiled and declared it "perfect!" It *was* perfect!

He had been able to capture and condense all the reasons it should be changed—beginning with the Committee's barrier theme—the old name was one of the biggest barriers to the very people they were all there to help, and people couldn't seem to see it. Maybe now they would. All he wanted was to help our Windy. I couldn't have loved the man more as I watched him be her protector and advocate. They were both my heroes, but even heroes need their sleep. So we three prayed, we called our sons and asked them both to be praying for her, and we went to bed. Windy slept soundly.

Another battle Lord? We thought we were coming to some small meetings to do some good as our Windy's support. We felt honored just to be here in the presence of these people. We had no idea about this on-going confrontational issue. We had no earthly idea we would be involved with any Committee business, in ANY way! Now we have lines drawn in the sand. Why? We don't know! We're so new to all of this. We didn't chose this battle—but we know You have a reason for it all. Please help us as we watch over her. Give all three of us wisdom in this whole thing. We need You in this Lord. Amen.

The next day, on September 24, 2000, (Windy's 27th birthday!) before the second day of the meeting began, David asked Sally and Madeleine if it would be proper for him to speak on Windy's behalf. They assured us that he had a right to speak for her, as he was there in the role of her Support Person, and so they said, "Certainly!"

When the meeting began, Madeleine recognized David, as he sat just to the right of Windy at the long table. He was so eloquent in his interpretation of our daughter's request. Some liked what he said . . . some didn't. It wasn't really presented to be liked or disliked, it was what she desired him to tell them. She was the only member (at the time) on the PCMR who had an intellectual disability. She had a right to voice her opinion and desires to people who had come to D.C. to help all Americans who had an intellectual or developmental disability. Her request had clout because of that fact alone.

Part of the minutes from the PCMR meeting of that day read:

Windy's father, Dr. David Smith, spoke to the Committee, on Windy's behalf. Some of what he said is found below:

Throughout Windy's life, she and her peers have climbed over many barriers and have gone on to achieve beyond what was predicted or expected of them. She feels that one of the greatest barriers is the stigma attached to the name of the very Committee that she has been asked to serve, even though the Committee was created to help people like her. How important is this? I feel this change is the foundation of all the other goals we are all trying to accomplish. Imagine if those who have gone before us would not have been willing "to live on the edge" to quote [HHS Sec.] Tommy Thompson. The name Mongoloid would still be acceptable. (Thank God it is not!) We ask this Committee to share our vision and potentially become part of a historic moment for the mentally challenged. We kindly submit this proposal for the Committee's sincere consideration."

A father had spoken for his daughter—a man couldn't show his love for his daughter any more than that!

After the meeting, as we three were walking down the streets of D.C. that afternoon, *several* people (strangers to us) walked by and said, "Happy Birthday, Windy!" They would smile at her, and she would thank them, and happily smile back. David and I were walking a few steps behind her, and he said to me, "It's just like in her theme song, *Windy*—"Who's tripping [walking] down the streets of the city, smiling at everybody she meets? . . . Everyone knows it's Windy!" *Happy Birthday, Windy! What a gift you have been to us!*

David smiled at me, and I remembered his sad face, that broke my heart, on her birth day. I couldn't help but rejoice now . . . for the joy she had brought to his face on *this* day! He was so proud of her, proud of how she had stood steady under great pressure. I *do* love that Smith boy as much as I ever did, and then some! *Thank you Lord for a wonderful husband, my best friend. He's such a great Dad!*

That night on the plane ride home, I sat next to Windy, and she was uncharacteristically agitated. I patted her leg, and said, "Honey, relax. We're headed home now. Let's take a break from all this."

"Mom, I'm going to fight this thing! I'm going to ask God to help me, and I'm going to write a letter to the President!" she said with determination, as she took her hand and made a fist, and socked it into the opposite palm for emphasis, as a display of her determination—to let me know that she was *not* going to give up the fight.

Oh, no! Here we go again! I'll have to watch her like a hawk. She could write something and send it off before I have a chance to read it. And she's not too happy with a fellow member who she felt was not nice to her Dad. No telling what she might have to say!

"Win, you write the letter, and I'll correct it. I *promise* I will let you send it—just *please* let me see it before you send it. *Promise* me?" I was begging here.

"Okay, Mom. I promise." Then—she must have felt she had done all she could do for the moment—she got out her drawing pad and began to sketch her fashions. God love her, she had become quite a Stateswoman to be reckoned with.

What fun these next four years were going to be . . . clashes, misunderstandings, false accusations, trials . . . and hopefully some fun and triumphs sprinkled throughout! It would take a miracle for a name change—

but we had seen them happen before, and we couldn't rule them out of her life, or ours. It was a miracle that she was on the Committee at all! David and I were happy enough with *that* miracle, but Windy saw the appointment as a beginning point—a springboard, if you will, to find ways to make the *whole* world better for *all* people who had intellectual disabilities. David and I were just thinking a bit too small, that's all. Just too darn *small*!

We had witnessed something miraculous on the day she asked for a name change. It happened quietly, and totally unbeknownst to all in that huge room, but to the three of us. It was a moment we will *never* forget as long as we live. She *was* born for this. She knew it on that day, and we did too. It was an epiphany moment if ever there was one. Windy has used her gifts and talents to the max!

I'm thinking if she hadn't been born with a disability, we *might* be calling *her* President right now—president of something: a company, a corporation, a country? (Who knows?) Instead, she has been called "The Honorable." (Her Poppie's favorite thing to call her. It really seemed to please him that his granddaughter, the one he had cried over at her birth "has now passed us all up!" He would often and lovingly address her as, "The Honorable". And, each time he did, he would chuckle with all the pride a grandfather can muster, as he shook his head in amusement and amazement!).

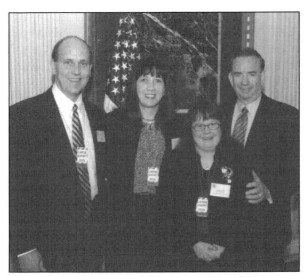

After being sworn-in with HHS Sec. Tommy Thompson

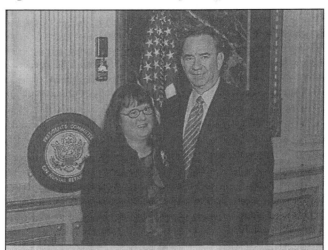

SPECIAL TO THE NEWS SENTINEL
Windy Smith of Blount County stands in Washington, D.C., with Tommy Thompson, U.S. Secretary of Health and Human Services. Smith is serving on the President's Committee on Mental Retardation.

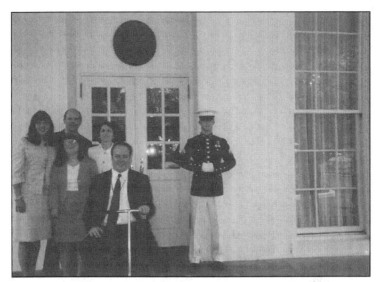
At White House with Madeleine Will & Troy Justesen

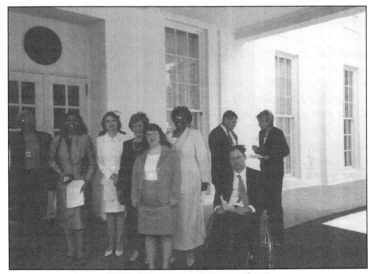
With fellow committee members

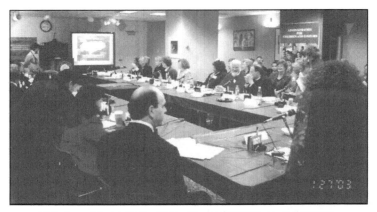
Windy and her dad, David Smith, at a PCPID meeting (2003)

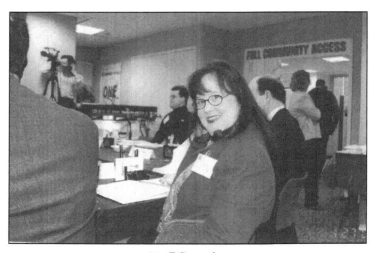
At a DC meeting

Chapter Twenty-Three
Proper Pleas, Persistence, and Possibilities

Windy *did* write the President another letter, and he did read it. This is another incredible happening in her life and when David has told it to some of his patients, even grown men have shed a tear. You cannot hear the facts without being moved. Letters don't just get to a President of the United States of America. The chances are very slim that they get to the Oval Office at all. For him to take the time to read Windy's letter himself, the chances were even less. This could not have just happened . . . it happened by Design.

We were told by Blake Gottesman, and Dina Powell, months later, in detail, all about the morning they hand-delivered Windy's letter to President George W. Bush. It had been quite a busy morning already for the President: He had *just* heard that North Korea had nuclear capabilities, and Ariel Sharon, Prime Minister of Israel, had just walked out of the Oval Office after an intense meeting with the President. The President's mind and heart had to have been occupied. It had already been an overwhelmingly heavy day of depressing and potentially devastating news concerning the world's population.

Blake walked in, and said, "Mr. President I have a letter from Windy Smith for you. Is now a good time to read it?"

Without any hesitation President Bush said, "Certainly!"

This was a man with the all the pressure of the Free World on his shoulders, and yet he greatly cared about the concerns of a young lady from Tennessee, who had been born with a disability. This speaks volumes about the true character and compassion of this man. He took the letter from Blake, read it, handed it back to him, and said, "Tell Windy we will get to work on this immediately." Wow! That was that. A bond of true friendship was so evident. A real friend will go to bat for you if you ever need them to. Windy, and every American who had a disability needed help, and they were going to get it! And, from the President of the United States, no less!

He turned to tackle the next item on his agenda for the day. Everyone in the room had been impressed with the way he respectfully considered her plight and the plight of all Americans who have disabilities. He proved beyond a shadow of doubt that he cared for *all* Americans, and that he respects all life and believes in the rights of all Americans—even those with special needs. They had as much right as any other American to his time and consideration! To us, it's what makes America so exceptional, and this one sincere gesture made President George W. Bush, an exceptional man to all of us. Forget politics, this had nothing to do with politics, except as a catalyst that brought him to this position. This is about integrity and honor. Our nation was at a place where we needed both.

> Our daughter knew this revelation right from the first. We know now God put this discernment in her heart so that she would be able to bless others because of her future friendship with a man that would be President of the United States of America. It was only a stepping stone to be able to be appointed to a committee she had no idea even existed. Her story is incredible. If God can use a young woman with disabilities to do wonderful things, it encourages all of us. God can use any of us if we will only make ourselves available to Him. He has jobs for each one of us to do to help many others. He's just waiting to hear from you—that you love him back, and that you are willing to follow Him—full out. To the

max! Windy knows it just takes faith and fearlessness. Another **WINDY LIFE LESSON**!

"Great works are performed not by strength, but by perseverance."

Samuel Johnson

Many months after Windy had written her second letter to the President, imploring him to give consideration to the committee name change, she received a phone call asking if she would please come to the White House for a private meeting during the time of her next scheduled Committee meeting in D.C. She was only too happy to say, "Yes." They gave her a time for the appointment, and she copied it down in a small notebook she keeps in her purse. She didn't talk about the invitation to anyone except her brothers and Kari. We knew she was all business about the subject . . . we found her in prayer many times over the next few days. We didn't know why she was asked to meet—but when the White House calls, you're going to show up to find out why, right?

Several days later, David and I accompanied her to her appointment. After going through rigorous security, we walked up to the doors that led into the waiting room on the West side. The military guards, who stood sentry, opened the doors for her to enter, and we followed her in. Windy told them "Thanks", as we passed through. She then walked up to a desk and checked in with the receptionist. She was told her appointment was with a man named Ryan, and that he would be with us shortly.

We were temporarily seated on a loveseat underneath a beautiful old oil painting. Windy glanced up, and over her left shoulder at it.

Instantly she was captivated by the painting and stood up to take a closer look. An Aide, who had watched her reaction from across the room, came over to explain to her who the painting was done by, the year it was painted, and what the painting was about. Then they began to walk around the room, as she told her something about each artist and their masterpieces. Windy stopped to look at each work of art with interest.

By this time David and I were standing with her to take in all the beauty and history. Patiently, the Aide described them all to us. There were innumerable and invaluable pieces of art in the room, and in the surrounding rooms. It was better than a trip to a museum! (The Norman Rockwell art pieces were some of her favorites; she saw those on her way to the Press Room when she was there on other visits. There were about eight or ten framed drawings by Rockwell lined up on the wall near the entrance.)

After our "private art tour", the young lady who was seated at the front desk walked over to us. They were ready for her to meet the man who had arranged the meeting. We were led down a hall, and we stopped at a doorway about halfway down. Windy once again, led us inside. We were getting used to following her now.

We found ourselves in a rather small office, and it was obvious that a tremendous amount of public service work went on within these four walls. The desk was piled high with files and papers, and several files were spread about on the floor beside the desk. A very friendly and respectful young man introduced himself as Ryan. He asked us to be seated, after he shook hands with all of us. Windy sat on a chair directly in front of his desk, where he had asked for her to sit. She immediately sat on the edge of her seat, partly so her feet would touch the floor, and partly out of anticipation for what he had to say.

"Windy, President Bush wants you to know that he read your letter requesting a name change for the PCMR." He went on to explain that he had been assigned by the President to work on this possible name change project, and that he and many others had been doing intensive research for several months. He spoke of all the work necessary to make such a change, and about the hundreds of people that he, his office staff, some of the PCMR committee members, and staff, had interviewed. He told her how they had documented the responses of Educators, Physicians, Advocacy Groups, and many others, all over the country. Then he said, "I think you suggested the term 'mentally challenged.'" (She had, it was her personal preference, and the word that she suggested the day she spoke to her committee members at her first meeting.) He asked her if his information was correct.

"Yes, it is," she answered him, as she looked squarely in his eyes.

He continued, "That *would* be a fine name change, but from the information we have gathered from all the people involved, the term that the majority of those asked had overwhelmingly voted for are the words 'Intellectual Disabilities.'" Ryan then asked her if the words, intellectual disabilities, were agreeable to her. She sat up straighter, thought for a second, then nodded her head, and answered brightly, "Sure! I like it! That's even better!" She smiled a genuinely, sweet smile at him. He smiled back at her, and said, "Great, Windy! Looks like that's the name it will be, *if* you and the PCPM committee members vote for a name change, and approve the new term."

He then went on to inform her of some very profound things—if the name change did pass committee. Ryan said the new term would not only be a new name for a Presidential committee, it would also mean the words, mental retardation, and mentally retarded, would eventually be changed to the words, intellectual disabilities in the federal, and individual states, laws of the land, and even in the new medical dictionaries, which were, by the way, due to come up for a ten year revision, just a few months after the proposed name change for the committee might take place! Talk about perfect timing! This was a very, *very* big deal! He then said to her, "Windy, President Bush wants you to know he is proud of the work you are doing for your committee. You have played a major role in helping elevate the lives of this segment of American citizens. A name change could lead to so many other older terms being eradicated in many areas and newer, better terminology replacing all of it."

With that, he thanked her for coming to see him, and said to our daughter, "It is truly an honor to meet you, and to be able to help you and your committee. I think your committee is going to be very happy with the results and feedback we have had about this possibility. Keep up the good work, and thank you for serving our country." He rose to shake her hand, and she stood up, all four feet and ten inches, and shook his hand back in a firm handshake. (She looked ten-feet tall to us.) We shook his hand, and we thanked him for his service, and for all he was doing to help all people with disabilities. We said goodbye, and then we were ushered out of his office, through the waiting room, and graciously escorted out into the foyer of the West Wing, where we exited through the tall, wooden double-doors, out to the driveway in front of the White House.

David and I watched as Windy looked up into the blue sky and smiled a thank you to the One she knew had orchestrated the wondrous things she had just heard. Amazingly, she *somehow* knew from the start, that it *would* be a big deal!

Almost with disbelief we quietly walked down the driveway of the People's House: this wonderful old Capitol that belongs to us *all*, no matter if we have a disability, or not. *Only in America*!

We walked on at a slow pace, as if there was no time constraint. Sure she had to get back to her meeting, but she had already been hard at work for them. We could take our time getting her back. We were still dazed by what had just happened. What a God-given moment, the respect and kindness that was shown to someone, some might say, was one of "the least of these", had been unbelievable. Here was Windy, born with an intellectual disability, involved in something of *this* magnitude. It was beyond our wildest dreams for her. Evidently it was exactly as the Lord had planned for her life.

We looked at each other in amazement. Would wonders ever cease? I pray never! At the edge of the grass we walked through the heavy iron gates and turned to our right onto the busy city sidewalk, contemplating again just what kind of person we had walking beside us. We travelled on in wonderment, pondering it all in our hearts.

If the Committee's name never got changed, we had witnessed so many inexplicable things already and would never question the outcome. God was in this, no mistake, and Windy's faith had already led us to unimagined heights.

Eventually the committee as a group embraced the idea of a name change. The new members, Michael Rogers, from Washington State, who was also an advocate (He still calls to check on Windy, and he calls her *his* hero every time he talks to her! He's one of the

Smith's heroes!), and another new member, a wonderful, friendly lady, named Zoraida Fonalledas, from Puerto Rico, jumped on board and were immediately ready to help change the name. Kim Porter-Hoppe was an advocate for the change, and she asked Windy to be her Co-Chair of the Public Awareness Subcommittee she was serving as Chair of.

Kim kindly kept Windy informed often about the many things taking place, and she worked long hours with others to help make sure the change happened. She had wanted it to happen before Windy had ever been asked to serve. So had many others. Many on the Committee and staff worked for months behind the scenes doing the necessary research, writing and creating the new pamphlet, and writing the exact proposal that would reach the desk of President Bush. Claudia Coleman, Zoraida Fonalledas and Vijaya Appareddy spent extra time speaking to Windy about their efforts on several occasions. She felt included and felt she was a vital part of the historic happenings because of the kindness and respect she was given. She was told Lon Solomon, the head pastor at McLean Bible Church, was doing his part in supporting the proposal. Many more members came to realize the change of a name would really change *many* things for the better. (We know there were more people involved in the efforts, but we don't know all the names. Their work was just as important and necessary for the positive outcome!) Coach Gene Stalling became a huge advocate for the change because he saw positive results coming from it, and he also helped it to become a reality. A great benefit from the united stance came as a surprise to us . . . Coach and Windy became good friends!

There are a few rare times in life when you feel for a moment that you know the very reason why you, or someone you know, was born on this planet, and put here at a particular time. It was like that for David and me, on July 25, 2003, with our fingers interlocked, standing in the middle of the Oval Office of the White House, beaming at our daughter, Windy. We were so proud of the bravery she had revealed, the compassion for others she had exhibited, and the determination and tenacity she had displayed when she proposed to her fellow committee members a name change for the Presidential Appointed Committee several month prior.

She was the reason David and I were there in the presence of the President, George W. Bush. (We had been invited to witness the event from the back of the room.) She stood next to his desk with her Committee members, looking over his shoulder as he signed Amendments to Executive Order 12994, changing the name of the Committee she served on to: The President's Committee for People with Intellectual Disabilities. The old name, The President's Committee on Mental Retardation, had been in use for over forty years!

(The committee was initially organized as a Blue Ribbon Panel by President John F. Kennedy in 1961, and later established as a Presidential Appointed Committee in 1966, by an Executive Order by President Lyndon B. Johnson. In 1974, during President Richard Nixon's term, new goals for the committee focused on deinstitutionalization, prevention and legal rights were established [for people with developmental and intellectual disabilities]. In 1996, a new set of goals was created by former President Bill Clinton encouraging full inclusion and citizens' rights. President George W. Bush introduced the New Freedom Initiative, in February, 2001, which was a comprehensive plan for the full integration of people with disabilities into all aspects of American life. The committee is under the Department of Health and Human Services.)

All in all, it was a worthy task to take on for them all. David and I had the privilege of watching them work out all the details and witnessed them changing history for future generations as President George W. Bush signed an Executive Order, on July 25, 2003. They asked us to be present at the signing. It was awesome and a great honor to witness. Can you imagine how we felt as Windy's parents? We had witnessed one miracle after the other as we saw God give Windy a desire to help other people and to have a dream, all her own, and to see it through to fruition. We were stunned, amazed, and feeling tons of humility and gratefulness to see so clearly the mighty power of God at work through our daughter and the hard-working committee she served on. Below is a list of those history-making committee members:

Madeleine C. Will
Chairperson
Chevy Chase, Maryland

Vijaya L. Appareddy, M.D.
Vice-Chairperson
Chattanooga, Tennessee

Nancy C. Blanchard.
Lakeville, Minnesota

James T. Brett
Dorchester, Massachusetts

Mary C. Bruene
Des Moines, Iowa

Claudia L. Coleman
Los Altos, California

Olivia R. Colvin
San Antonio, Texas

Zoraida F. Fonalledas
San Patricio, Puerto Rico

Kathy Hargett
Potomac, Maryland

Brenda A. Leath
Washington, D.C.

Kenneth E. Lohff
Milton, Wisconsin

William E. Lori, S.T.D.
Bridgeport, Connecticut

Edward R. Mambruno
Waterbury, Connecticut

Alvaro A. Marin
Huntington Park, California

Kim M. Porter-Hoppe
Ypsilanti, Michigan

Michael J. Rogers
Kenmore, Washington

Windy J. Smith
Knoxville, Tennessee

Lon Solomon
Fairfax, Virginia

Karen L. Staley
Beaverton, Oregon

Gene C. Stallings
Powderly, Texas

Annette M. Talis
Madison, Wisconsin

The letter written by PCPID Committee members in wording anyone could understand was printed in the booklet, *A Charge We Have to Keep*, printed in 2003, by the PCPID, is below:

Dear Americans,

The United States is a nation that cares about everyone's success.

The President of the United States has a special committee that studies ideas and government programs that are important to people with intellectual disabilities. The Committee includes people with intellectual disabilities, their families and others. It also includes important leaders from Washington, D.C. This year, the committee sent a report to the President.

The committee's recommendations address many of the challenges and goals for people with intellectual disabilities as outlined in our President's New Freedom Initiative. This initiative was signed only twelve days after President George W. Bush was sworn into office in 2001. It was obviously very important to him.

The New Freedom Initiative was designed to ensure that Americans with disabilities, including people with intellectual disabilities, have the chance to learn, develop skills, work, make choices about their daily lives, and be included in their communities. Providing ideas to make these goals a reality is what motivated the Committee.

The President's Committee for People with Intellectual Disabilities, to quote the booklet:

"In July, 2003, Americans celebrated the 13th anniversary of an important law called the Americans with Disabilities Act. President George W. Bush celebrated the important day with a special announcement on the radio and an important decision: the President asked Americans not to use the words "mental retardation" anymore. He said everyone should use the words "intellectual disability" instead. The President believes that the new words will make a difference in people's lives because the old words were connected to the wrong idea about people with intellectual disabilities. To get America started, President Bush signed an important document which gave the President's Committee on Mental Retardation a new name. From now on that important committee will be called the President's Committee for People with Intellectual Disabilities. He invited the committee members, who asked for the change, to the Oval Office as he announced his decision."

This is what President Bush said the day of the signing:

"We are making good progress toward ensuring that persons with disabilities know the American dream is meant for them . . .

more and more individuals with disabilities continue to become full participants in the American life."

President George W. Bush, July 25, 2003

From this day forward, a new term (Intellectual Disabilities) would be used to address people with intellectual disabilities. Most thought the old term (Mental Retardation) could never be changed, that it was 'written in stone' . . . but not our daughter! She had seen an opportunity, months before, where she could help thousands of people, and she boldly went for it. The implications of such a strong word change were slated to become far reaching: in public policies, as well as, in the everyday lives of all Americans with a disability.

That July afternoon, Fox News Channel announced the name change on the headliners at the bottom of the newscast screen. We watched in amazement as it came on about every six minutes. Windy could *not* be distracted from her spot on the floor in front of the television, at the home of our friends, the Rectors, in Virginia. Each time the news traveled across the screen, she let out a euphoric holler and motioned for all of us to come see the triumphant news: the hard-won victory, now in printed words for all the nation to see. She was ecstatic.

This new name was not just a cosmetic change; it was a necessary change to help alter the world's view of people with disabilities. Hopefully, now they would be seen as people with legitimate needs, hopes, and dreams like everyone else. They deserve respect and compassion. We, parents, siblings, and friends, have always known this. Now everyone else would too, because our government was making laws that insured they would be treated with dignity and honor. This change was a huge step in the right direction.

On that day, as well as the day we watched her make a proper plea to the committee, we knew why Windy had been born. Not that we had ever questioned her birth, only the way she had come into this world. We would never have given up the years we had been blessed by knowing and loving her. But to be quite honest, there have been times in her life (especially on the day of her birth) that we have asked God why she was born with a disability. It had been a great mystery until the moment that led up to her presence in the Oval Office. We knew that she had been born for *this*—to help the other disabled Americans, whom she represented. She could understand, to the fullest capacity, what it meant to live with a disability—day in and day out. She had a deep compassion for those who also had a disability. Through the years her unique personality has been shaped by her strong faith and by her belief that through Him she can do all things—especially as she attempts to help others. This important day was thrilling to us, yet it was impossible to forget the costs involved, which had led up to this point.

On one of Windy's trips to Washington we decided to leave early and spend the night with Mikey and Kari in Lynchburg, Virginia. He had been accepted in the first class of the new Liberty University Law School, and Kari was an operating room nurse at one of the local hospitals.

With bags packed (and I do mean bags in the plural) and the car loaded down, we headed north to Virginia. David gently chided us, saying that we had packed way too much stuff. We reminded him that we had to be prepared for all weather conditions. We had clothes for the cold days and clothes for a possible warming trend. Windy also packed early Valentine gifts to give her little brother and his wife. As usual, she had picked out the perfect items according to their individual personalities.

She bought a red toile backpack for Kari (She loves red toile and had decorated their new dining room in that fabric.) and a tie for Mikey with several breeds of dogs, including one similar to their beloved Cowboy, a short-haired pointer. (He had to wear a tie to law school classes on many occasions, and a fun print would make the wearing of a tie more bearable, she believed. We can all feel his pain since it wasn't so long ago that he could wear shorts and a nice tee shirt to work in a church sports ministry. Soon he would be the epitome of the conservatively clothed gentleman, Windy felt, albeit, in a tie with a small wink in the face of tradition.)

The weather got colder and wetter and darker as we traveled on the long trip to Virginia from Tennessee, and we make it just in time to eat dinner with our kids. We related the possible trip to the White House, and Mike was ecstatic. As he was studying law, and how the Founding Fathers formed a great nation out of raw documents, and strong beliefs and ideologies, he has a great fondness for D.C. and for the freedom of Democracy that it represents. He also has a fondness for the historic White House, and especially for the Office of the Presidency. (A love of anything to do with sports and basketball didn't hurt either.) Windy said in her quiet, sweet, but convincing voice, "You should come with me, Bud. You need to be there!"

He looked at us incredulously, "Do you think I could?" David said he thought it would be all right if Windy called and asked Michelle and Ashley, the two ladies who set up the visit. She was excited about the possibility of him going with her, and phoned them immediately. They had to ask permission they said (from whom we don't know) and put her call on hold. They came back to tell Windy they would love for her brother to come. In ten minutes it was a done deal!

Mikey felt like another impossibly wonderful event was about to take place, and he thought that missing a day of school would be worth it for a lifetime opportunity like this. (I think it was the only school day he missed in three years!) With Kari's blessing, he packed to go for the day to D.C. with us. She had to stay behind to work; we were all sorry she couldn't go. David and I were acutely aware that Windy's first pick would be Kari and Mike, or her brother, Dave, to accompany her, at any time. We admittedly, were a poor second, but would have to do. At *least* Mikey, coming along with her for a day and night, helped her cope with her parents. The parents, who were always cramping her style! She never said this to us, but I'm pretty sure she has admitted this to her brothers and sisters-in-law . . . we've just got a feeling about it.

Sunday morning, our traveling day, we woke up to ice and snow on the road, and even church services had been canceled. We decided to leave earlier than planned because of the weather. It could possibly take longer than the three and a half to four hours to get into the city. Reluctantly we kissed our daughter-in-law goodbye and headed out. Windy rode shotgun in her brother's car, following us. This time together is invaluable to the two of them, brother and sister. They have been *so* close, and now the many miles between our home and theirs was hard on Windy. She missed their talks and time spent together.

As the miles clicked away on the odometer, they shared their adult hopes and dreams and encouraged one another. I looked in the rearview mirror and saw Mike laughing hard at something, and my initial guess, I learned later from Mikey, was correct. Windy has said something so quick and direct that it sent him laughing. Had she been born normal, would they have loved each other more or had a better time together? I don't know, but somehow I don't really think so. Only God could know, and apparently He wanted it no other way than what it was today. It was not ours to question, and we smiled at the two of them talking away. What a blessing siblings are, or at least, are meant to be, to each other. They have a bond even a parent cannot share.

We got into the L'Enfant Plaza Hotel just before seven p.m. that evening, and Windy walked right up to the front desk to register. As usual, they look at us, standing behind her and expect us to announce who we are, and what we are there for. As usual, at her meetings, we stand back and let her be in charge. After all, we're there because of her. She *is* in charge! She states her name and that she is with the PCPID. They look a bit taken aback at the speaker and then proceed to check us in under *her* name on their guest list on the computer screen. Language comprehension is a small struggle at first because of Windy's American Southern vernacular and the reservationist's accent from another country. They communicate deliberately, and precisely, and smile at each other in the process. In a relatively short passage of time, she is graciously welcomed as the hotel's official guest and handed a room key, or more aptly a room card, and we head for the elevator.

Unfortunately, the bellman assisting with all our luggage, inquired how long we would be with them. When we told him only two nights, he was amazed at the amount of suitcases we had with us, and Windy and I started to giggle. The look on David's face was priceless. He was right (again) after all. We had packed *way* too much stuff. It was hard to get the five of us, and the rolling luggage cart, on the same elevator. We'd try to work on down-sizing the "packing thing" *next* trip, we promised. That thought stopped our giggling cold. That would be a difficult task for both of us. It was very sobering!

We had just enough time to throw the stuff in the room and change out of our jeans and into dressier clothes for dinner. (The dressing up for dinner was her idea.) Windy had a favorite special place she wanted to take Mikey to eat, and it closed in one hour, due to their winter hours. We rushed back down to our car and took off for Hotel Washington. Mikey had never been there before, and Windy loved to take people to see the view that she loved to look at, high above the city, and to watch their reaction. (It is high, at least for D.C., as nothing can be built higher than the Capitol.) In daylight or dark, the bird's-eye view of the White House to the east and the Washington Monument to the south is spectacular.

Mikey was quiet as he gazed out into the night sky, with the lights of D.C. glowing below. Windy almost whispers, "It's nice, isn't it, Bud?" He agreed wholeheartedly, as he slipped his arm around her shoulders. The hostess seated us right next to the railing and only a thick plastic window blocked the cold blowing wind. We hardly noticed the cold; it was as if that glow from the city all around us warmed us. Before we ate our dinner, Windy told Mikey that he had to share a Piña Colada with her. "Two straws, *without* alcohol," she added quickly, just like she did with her dad, the first time she came to D.C., and just like she shared with her older brother, Dave, when he drove her for up for a meeting once. It was now an official tradition.

This restaurant was the place she first met her fellow Committee members at a lovely formal reception held the night before her first meeting on the PCPID. It was the perfect location to view the Capitol city, and to be introduced to the magnitude of their Presidentially Appointed duties. (We have seen Washington, D.C. from that very vantage point countless times now. Some stand out in our memories for various reasons. Windy taking both her brothers there for the first time was so sweet to us. Seeing the city on her first night in D.C. at the Committee's Reception was a 'dream-like' experience. Taking in the view in the daytime and feeling the gentle salty air blowing in your face, as you gaze out to the Washington Monument in the distance is breathtaking. Seeing police snipers positioned on top of the White House roof, on the first Anniversary of 9-11, was frightening because of the reason behind the necessity, and yet it was reassuring, simultaneously. We have enjoyed each visit. The pulsebeat of the city can almost be heard from up there!)

While we waited for our food, Mikey called a couple of friends. The first person was Brady Tarr. We were all so aware of what a miracle it was to talk to him at all since it had only been ten days since his skiing accident. Brady is the youngest son of our dear friends, Bill and Deirdre. He was in Breckenridge, Colorado, on a skiing trip three days before he was to attend a college semester at Focus on the Family's Institute in Colorado Springs. He was found by the Ski Patrol lying on the frozen ground with a serious head injury and taken to Craig Trauma Center. There he was watched over by physicians and family for a very traumatic first week as he slowly regained his physical health and memory. That Brady *could* speak to us over the phone was a real praise! We were all delighted by his recovery, although a complete recovery would take many more months. (Brady is now married to a wonderful girl, Ryan, and they are parents to darling little children. They now live in the city where Mikey made the call to check on him. He's a pastor in D.C.)

Next, Mikey phoned a childhood friend of his and Windy's, Nolan Sherrill. Nolan was living in D.C.. He was pleased to hear the voice of his old buddy from home, and he arranged to meet us for dessert at our hotel's restaurant.

When he arrived, we hugged Nolan and enjoyed catching up. It was amazing to see the three of these young people sitting with us and seeing God's hand upon their lives in such mighty ways. Mike was in Liberty Law School, Windy was a part-time special employee of the Federal government serving on a Presidential Committee, and Nolan was working for the Department of Defense in the Pentagon, as a fellow for the Deputy Secretary of Defense, Paul Wolfowitz. They'd come a long way from CAK and Farragut schooldays! Mikey and Windy told Nolan of the upcoming visit to the White House. He thought it was so neat that they got to see the President *and* the Pistons. "How in the world did all this get to happen?" he asked. Mikey pointed to his sister and then Heavenward. Nolan nodded his head in understanding. This was all way bigger than us. But it always had been.

We asked about his recent ten-day trip to Iraq and were in awe of his recounts of the dangers, including his landing in a Black Hawk helicopter. David and I exchanged a big, amazed look between us. Who would have thought these kids would grow up to help shape, in some small way, the future of our country? Here we were talking to these grown-up kids, adults now, about the current events they were involved in, and on such a grand scale. Who would have believed that Windy would be there right in the middle of these guys? Just when we thought it couldn't get much better, Windy threw down her napkin and said that she'd be right back, excusing herself from the table. David and I watched her go over and boldly pat someone on the back, and then give a bear hug to him as he stood to hug her. She came back smiling a big smile and told Nolan and Mike that someone was coming over to say "Hi" later on. She smiled at David and whispered behind her hand, "Gene is coming by!"

A few minutes passed before a tall gentleman strolled over to our table to stand behind Windy and place his big hands on her shoulders. He said he had promised her that he would come over to meet one of her brothers and her good friend. Windy looked up, and back, to smile at him. Towering over her head stood Gene Stallings, former Texas A&M University football player under Coach Bear Bryant, who later became the former, award-winning football coach of Alabama, Texas A&M, Dallas Cowboys, St. Louis Rams, Phoenix Cardinals and a fellow Committee member. Our men stood up to meet the legendary coach, as Windy made the introductions around the table. (Gosh, I was proud of the way she flawlessly introduced family members and a childhood friend to a relatively new friend!) He spoke to us for a bit, and then bid her goodnight, as he explained he is going to get some rest before their meeting early the next morning. He gave her a hug before leaving. We all watched him walk away.

Nolan looked at Windy, and was astonished, "Wow, that was really something! Thanks!" We were struck by the always miraculous events like this that Windy seemed to provide for all of us. Great surprises happen when you hang out with Win. Here was Nolan, with all he had done in this city, and all the people he had seen, still able to be impressed with Windy's grace and ease as she introduced one of *her* friends. Here were these two young men that cared about sports, and sports figures, and she happily proved she knew a person or two in the sports world herself. God does have a sense of humor. The situation was so funny, and so cute. It was so memorable. Such a *Windy* moment.

The three of us took the elevator to our hotel room and left Mikey and Nolan talking on into the night. They had much catching up to do. Windy had to be talked into turning in early to be fresh for her meeting the next morning. She went to bed, but her heart was with the guys she had stayed up with on many a night in the years before. She had learned that active Statesmen, or in her case, Stateswomen, sometimes had to skip fun for duty. Duty first. The fun would have to come later.

Here's the rest of the story about Windy and Coach Stallings. It's remarkable on several levels. She thinks the world of him, despite their rocky first couple of meetings (a story she thinks is funny, and loves to tell about how they met now). They have a lot in common! They share a love for people with Down syndrome (DS). Besides having DS herself, she cares deeply for many friends, and for people who have DS. It is something Coach Stalling's family is very familiar with since Gene's son, John Mark, was born with the same syndrome. The love for his son and for these people runs deep with Coach Gene and his wife and daughters. Another commonality is, Windy and Coach both love America and enjoy volunteering to help in many ways to help make a difference.

Windy believes Coach is a great man. So do we because now we know the real man behind the legend, know his soft heart, and the exceptional kindness behind the gruff Southern accent. Knowing the following story makes us love him all the more, and you will love him, too, after you read this tender story. (This father's love runs deep. He has mentioned his son to Windy *every* time she's spoken with him.)

This *Online Athens, Athens Banner-Herald*, under the Sports heading says it best of all.

> Gene Stallings visits Athens Touchdown Club
> updated Friday, September 14, 2012-9:28
>
> "Whenever he stands at a podium, Stallings always finds time to tell his audience about his late son, John Mark Stallings, who was born with Down syndrome. Everything becomes hushed as Stallings goes from a Bear

Bryant vignette, which provokes uproarious laughter, to an on-going eulogy of his only son. The coach will proudly tell you about the buildings, memorials, streets and scholarships which have been established and carry the name "John Mark Stallings." Eternally reverent and respectful.

On John Mark's death bed, a heartbroken father lay down beside his son and asked, "Johnny how you doing?" Johnny replied, "I fine." With that, Bebes Stallings [a nickname close friends and family call him], a plain spoken man, reminds his audience, "My complaining days are over."

Shouldn't your complaining days be over? Let's quit complaining and try to make the world a better place for us having been in it. It's what people like John Mark and Windy excel at . . . teaching us to be grateful for all the blessings in our lives and to follow God all the days of our lives. *This* is a life well lived and one to emulate. What examples the Lord has put right before our eyes! *Thank you God for these special, special people!"*

Eight a.m. meetings, we decide, are extreme attempts to help a large group of travel-weary people focus early in the day, so that by the afternoon, before everyone is too tired to think straight . . . they will have a unified vision of the direction they hope ultimately to be going in, for the remainder of the sessions.

Windy's meetings *always* started early, and were very effective. At least it was so with those particular PCPID Committee members, the ex facto members representing the various government agencies, and the Staff and Chair, of the PCPID, that our daughter was privileged to work with. They were an exceptional group of people. They represented diversity in myriad ways: their race, culture, religion, political affiliation, the many different geographic places they lived, and in their education. They were a good, strong representation of the country as a whole. Most importantly, they were very united in their individual, as well as corporate, goals and hopes to help the intellectually disabled citizens of the United States of America have the opportunities, protection and respect offered to all other citizens regarding housing, education, healthcare and good jobs after their graduation. Their hearts were in this 100 percent, no question. Period.

Everyone came to the table with either a lifetime commitment of educating people with disabilities in some capacity, or through working with children or adults in a variety of ways to improve their lives and lifestyle. Most came with something deeper than a desire, they came with a heart for a special person in their life, who had a disability: a son or daughter, a sister or brother, a friend, or for two of them, a personal experience living with a disability every day. It is this common bond that transcends all the differences they had and pulled them together in a strong bond.

There are many Presidential Committees working for various causes and reasons on a daily basis in D.C., but I venture to say that not another group had such an enduring bond as the love that bound this particular group of individuals together. They may have had personal agendas, (I didn't say they were *perfect* people on the *perfect* committee), but they all seemed to have this central common goal. Their work, and resulting concrete evidence of that work, is on record for all to see. The very fact of the name change of their Committee is the ultimate realization of the changes they were making for a better future for people with disabilities.

They have helped remove some big barriers, and they made great strides in a relatively short amount of time. But there is *so* much more work to be done. So many changes need to take place before we can all agree that full equality has taken place in all aspects of the life of a person with a disability.

During planning times they voted on possible dates for the next meetings, and for the topics to be taken up for dissemination and discussion. Windy listened to the proposals, and her hand always went up for the count, along with everyone else's. That's the ultimate, her vote *was* recognized and *was* counted. Everyone in those meetings is to be commended for setting the standard for Americans who have a disability.

It is evident to us that Windy *was* born for this!

Monday morning, the day of her meeting, begins for us very early. Windy and I rise two hours before the 8:00 starting time, so we can do our hair and dress without too much rushing, to get out the door on time. (It takes me a while to roll her hair, and mine, and to polish fingernails.

A quick walk to the outside, down some concrete steps, and across a busy street, and we entered the building we were looking for, where the U.S. Department of Health and Human Services Administration For Children and Families offices are located. We stopped at the guard station while she showed them her government badge. David, Mikey and I presented our papers. Soon all our names were checked off their list, and we were given permission to pass through Security. After receiving clearance from Security, we took an elevator to the designated floor.

We got to the proper door and went in. The committee meets in a room where the members sit behind their nameplates at large tables that form a rectangle so that the members are all facing in and toward one another. Windy went in quietly and assessed the room, as is her way of processing who was there and where she was to sit. She spots her nameplate and deposits her purse and the black and hot pink briefcase with a large pink W on one side, down beside her chair, within easy reach. She looked around the room. Her face lit up as she recognized faces, and she quietly began to go around the room, walking up to people as she bid them, hello.

We watched her as we found a seat in the row of chairs provided for visitors. She shook some hands, and gave hugs to others on her way to the coffee and refreshment table. She felt needed and happy at these times, and although very quiet, we know her to be, at the same time, very alert. She listened to everything being said and was usually vocal to us afterwards about her opinion on something she had heard that day. It takes time for her to mull over the whole thing and to process. Believe me she *does* process it.

We wished she would tell them out loud what she said to us in private. But, she probably never will. It is just her way. I think she feels it might not be nice to speak out and say what she thinks in a crowd because she might hurt someone's feelings. She, who has had her feelings hurt in many situations, is very hesitant to regale her own opinions to someone else. In a way we wish more people had as high a regard for others as she does. She has taught us another "pearl," an important thing in life to know: Never mistake a soft or a quiet response from someone as a sign of ignorance. You may be very sorry, and you may miss an invaluable opinion that impatience (and impertinence) can cause you to miss. Truly a wonderful **WINDY LIFE LESSON.**

This particular meeting was called to order by the Executive Director, Sally Atwater, and Chairperson, Madeleine Will. (Madeleine, and George Will have a grown son named John who was born with Down syndrome. Her heart was in the committee's workings, one hundred percent, for obvious reasons.) The members quieted down and took their assigned seats. The committee seemed ready "to roll up their sleeves and get to work."

The speakers, who were asked to come and talk to them that day, begin presenting their programs to acquaint their listeners with their various concerns for the people with disabilities. They came in hopes of having the committee focus on some of the greater national needs, to educate them about the needs, and to tell of some of the ways the government might be able to help them come up with better solutions to some of those needs. They hoped to improve the lives of people with disabilities in specific arenas. Many people came representing many groups, who have worked hard through the years to help those who can't help themselves. It was evident that much work and research had gone into the presentations, and we learned so much. Twenty committees couldn't possibly get the work completed on all the needed areas, yet gallantly, the members began to discuss and to vote on the ones they tried to prioritize.

Lunch break came and they adjourned for one hour. We got up, and Windy motioned for us to come on, as she tapped her pink, digital wrist watch—her way of letting us know we had to hurry and leave for her next appointment. Michele Tennery, who Windy had invited to go with us to lunch and to see the Pistons, came alongside the four of us. Sally Atwater waved to us as we walked out of the door, and we stopped to allow her to catch up with us.

Sally said, "Windy, I know you're leaving in a minute to go over to the White House. Would you like to take a copy of the Committee's new booklet and the companion pamphlet with you today?" Windy had already asked her permission to miss part of the afternoon meeting, in order to attend the special function. Our daughter replied in her forever positive and enthusiastic tone of voice, "Sure!" Quickly spoken, but not said without some thought. She was extremely proud of the concrete evidence the booklet represented of all the work of the PCPID Committee on which she served. "Maybe," Sally suggested to her, "you might have a chance to give it to the President. If you do get to see him, it's all right to hand it to him."

At this revelation David and I exchange glances. We feel somewhat uncomfortable with this suggestion and talk about it later with Michele over our lunch. We hated to think that President Bush might feel that Windy was being too pushy, or that he might believe she was being manipulated by someone else. We fully trusted Sally, but we wanted to be sure about this. (The last thing we wanted was for Windy to try to hand something to the President, and the Secret Service step up to stop her, as they protect him.)

Michele assured Windy that it was perfectly *fine* for her to give it to him if the situation should arise and if she had a chance to hand it to him. It was the way things were done in D.C. We trusted her protocol knowledge, but we weren't convinced in our own minds that it was okay for our daughter to do this task. We, too, were proud of the Committee we had the privilege to watch in action, and we knew the work, and many hours that had been poured into that booklet. It was a great testimony to the dedication and sacrifices made for the intellectually disabled citizens of America.

If the President did have a chance to see the booklet, it would be a fabulous opportunity for everybody. It was worth taking a chance on it being misinterpreted, we decided. We asked Windy, (who had been listening to every word Michele had said), if she felt good about it. In typical Windy style she quipped, "I *want* the President to see the booklet! Now let's eat some lunch!"

Guess we knew how Win felt about it. She had already decided she was *going* to pass this on to her friend, George W. So much for thinking we had helped her in her decision! That girl had already made up her mind. She believed the job she had been given was an important one, *and* she was a ready and able servant. I was impressed and humbled.

Thank you God for a daughter who is able to show us all how to live a God-led life. Thank you for another ***WINDY LIFE LESSON****!*

Windy held tight to her papers, and we left the building to hail a cab. One stopped for us, and the five of us squeezed in. We were used to having many family members in close proximity for times such as this, and thankfully, Michele was a real sport, being one of seven children in her family, she squeezed right in with us. (It was a privilege to call Michele a friend. She would email us one day with the news that her beloved sister, Kathy, had died at the age of fifty-eight. Kathy had been born with Down syndrome. We were sure she would be sorely missed by all those who loved her so very much. Our hearts truly grieved for them. Michele was so sweet to Windy. Her compassion was real because she was a sibling of someone who had been born with a disability.)

Since we had two hours for lunch the day of her special invitation to see the pro basketball team, and plenty of time before we had to check in at the White House's East Gate, we went to one of Windy's favorite eating establishments, the well known, 'Old Ebbitt Grill'. There is so much history surrounding the place. Past Presidents, Statesmen and Stateswomen alike, have been patrons since Presidents Grant, Cleveland, Harding, and Teddy Roosevelt began going there for food and ale. It's still a popular place to meet for those who are political insiders, authors, journalists, and celebrities. You never knew who you might see as you walked through the restaurant. It was also within a short walking distance of the White House.

It was in this place that we had a good visit with Michele. She gave us a crash course, a brief 101, on government processes. She told us about how there are so many bills and official documents that any one President could not possibly see them all. They are all read and studied, but not necessarily by him personally. Very few are read by a President. His Staff's job is to study the reports, and then in turn, educate the President by conference, email, and messenger-representative, on the contents of the reports. He attends *many* briefings during a day. The PCPID's booklet and companion booklet (written for those who have a disability, so they can easily read and comprehend it) had already been sent to the President, and previously reviewed and been approved for publication. It probably never got as far as actually being in his hands.

This was a great opportunity for the President to see and read the PCPID's material for himself, she assured Windy. And we thought this day and invitation were going to be a fun time at a special social event. We were now aware of another mission that she had been called to do, a serious side juxtaposed to the fun. It seemed benign enough, but it could have huge implications for those who needed help.

> On a deeper level, when you pray for God to use you, don't be surprised when He calls you into action. You can rest assured He has worked out *all* the details, to the tiniest degree, even if it *is* all a bit of a surprise to *you* when the events unfold.

We have wondered if maybe Sally, Madeleine and Michele had arranged all this so Windy would at least have the opportunity to give the President this booklet. Even if they had arranged plans to this point, there was no guarantee she would get to speak to him. It was a gutsy move on their part, if that's what had been conspired, but it turned out to be a *real* gutsy move on Windy's part, to carry through with it. If she hadn't believed it was for the best, she would have refused to pass it along. That much we *do* know!

At two o'clock sharp, we were standing on the sidewalk with a small gathering of people. We were at a locked and guarded, black iron gate that led into the East Wing of the White House. It was freezing cold, and we moved about to keep the circulation going. I showed Windy where to stand to take every advantage of the weak, pale sunshine. We were too excited to let a little cold weather take away our joyfulness. Who would have thought David and I would again be following a child of ours through the doors of the home of a President? That surreal feeling, as if watching everything on a movie screen, and not actually a real participant, came to me as it does on moments such as this as the gate swung open, and we filed in one at a time as they checked our ID's and directed us to pass through the metal detectors. Security was very tight.

As we came out onto the driveway, we saw other people heading to a specific door, and we followed. We had never walked on this side of the compound, and we enjoyed seeing the grounds from another viewpoint. Windy walked faster than she normally does and told us to hurry up. She and I both had on leather boots with high heels, and you can only walk just *so* fast in those things. We wound our way down the drive to a sidewalk, and then up a series of stairs to the large, glass-paned double doors. We were greeted by White House Staff and the Military Personnel assigned to this event as they opened the doors for us.

Our coats were checked at the second door down on our left, and we entered a great hallway. We were busy taking off our outerwear and trying to take in all the surroundings, simultaneously.

There was *so* much to see: The majestic doors and trim, high ceilings with oversized crystal chandeliers, hanging about every fifteen feet. We all remained clustered in a group until a Staffer directed us to the large marble staircase.

Just before our group ascended the stairs, a friendly young man said hello to us, and told Windy that the President was delighted that she and her family could make it today. He said he worked on the Staff and had been watching for us, and that he wanted to usher us to our seats. We followed him up the stairs. We stopped at the top, as some of the Press made their way past us as they entered the East Room.

The bright lights of the television crews were beaming light and heat into the room from their position along the front walls. The rows of chairs were filling up with family members of the Pistons, the Mayor of Detroit, and the Governor of Michigan. We were surprised as the kind young man led us *all* the way up to the third row from the front, where our seats were waiting for us, indicated by each of our names on a printed name card placed in the chair seats. Since the rows were placed on a slant, Windy's seat looked directly onto the stage and podium before her. She would have a great view of the ceremony. She was shorter than most of the people in that room, especially on that day with the extremely tall gentlemen who occupied the room. She could not have possibly seen over anyone's head form a seated position. Someone else had thought ahead about that for her. She was on an aisle seat. If the President walked down the aisle, she would be close enough to see him face-to-face.

We filed in, first Michele, then David, then me, and next Mikey, with Windy seated on the outer aisle seat. She picked up her place card and handed it over to me and sat down. We began to look at our surroundings. This was the first time any of us had been in the East Room. It was a gorgeous and elegant room. We tried to take in all the details. The ceilings were super high, and the tall walls were heavily trimmed in painted, thick wooden molding. The voluptuous gold fabric, on the floor-length drapery at each window, was outstanding. The gigantic oil portraits looking down on us were all familiar faces of past Presidents, and their respective First Lady. We were sitting in front of the famous portrait of George Washington, painted by Gilbert Stuart, *the* one that Dolley Madison had yanked off the wall and saved as she fled in haste, during the raid and subsequent burning of the White House by the British Army in the year 1814. (During the War of 1812, we looked it up later so we could tell Windy all about it.)

We felt like we were sitting in on a History Channel Special as we looked up at the picture. How beautiful the White House and all its national treasures looked to us. How awesome that this lovely house belongs to every citizen in this great nation.

Right on time, and maybe a few minutes early, the Detroit Piston team members began to file into the room, and the camera shutter lenses could be heard as they began to click profusely around the room. The tall, giant-sized men filled the bleacher steps up on the stage. Their coach, Larry Brown was almost dwarfed by these men, who had played their hearts out and won the 2004 World Basketball Championship. They were there to receive the award presented to them by President George W. Bush in recognition of their tremendous accomplishment. Windy sat up straight with her hands folded in her lap as she looked at the President and the team with rapt attention. She did look back at Mikey and smiled once, and then quickly turned back to the happenings before her. She knew he was enjoying all of this with her. She is always respectful and shows great dignity at such times as this. We are never concerned that she won't act appropriately.

After the President spoke and presented the award in the short ceremony, he walked up into the bleacher steps, where the team was standing, and the photographers went wild. He made a point to shake every team member's hand and said things to them personally, that only they could hear. After a few minutes of photo moments with the team, he stepped off the stage and into the audience, that was still standing at their chairs. He went around shaking the hands extended to him and stopped to talk and laugh with some, as he made his way slowly down the aisle.

Windy was standing up and clutching the booklet to her chest. David and I watched as Blake, the President's Aide, saw Windy and smiled, and says, "Hello, Windy!" and he came to stand right at her side. He was there for the President to move his way, as he slowly proceeded to the back of the room. David and I said almost at the same time, "Give it to Blake, Windy, give it to Blake." We thought it was a wonderful opportunity to hand the booklet over to his personal Aide, who was now a personal friend, and an e-mail buddy of Windy's. They had been e-mailing each other occasionally ever since they met in the Knoxville airport. (During President Bush's first term, she would write a quick note just to check up on George W., and Blake was kind enough to answer her, each and every time, no exception, and pass on her message of encouragement to the President.)

We thought she would hand the booklet and committee's letter to Blake. No deal! She didn't even look our way, just shook her head no, and kept her eyes locked on the President. She hadn't put in all that hard work from her heart for the President's Aide, much as she liked and respected Blake. It was obvious to us that she was waiting for the 'Big Man' to give her Committee's booklet to. Finally, the President got to our row, Blake a few steps in front of him, with the Secret Service surrounding him, and he stopped and looked right into her upturned face, and exclaimed, "Windy, how are you? It's great to see you!" He hugged her and kissed her on the cheek. He continued by saying he had heard she was in D.C. for a meeting. She said, "I am! And I would like to give you this!", and she handed him the booklet from the PCPID. Her smile was big and real.

When he left, he had a copy of the committee's report to read and to look over. It made her happy for him to know that The President's Committee for People with Intellectual Disabilities had been busy doing good things for Americans with disabilities. (It was so exciting to Madeleine and Sally when they heard the whole story. It was rewarding to them to know the sacrifice and hard work of the PCPID had not gone unnoticed.) It had been a good afternoon for her, *and* for the PCPID, for sure. (PCPID's staff was also pleased— Sheila Whittaker, was always sending Windy the Committee's info, and somewhere on the pages, she would draw a smiley face or pen a short, friendly message to her. It showed an outstanding, kind spirit behind the sober professionalism she portrayed at the meetings.)

The guests were then allowed to move about the room and meet the Piston team members. They were kind enough to stand for pictures to be made with them. Mike and Windy enjoyed meeting many of them and getting some pictures.

We have a great photo of Windy and a White House staffer, Katie. They are both smiling at the camera, with the game ball that had been presented to the President. Katie had been instrumental in getting Windy to this exciting sports event and had been so kind as to allow Windy to be included in the special pictures and tours of the White House. As we left the East Room, we were free to walk into the beautiful rooms to our left, and to our right. We were escorted by the many military personnel dressed in their uniforms and serving as "guides" who followed closely behind all who entered the rooms on view. It was awe-inspiring to walk about in the footsteps of our past (and present) Presidents and their families.

I whispered to Windy that I'll bet even 'George and Laura' still feel the amazing feeling you get when you walk and live 'smack dab' in the middle of history. It's not something that one would forget or become used to I'm sure. She nodded a big "Yes". We followed her into the gorgeous Green Room where the silky damask-like fabric on the walls make a fitting background for the stately, gold-gilded frames of the massive portraits of Andrew Jackson (another Tennessean!) and of Benjamin Franklin. One of the military personnel informed us that the room is referred to as the twenty-dollar room because of the wavy green color and design of the wall covering, with Jackson's portrait on the wall. Windy stood back and looked up, and then, smiled and said, "Oh, I get it!" You do feel as if you are looking at a giant, twenty dollar bill.

We went into the next room, where the State Dinners are served, and we were surprised at the understated elegance of the room. It is an immense room, sparely furnished with a large, long table in the middle of the space. The real glow of the room must come from the people who attend the functions held there. The chandelier overhead and the large fireplace, with a prayer engraved in the white marble, must have paled in comparison to the lively personalities who have graced the place in the antique chairs surrounding the grand old table. Windy and I said we could almost hear the buzz of past conversations and the gentle clinking of fine china and crystal, during the dinner courses served to so many influential people down through the years. It was fun to imagine.

We also walked into the President's Working Library. It had the warm, inviting smell of ancient book leather, almost beckoning one to walk over and pick up a book, to read the hidden words within. We didn't touch the books however, *or* the walls *or* heavy wood molding that surrounded each doorway and window. We kept our hands to our sides as we "touched" everything with our eyes. The temptation to feel for ourselves was strong, but not permissible. We wanted our grandchildren and everyone else's grandchildren to be able to come back and see the very things we saw, to see what our predecessors put in place for America to own together. It wouldn't take too long for the wear to show if everyone who entered rubbed the wood or touched a painting. Restraint is often a good thing!

It was getting time for all guests to leave. There was no spoken word, but we grew aware of the "guides" behind us closing ranks and slowly and purposely directing us to the stairway we had ascended earlier that afternoon. Those who remained walked as a loosely gathered group down the stairs to the room used as a large coat and outer wrap closet. We handed our ticket stubs to the men who had checked our things, and we received our coats and scarves. Wrapping up to combat the intense cold weather waiting outside, we walked down the sunny hallway where we could view the White House grounds and landscaping just outside the wall of windows. Everyone was silent.

David looked lost in thought as I watched him walk ahead of us. I saw him slow his steps as he looked to his left at a larger than life statue of Abraham Lincoln. I watched him take it all in, the deep thought-provoking look chiseled into President Lincoln's face, the pain so palpable in his brow and eyes as he seemed to look out beyond his time and space into a future time for all races of people in America someday. (I instantly feel *David* is larger than life. He is such a wonderful husband to me, and father to our children. I am reminded of my deep abiding love for the man before me. It was a precious moment for me.) An unsmiling man in the Secret Service, standing near the statute, kept his eyes on the group walking by. We like the fact that there was no doubt he took his job seriously.

We walked outside and breathed in the cold, fresh air and tried to clear the 'dreamlike' feeling we had after walking out of the White House. It almost didn't seem real that we were just inside those walls and in the presence of the President of the United States. We walked out of the tall, wrought iron gate onto the main sidewalk that surrounded the block. "What do you think, Mike?" Windy wanted to know what her younger brother thought about the trip his sister took him along on. For once Mike was speechless. "Well, Sis," he finally spoke out, "that was something! Certainly worth skipping a day of school for. Thanks for asking me!" They hugged as David and I stood on the street, grinning at the two of them.

(There was an old flowering bush that grew on the Clinch River bank at the home we bought from Mrs. Bond, when our children were younger. She had wandered through the landscaping with us as she educated us on the names of the various plantings she and her husband had laboriously tended to for fifty some years. There was a particular plant that had always stayed in our memories because of its colorful descriptive name, it was called "Hearts Bursting With Love." That name was a perfect description of how we felt right that moment on the sidewalk in D.C.)

We walked back over to the Aerospace building just as the PCPID Committee meeting was breaking up for the day. Windy had missed all the first afternoon's speakers, but we knew she had been on her own mission for the Committee, a mission only she could have carried out. The President had a copy of their report in his hands! That was awesome!

There are many Committees, and the President can't possibly see, or read all the reports they work on. It was fantastic that he would see this one with his own eyes. An important document *"Signed, Sealed and Delivered."* What a job well done, and yet we only quietly told Sally, Madeleine, and the Staff who worked for the Committee, that she had been able to "pass it along". We wondered when they would tell the others. We had no doubt Madeleine and Sally would tell them when the time was right, and when the focus would not be on Windy. She certainly didn't do it for praise.

We did hope they would all know how far their hard wrought efforts had gone, and by way of the very hands of one they were all there to help. Could it happen again? Probably not in a million years. You can't just hand the President something and not have the Secret Service down on you like *that*. The timing had to be just right, and we could not have *made* any of this happen. We were told it was a miracle . . . but we were not surprised at that. We have witnessed many miracles with our girl. Many.

We asked Michele to join us for dinner, and she said she had promised to take Michael Rodgers and his support person, Lisa, to dinner at a seafood place Michael has asked to go to called the *Seafood Market*. They asked us to join them, and we were pleased to say yes. Michael is a delightful person to be around. He was the only other self-advocate, besides Windy, serving on the PCPID, and they traveled all the way from Washington State to attend the meetings. Michael is almost completely wheelchair mobile. He cannot read the written word, but he was a whiz with new technology—a computer program that reads aloud his emails and reports. He holds a job with the state of Washington, in a self-advocacy role, advising the government agencies in the best interest of people with disabilities. He has a "cut to the chase" attitude, and wraps it successfully in a great sense of humor.

He also has great discernment. He knows if someone is sincere, almost the moment he meets them. To his displeasure, he makes the trips without his wife, Emily, who has to stay home because of her job situation. If life had been different for him at his birth, if he had not been born with a disability, undoubtedly, Michael would have run for office himself. He's just that type of fellow. An overachiever with a drive to be the best he can be! Be assured, Michael Rogers *is one of* the best!

Lisa is a very sweet, soft-spoken woman in her thirties. She accompanied Michael to the meetings as his Support Person. She might be called to read a handout to him, or she may do something as simple as getting him a drink of water. She has a full-time job back home, and is a singer with a band. (She's a great singer. She sang, *Somewhere Over the Rainbow,* a cappella, for us one evening!)

The six of us sat and enjoyed our visit together. David said our blessing, and we all shared about how our faith played such an important role in our lives. We were all blessed to get some down time with such special friends. Michael and Windy both spoke brightly of their hopes for the direction the new report would take the country for people with disabilities. Their enthusiasm was contagious. They just hoped the word got out and that many people could be exposed to the good things being done, in our government, on behalf of this group of citizens. We all agreed and started suggestions, as we went around the table, on how the facts could be made known. Windy and Michael suggested newspapers or magazine articles, and we all wondered how this might be accomplished.

All of a sudden Michele looked up and said to us quietly, "You're not going to believe this, but a reporter for a national magazine just walked in, and he is sitting at the table in front of us!"

"That's it!" Michael Rogers exclaimed, "Let's go over and ask him to write a story on this!"

"I'll go with you, Michael," Windy chimed in. "Give me my lipstick, Mom. Quick!" she said, as she frantically shook her free hand at me to get her lipstick out to give to her, while wiping her mouth off with her dinner napkin, with the other hand. She was prepared to do her part for the cause she held dear to her heart. I complied with her request as David stood up to help Michael get his suit coat back on. They were going to present themselves in proper attire. Michele ran to her car, parked just out front on the curb, to retrieve a copy of the PCPID's new report to the President, so they would have a hard copy to give to the reporter.

It was inspirational to watch the two of them, Windy helping push Michael's wheelchair over to the writer's table, where he sat alone. We sat there in silence, and in immense admiration for Michael and Windy. It took guts to go over to him cold turkey, and make their introductions, and inform him of their Committee's work. Being a powerful writer on the triumphs and perils of the human race, I hope he now realizes how much gumption it really took for them to approach him.

Actual words could not be heard, but we could see that they had an attentive listener, and after handing him the PCPID's report, they turned and made their way back us. We smiled at their contagious smiles, spread from ear to ear. They reported the writer had been nice and promised them he would look it over. They could both see in their mind's eye a big spread, possibly in the next issue. (Michele told them he wrote for the magazine and for other publications that could help educate people, and eradicate the many barriers that stand in the way of full inclusion of all people with a disability.) It would have been a wonderful, helpful, and touching article for many people to read and see . . . but it was not meant to be. Although Windy and Michael searched every issue of the magazine for some sort of mention for weeks later, there was never a word about it.

The tenacity and courage of Windy and Michael Rogers was tremendous. They were real heroes. The two of them were as responsible for the word change as anyone else in many ways. They had lived under the old terminology and had helped to erase it and usher in a new day for everyone with an intellectual disability. This had been a victory for all Americans who have had to live with the "R" word all their lives.

When we were finished with dinner, we all left the restaurant and went our separate ways to our respective homes . . . our demographics involved interior states, and states from coast to coast.

Federal governmental meetings this high up are: invigorating, encouraging, exasperating, exhausting and exciting—simultaneously. Washington, D.C. is the arena the entire world watches to see our freedoms and governmental process in action. And to think our daughter Windy played such a gigantic active role on a Presidential Appointed Committee! It is almost too much to ponder as we head out of the city on our way back home to Tennessee and Mikey headed his car toward Virginia.

This trip was full of special "Windy" moments, and David and I talked over some of the highlights with her as the views out the car windows turned from cityscape to a more rural scene. From the backseat, Windy put one hand on her dad's shoulder and one on my shoulder and pated us gently. "Thanks for bringing me to my meeting, Mom, Dad." We said an empathic, "You're welcome!" as both of us thanked her for allowing us to come with *her*, as her supporters. She got a little teary eyed as she looked back in the direction of D.C. and said, in a quiet, low voice, "I hope I see the President again sometime soon. I am going to be praying for him and Miss Laura and their whole family, and that I get to visit with them again." Then she turned, and fixed her eyes forward, as she placed her headphones on her head. It wasn't long until she was asleep, resting in that peace we all try to obtain. She leaves her request at the feet of God, and has the unwavering faith to believe He knows what is best.

Our daughter has likes and dislikes like anyone else. She loves sports, especially being there in person, watching or participating. She enjoys basketball and football games and anything the University of Tennessee is playing. She loves it anytime someone asks her to attend a game with them.

She likes helping others and always prays for our troops. She has written letters of encouragement to soldiers, and has bought, packed up, and shipped off socks, gum, energy bars and powered drink mix through the years. Often when she sees a soldier on leave at an eating establishment, she will not eat until she has spoken to the person waiting on them, and then either pays for his or her meal, or asks us (her family) to pay for their meal. She never reveals to them who paid for the meals, just smiles and has a joyful heart as she eats her dinner. We do, too!

She likes the Broncos because she likes Denver and Payton Manning (a former UT Vol). She likes to watch the Lakers sometimes. We don't know why they are her pick, but they are. She also enjoys a Braves and Rangers game on television from time to time. The Braves because it is her sister-in-law, Treva, and big brother's favorite baseball team. The Rangers because of George W.'s involvement with the team, and because she knows one of the strength and exercise trainers for the team, Jose Vasquez. Jose married Anne Campbell, a friend of Windy's from CAK school days. They have told her they see the former President at the games sometimes. If Jose or Ann ever get the chance to tell G.W. that they know Windy, I'm sure he may wonder just who this woman named Windy is and how she knows *so* many people!

A couple of years ago we ran into a friend we had not seen in years, having dinner at a restaurant. Windy, David, and I walked by his table and he stood up to speak to us. He talked for a while and then suddenly, he said, "Former Governor Don Sundquist and his wife, Martha, just walked in. I happen to know them. I'll introduce you all to them if you'd like to meet them." Before he had gotten all his words out Windy rushed over to say hello to the Sundquists, and we all heard the Governor say brightly, "Well, hello, Windy!" She hugged Don first and then Miss Martha. Our old friend turned back to us and said, smiling, "Well, I should have guessed that she knew them, or to be more accurate, that they knew her! Cool!"

She's like the cute little character, Goldbug, in the children's book series, written and illustrated by Richard Scarry, called *Busytown*, and *Cars and Trucks and Things That Go*. We used to read those books to our kids and they loved to look for the tinny mouse that's hard to spot, but always present, on each brightly colored and busy page. You never know where you will spot '*Goldbug*' or our Windy, enjoying life to the fullest! She loves being where the action is. (She especially likes going to her nephews' soccer and basketball games. She loves to cheer them on!)

She has become a workout fanatic and is very disciplined in her adult years. She works out with weights, and exercises aerobically on an elliptical or a treadmill several times a week. We never have to tell her to go get some exercise. She doesn't like to miss a workout, and plans her day around it. She's gotten into great shape now and can walk great distances without getting winded. She still isn't interested in hiking, but she goes anyway and hikes without complaining. She knows the rest of her family members like it.

She has hopes and dreams for her life like we all do. She would love to meet the man of her dreams, *after* she meets her current crush. She is crazy over actor Zac Efron. No matter how many times we have told her she will probably never meet the guy, she is eternally optimistic about their first meeting.

She also hopes to meet Dolly Parton in person and talk to her about all that hair and fashion and frilly pink stuff. She likes Miranda Cosgrove and Debby Ryan and thinks that if they were introduced they would hit it off and become BFF. She dreams often of becoming an actress. She can just see herself starring in a guest appearance role on a Disney sitcom. She is never a Drama Queen in real life, but we know she'd make a great actress and could portray a wonderful Drama Queen!

She loves music, especially Christian music. She listens everyday to the radio station *Air1*. Some of her favorite musicians are: David Barnes (who went to her high school!), Nichole Nordeman (who she got to meet in person), Jeremy Camp (met him backstage once), Danny Gokey, and David Archuleta, and Matt Kearney. She also likes Train and Big Time Rush.

She still wishes for a car of her very own, specifically a VW bug painted a lovely shade of bubblegum pink, of course. If she could wrangle up the funds she'd have one in the driveway right now! (We think she'd say she was ready to drive if she had one!)

Windy loves to bake and has an interesting collection of aprons she has bought or people have given her. She rotates wearing them each time she's cooking. She loves to watch the Food Channel, especially *The Pioneer Woman*, Ree Drummond. Ree can do no wrong in the kitchen, and she cooks everything just right in her mind, as she watches Ree make exciting culinary creations. She asked me if she could be a guest on Ree's show. I know what my daughter's thinking. She can just imagine herself mixing up cupcakes alongside of Ree, talking and laughing about clever things they'd say to each other, as they mix batter with abandonment! A horse ride on the ranch before the ovens heats up, and right after the aprons are untied, wouldn't hurt a thing, either, we're thinking!

Windy *adores* fashion. Anyone who knows her knows she is always dressed up and dresses very fashionably and put together. She dreams of starting her own clothing line and still draws and designs fashions all the time. (She's really good at it, too! She has that "certain something".) She'd like to go watch the models walk down the runway in the latest styles. She's quick to tell me what looks good on me, her grandmother, and her sisters-in law. She's usually right!

Windy Jeanne is adamant about her hair and her clothes, and she certainly has a flair for decorating. She loves, loves, loves, the color pink, and always has a touch, if not a complete outfit of the color on every day. She wore pink in 2000 to the White House when it was not exactly the perfect color choice of the masses, who worked in D.C. at the time. Black was the accepted color choice for most. She confidently (and adamantly, at least when she opposed my wardrobe choices for her attire), wore pink, or pink and black, and always with cute dress boots, or cowgirl boots. When I questioned whether she should wear the boots to a meeting, she told me, "Sure, I should. Our President's from Texas. He probably has them on right now!"

Always she looked like a 'doll' at her meetings, and people couldn't help but comment on how darling she looked. As her mom, I have had many discussions with her on what she buys, what she wears, and how she decorates her room. (Mothers of daughters know what I'm talking about here!) Usually at these times, I lose by default, or exhaustion. After all, she is an adult, and her strong opinions are partly my doings. I am directly responsible for making her so darn independent!

She is never theatrical, (now that she is an adult woman) and is completely without guile. Many times people are drawn to her refreshing sweetness and upbeat personality. A few times (thankfully, rarely) some people do not know how to interact with a person who has a disability. They back off, and back out, of any interaction with her. That's okay. It's their loss. God's timing is perfect. There may come a day when they will be able to get to know someone with a disability, and they will be surprisingly grateful for the time spent with them.

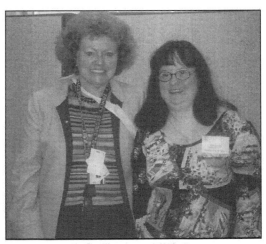

Sally Atwater and Windy

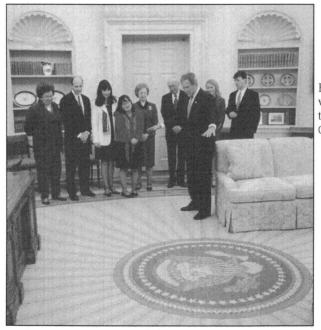

Family visit to the Oval Office

PCPID Committee in Oval Office

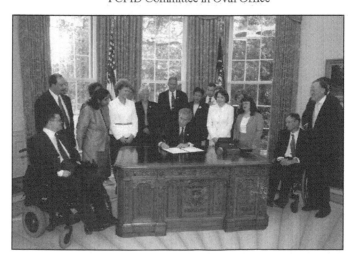

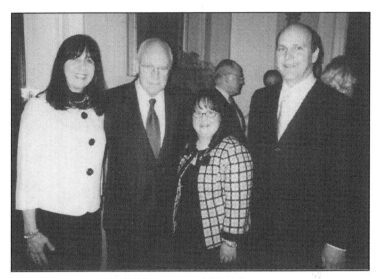

With Vice President Dick Cheney

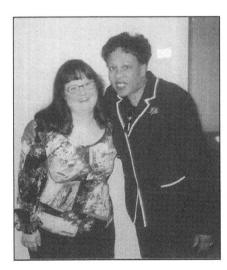

With Kim Porter-Hoppe

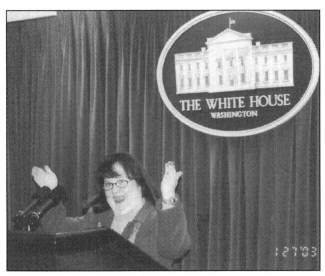

At the podium in the White House newsroom

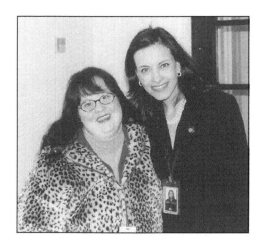

With Dina Powell

Chapter Twenty-Four
Windy Moments

Windy was asked to speak before thousands of students at Liberty University's Convocation in 2007 by Jerry Falwell. As the Liberty Journal, the Winter/Spring edition, described the speakers, "Liberty University continues to bring speakers of global significance in every sphere of society to address its student body in a thrice-weekly Convocation—the largest weekly gathering of Christian young people in the world." Pretty heavy. (Some of the past Convocation speakers include; Pastor and Author, Francis Chan (2011); Author and Founder of Joni and Friends, Joni Eareckson Tada (2010); Television Stars of Nineteen Kids and Counting, Jim Bob and Michelle Duggar (2011); Pastor and Author, John MacArthur (2011); Celebrity and real estate mogul, Donald Trump (2012); World-famous Pediatric Neurosurgeon, Dr. Ben Carson (2012); Veggie Tales Creator, Phil Vischer (2012); Best-Selling Author, Frank Peretti (2012); CEO of Focus on the Family, Jim Daly (2012); and NFL Standout, Tim Tebow (2013). The list goes on and on, but you get the incredible level of speakers that Windy was included in. (Not bragging, just stating facts so you can see how awesome it was for her to be included in this list.)

She jumped at the chance to speak at Liberty. She got to speak to several thousand students about her faith. She hoped to encourage them, *and* she got to visit with her brother, Mikey, and his good friends: Willie Roach, David Robinson, Ryan Lane, Daniel White, Matt Krause, Josh Dorsey and Gil T. Leon. These young men were all getting ready to graduate from the first class ever to graduate from Liberty Law School. These guys, along with all their classmates, were to be commended for persevering through the past four years. We admired their faith, drive and determination that had gotten them to this point in their lives.

We were in Lynchburg on the day Dr. Falwell died, and Windy said, "Oh, no, Mom! I know he's with Jesus now, but it makes me *so* sad for Liberty!" Tears coursed down her cheeks, right in the Wyndhurst area restaurant where we were having lunch that day. We saw the news of his death on the flat screen television on the wall above our booth. There was hardly a person in the entire restaurant who wasn't affected by his passing. So many of the servers working there that day had been, or were, students at the school. Strangers instantly became united as everyone stood before the newscast and mourned together. We immediately prayed for his family, for the school, and for Thomas Road Baptist Church where he had been the Senior Pastor.

Windy loved the little time she had spent in Pastor Falwell's presence, and she really enjoyed his sense of humor. She liked the stories Mikey and his friends told her of how he would often drive around the campus and stop to speak to the students. She cherishes the time he pretended like he was going to drive by, without stopping at the cross walk, as she crossed the street one day with her brother and his buddies. (Going about one mile an hour, or less!) He had hollered out his car window in greeting and waved a hand as he pretended to stop quickly, and he gave a big old smile to all those crossing the campus streets. Then he would stop and converse with the students about their majors, their instructors, their future employment, asking them where they were from, and where they were going when they graduated.

Someday, some of these students, who were in the audience when Windy spoke, will undoubtedly be faced with a decision when they find they are expecting a child with Down syndrome, or some other type of disability. We hope and pray they remember seeing a brave and sweet young woman speaking to them at their Convocation. We hope that memory will help them to bring that baby to term, and to follow the Lord as they raise their child. We think that's why she was there—to reach out, and give hope to the young women and men who heard her.

Ten years after she spoke at the Convention, Windy was invited to attend the Groundbreaking for the George W. Bush Presidential Library at Southern Methodist University campus in Dallas, in 2010. Don Evans hugged her and told her how honored he was to know her, and said what a huge part she had played in all of their lives. He asked her to please come to the Opening of the Library in 2013, again holding her small hands in his big hands, with a big smile on his face. She said she would be there. They hugged and said goodbye for the time being. Before we turned to go, he asked David and me if we would please bring her to the opening. We promised that we would try to be there.

Andy Card also visited with her at the Groundbreaking and expressed the same kind greeting, and invitation. His words to us about our daughter were so complimentary of her and of what she had meant to all of them. He spent several minutes catching up on how Windy was doing.

Dana Perino, Fox News Contributing Reporter, gave her a hug and greeting. Windy has had an indelible influence upon so many people. David discreetly pointed to the sky. I nodded in agreement, and bit my bottom lip to keep from crying! We know from whence our blessings had come.

Years later Windy's picture with Josh and Flo Jo still hung in the Knoxville Sports headquarters. A photo of Windy with President

George W. Bush hangs in a Farragut restaurant called Sam and Andy's. She loves to eat there, and they love her and put her picture on their wall. Her picture also hung in the West Wing of the White House for a while. It was a large color poster of the first Lady, Laura Bush, with her mesmerizing aqua blue eyes, with our Windy beside her, at the President's First Speech to Congress. That first public photo in the Memphis paper *was* the start of many more to come! Who could have guessed this all would have taken place? God had a plan. We just couldn't have imagined it or planned it this BIG!

Once, during George W.'s Presidency, Windy was called on her cell phone by an aide with the invitation to greet the President as he got off at Knoxville's airport to give a speech. He had requested for her to be there. (He never forgot her! Or maybe, Miss Laura had reminded him that Windy lived in one of the cities he was visiting that day? The end result was the same—she got the opportunity to visit with the President again. How sweet is that?) She told them she would love to come and she asked if they would speak to her mom about it. She handed the phone to me in the middle of an aisle in Wal-Mart—we were there with a "to do" list. Finding a quiet place where there was no talking, no music, and no announcements over the loud speakers was a difficult thing to do. (Try it some time.) We found a more private corner. We looked like prime shoplifters—leaning over and covering up something in our hands—the phone—but it was hidden from view—and then stooping over to talk quietly. We looked rather suspicious. Never-the-less, it had to be done. With calls like that you hesitate to say, "Hey, we're sort of busy right now. Would you mind calling us back in a little while?"

After opening our purses in a panic and digging up a pen and paper, we jotted down the date and time. Some lady, supposedly shopping, or maybe a plant to catch shoplifters, was beginning to lurk around us attempting to catch us in our mischievous deeds. I'm sure she was thinking she had two characters in range. I wanted to say, "Excuse me, the White House is on the phone, if you don't mind! I didn't say it though. Who would believe Windy was talking on her cell to *them*? Sometimes God's surprise blessings surprise even the one being blessed, and especially those around that person. After I spoke to the woman on the phone, Windy got back on and said, "Thank you for asking me. I can't wait!"

On the day of Air Force One's landing, we got up early, really early, to get dressed and get to the airport. Of course I knew how to get there. She kept asking me if I was sure I knew how to get there. I reassured her that I did (She knows I get lost very easily. She has helped me navigate in every major city in our home state, and in all the others we have visited. Okay. I get lost more times than not. Our GPS is not much help to me at times. I have been known to turn a seven hour trip into thirteen hours. No problem. So you can understand her concern here.) I told her that we had plenty of time. I drove into the small parking lot of the even smaller private jet airport. (It stands next to the main McGee Tyson Knoxville airport.) We parked the car and started walking to the main door. We were two hours early like they had asked us to be.

A bus pulled in and the door swung open, and the driver, a lovely African-American, named Maxine, a friend of Windy's that used to work with her at Goody's yells, "Hey, Windy. How *are* you?" You could hear joy in her voice as she greeted Windy. Windy was thrilled to see her as she had not seen her in months. Maxine had taken a new job, and Windy no longer worked at Goody's since she had been let go in a downsizing of her department (Several people, and I do mean several, were so angered by her being let go that they called us at the office to tell us they had "cut up their Goody's charge cards and were never going to shop there again." At least she didn't have to worry about those potential broken fingernails anymore!) Maxine and another African-American lady, Edna, had been so sweet to Windy and she loved them both and prayed for them on a regular basis. David asked her once who they were after hearing her speak so highly of them, and she answered, "My best friends, Dad. I work with them."

As soon as Windy recognized her friend, she said with a yell, "Maxine!" Windy ran up to the bus door, climbed up the steps, and met Maxine halfway. They hugged each other. Windy was every bit as thrilled to see her as she was to see the President later that morning. They were totally equal experiences in her estimation. She was blessed to see two friends, and it made her day. That thrilled *me*. Windy sees any, and everybody, on equal terms.

> (Why, oh why, can't we all see each other as she does? As God means for us to see each other, as He sees us? This is the confusing part: who has the handicap, the disability? Tell me again please, is it people like Windy or is it people like you and me? Why can't we love unconditionally like that and put our prejudices and degrees and agendas behind us, and go forward with a love for our fellowman? That is a **WINDY LIFE LESSON** we could all use!)

After the brief hello, Windy and I headed into the doors of the airport. There were several people milling around. Windy said, "Now what, Mom? Do we tell somebody we're here?"

"Sounds good, honey. Why don't we look for someone who looks like they might be in charge?" We eyed everyone in the small room. Lots of young aides coming and going quickly out of the room, but we were unsuccessful in picking out *the* person in-charge. It was hard to tell. Finally a guy came in, who looked our way, and

Windy and I walked up to him. She introduced herself to him and told him that she had been invited to greet the President at the plane. He was kind but understandably busy with all the details it takes for White House Staff to arrange a successful visit for the President. He told us his name and position. He said he had to check with the staff in charge of seating the people who were coming to hear the President speak, in the enormous airport hanger, just behind the wall where we stood. He asked us to take a seat, and he would send someone to check in with us soon.

The minutes ticked away as we were joined in the room by dignitaries, local and state, who were to fill the bleachers behind, and beside the President. Windy introduced herself and her mom to them as they filed by us to introduce themselves, shake hands, and then take a seat in the room. Rep. Marsha Blackman was one of the people we remember. She was cordial, but very quiet. She probably had a lot on her mind. Windy didn't know her, so she punched me with her elbow and quietly inquired who she was.

She asked me for about the tenth time if we needed to get her out to the plane. She was fearful of missing the arrival. So was I, now. We had asked someone about every thirty minutes or so where we needed to be, but without receiving any instructions. Everyone told us they would go find out, and then they just got busy with more pressing things and forgot, we supposed. We were trying to be polite and yet, felt time was of the essence here.

"Mom, I'm going outside to see if I see the plane."

"Okay. Let's go ask someone out there." So we went out the back doors leading to the smaller runway. There were many men in dark suits, white dress shirts, with an earphone in one ear, standing all over the place. There were also many police officers standing on duty out there. One particular Secret Service agent caught Windy's attention. He was tall, handsome and distinguished-looking with short cropped silver hair. She remembered seeing him once before and left me to walk up to him and introduce herself. I stepped up, and we explained our dilemma. He told her he remembered her, listened to our quick story, and then he said, "Ladies, please step back over here while I find out where you should go," and then he started telling our plight to someone over his microphone.

After just a few minutes a police car pulled up to the entrance, and the same agent came over to us and told us our ride was here. He explained that Windy was indeed supposed to be at the plane and that we had no time to waste—the plane was scheduled to land in less than ten minutes. And, by the way, we were at the wrong airport . . . we were supposed to be at the Naval Base across the tarmac from where we were! I had us in the wrong place? Windy would never talk to me again if I made her miss this exciting opportunity. I wouldn't blame her. I felt terrible about it.

The Secret Service agent quickly introduced us through the open passenger window to Officer Loundland (at least we think that was his name) who was in the driver's seat. He then opened the back door of the police cruiser, and Windy and I hurriedly climbed in. We thanked him sincerely for helping us. He said, "You're welcome," and then he leaned down and looked us in the eyes, and added, "Remember, ladies, the White House Staff may let you down sometimes, but President Bush's Secret Service will *never* let you down." With that he surprised us with a big smile (We didn't know they were allowed to smile on duty!), and he shut the door and we took off. The officer driving was a bit nervous. Okay, more than a bit. We could see the sweat beads forming on his brow. He had been given a huge assignment: beat the plane to the landing site!

We remained silent. All he needed was for us to start asking questions. We were speeding across the main airport tarmac with the possibility of Air Force One barreling down on us any second. Windy and I looked at each other and smiled weakly as we reached out for each other's hand. Would we make it in time? It wasn't looking good. I could hear her apprehensive intake of breath as the officer communicated with the control tower personnel. I was holding my breath. They were telling us to go back, and fast, because the plane was coming in, and we had to clear the runway, ASAP! Oh gosh, we were out there on the runway! Whatever happened to the boring life I envisioned for us after her high school years? I asked myself as I felt the palms of my hands start to feel clammy. She and her exciting life happened, that's what! Boring wasn't on the radar for us, but an in-coming plane certainly was. We raced right back to where we had come from. We made a U-turn, the old "Duke boys" in their car "The General" would have been proud of! Soon we were pulling up to the same door we had just left.

We thanked our driver for giving it his best effort, and then we both turned and tried to open our doors to get out. He had given it his "best shot". We were grateful for his gallant attempt. Silly I know, but we kept trying the door handle without avail. We didn't know you couldn't open the back doors of a police car by yourself. We know now.

Two officers came over to let us out, and then they escorted us several yards away from where the President's car, and his entourage of cars, would come through in the next few minutes. There we stood, not able to get back inside—our request to reenter the building had been denied emphatically. They were only doing their job, but we knew we were supposed to be in there, even though Windy had missed her chance to see George W. Bush. I looked over at her, and she wasn't smiling. She bit her bottom lip to keep from crying. She lifted up the edge of her glasses, and wiped away a tear. Then she straightened up and watched all the black SUV's and cars pull up and let the passengers out. There were so many people there to protect them that it was impossible to see who they were. Soon they were all in . . . and we were definitely out.

Forbidden to enter. Now what? Surely she would get to hear the President give his talk, even if she had missed her opportunity to actually get to see him and speak to him. There were places to stand where she could listen if we could only go in somewhere near the back. I had to try again for her sake. She was standing there looking so dejected when she had been so excited a few minutes prior to our mayhem.

"Windy, let's ask one more time, okay? Start praying!"

She squeezed her eyes tightly closed, "Go for it, Mom!"

The officer that had driven us on our wild tarmac ride walked by us. I asked him to please try to get permission to escort us back inside. His face turned a slightly grayer shade, but he said he would try. I think he felt partly responsible for her missed appointment but it hadn't been his fault. It wasn't long until he came back with another officer, and they took us back into the room, past the heavily guarded entrance, where we had waited all those hours. At least we were back inside.

Windy and I sat down. I was reflecting over the last few days. Hadn't God given her a once in a lifetime opportunity? Now was it a missed Divine Appointment? We both thought it was. So many times when everything looks hopeless, God shows us that He had something else in mind for us. Something that would be even better than we could imagine in our wildest dreams! We know this, have experienced these supernatural surprises, but we thought it couldn't happen *this* time. We had missed the plane, and the President would be whisked away for his next event in another part of the country. We sat slightly bewildered as to what we should do next? Remain seated in the almost empty room? Walk out the front doors to our car and leave? Then we saw a side door open.

"Windy. Mrs. Smith." We heard a young man's voice say, as he walked into the room, "I'm with the White House Staff, and I am so sorry for the mix up here today. We should have come looking for you all and gotten you to where you belonged. Please forgive us for our mistake."

Windy turned to shake the aide's hand, and then she said, so appealingly and sweetly, "Would you please explain to President Bush why I wasn't there? I hate to disappoint him." He looked at her upturned face, smiling her smile that says volumes without having to use words, eyes sparkling (with the aid of a few stray tears), and a wisp of Nina Ricci perfume wafting in the air as she moved towards him.

He was smitten. With real compassion he said, "I sure will. That's a promise. You just stay right here, and after his speech he may have a second to talk to you. I can't promise that, but I'll see what I can do. Sit tight for a few more minutes."

More waiting. (We could do "Wait". We had gotten good at it many times in our life. This was baby stuff!) After about twenty minutes, we heard the distant clapping and knew President Bush had finished speaking. More minutes ticked by as we knew he would be speaking and shaking hands with the many people who had come out to see him. Then true to his word, the young man finally came back to motion for Windy to come to the door that led to a long, narrow hall where he said they were leading the President out to a car, that would take him to the plane. "Stand right here, and the President will see you as he leaves."

I said, "Thank you", and patted him on the arm. I was so grateful. Windy would get to see the President after all, albeit probably just a wave goodbye. She would be satisfied and happy that she got to see him as he walked to the plane. That was wonderful! We were the only citizens in that hall except for several armed police and armed Secret Service at either end, and at each doorway. It was very quiet. She stood shifting her weight from one foot to the other. She was feeling the pinch on her feet from high heels and probably was moving a bit as a way to release some nervous energy. Her face sure didn't show any nervousness. She looked calm and collected.

All of a sudden her face lit up . . . she saw George W. step through the door on the far end of the hall, as he followed Secret Service people ahead of and closely behind him. He was walking briskly towards the exit, and would soon be passing directly by us.

"Wave, honey," I said to her as she stood perfectly still, refusing to lift her hand in a wave. I just stood still, too. Looking back, I think she knew he wouldn't just walk by and wave goodbye to her. She already knew him well enough to know that. I didn't, and I didn't have a clue as to why she *wouldn't* wave goodbye.

He stopped right in front of her (everyone with him came to an immediate stop) and he said, "Come give me a hug, Girl! You missed the plane didn't you? Well, I'm sorry, but I'm sure glad I got to see you today anyway!"

"Me too!" she said. "I'm still praying for you and Miss Laura!"

"I know you are, and I thank you. We need *everyone*'s prayers. Keep it up! How have you been? You're looking great. Are you exercising?" She had lost weight, several pounds, in fact, and beamed when she realized he had noticed. She was so proud that her hard work had paid off, and, that all her effort was recognized by the President was beyond fantastic!

He told her he had been running every day. She told him she thought that was great. He asked her how she was getting in shape, and she told him she was working out with weights and walking. He encouraged her to continue. How kind is that? He had the weight of the world on his shoulders, and yet he was spending what looked to the observers as unhurried time with a dear friend. He was as special as she thought him to be, and the feeling must have been mutual. I was in awe . . . of him, of her, of the situation, and especially of God! What a God moment . . . a private conversation with the Leader of the free world.

"I'd like you to meet my Mom, Vicki," she said with grace, and impeccable manners, as she included me in on her moment by stepping *slightly* to one side and waving her left hand in my direction. I moved towards them and extended my right hand to him as I saw his motion to shake mine.

"Hi, Mom!" he said as he shook my hand with firmness. "This is *some* lady!" he said of my daughter, as he looked back at Windy, and smiled. "We all love Windy!"

"She loves you all! Thank you for everything you have done for her."

"We thank *her* for everything she's done for us!"

One on one, he was very impressive. So alive. So energetic. And so funny. He smiled lots and seemed to love to joke with people.
"Have you ever been to the White House and seen the Oval Office, Windy?"

"Yes. Once I looked in the roped off room." She was led on a private tour on her first visit to the White House. The President was out of town for the day. Someone on his staff and Tennessee Rep. Jimmy Duncan, had planned a wonderful special tour for her of the White House and the Capitol. (Congressman Duncan was a friend of Windy's, and has been for a long time. We attended the same church in Knoxville, and she and Mikey had attended school with his daughter, Whitney. He was so kind to give her an educational tour of our nation's Capitol, and he took her to eat in the Congressional Dining Room during that same visit.)

"Well, you need to be able to *walk* into that room. It belongs to you, and to every American. It's the People's House. Blake, give Windy your card with your cell number on it." At that, a tall, really cute guy (I thought Windy might swoon!) stepped up, reached into his inner suit coat pocket and quickly jotted down his number. He reached out his arm, and Windy reached up to take it from him. They shook hands, and he smiled kindly at her.

"Get Mom and Dad to bring you to D.C., and you call Blake, and he'll arrange for you to come and see me at the White House, okay?'

"Sure, I'd love to!"

"Now, come and give me a hug goodbye. I've got to go hop on the plane, and give another talk in another city in this beautiful state of yours. I'll tell Laura I saw you today. That will make her happy." She obediently fell into his open arms, and they hugged tightly.

Blake looked over at me and smiled, and told me to please have Windy call any time. He had such fine manners, and seemed to be a really good guy. (We found out later he was a great guy! He and Windy became friends from that moment. He was always really respectful and sweet to her.) Everyone around this man, this President, had been super nice.

Windy and I smiled, and she said goodbye, and they began to walk away, and then—she waved. The President waved back! He and his entourage filed out. The door at the far end of the hall closed behind them.

First impressions do count! President George W. Bush was so energetic and at ease with people. It was obvious that he liked getting out and meeting people. When someone with that much of a lively personality leaves a room, the silence is all the more evident. Windy remained quiet. So did I. (I couldn't believe what had just taken place!)

We waited a few minutes until we got the all-clear, someone's voice on the other side of the closed door came over a walkie-talkie, and we were told he was out of the building, and on the way to the plane. The police, who had remained on duty in the hallway, began to file out.

One woman, a plain clothed police officer, or a security guard (we didn't know which), was on special security duty that day, and she hung back to walk out next to us. She looked over at me and said, "Wow, that was something! *Who* do you all know?" (Even she had been impressed with the rare conversing she had just witnessed!)

"Well . . . we, my husband and I, don't know anybody," I admitted to her, "but, *she*," and I gestured my head and my hand in Windy's direction, "*She* knows *him*!" and I pointed to the door where the President had walked out, only moments before.

"I *guess*!" she declared heartily. All three of us laughed at her statement, as we walked out the door and headed outside to feel the sunshine's warmth.

> *Heavenly Father, we thought we had missed the important moment and yet, You orchestrated an even better moment. What a Divine appointment and with a promise of another visit for Windy! How exciting for her. Thank you Lord, Thank you!*

"Mom, wait till Dad hears this! I can't *wait* to tell him! He'll be so surprised!" The bright daylight had stimulated her flow of conversation.

He was. Very surprised. And very grateful to George W. for befriending her. Our President had our respect because of his overwhelming kindness to our Windy.

President Bush kept his promise to her. She visited in the Oval Office *five times (*We think five but we really lost count!*)*, sometimes on official Committee business, and sometimes for a short personal visit by personal invitation of the President. She was responsible for taking along her parents, brothers, a sister-in-law *and* her grandparents with her on some of those trips. At her birth, David and I had been told that she might never walk. Well, she did learn to walk, and then years later we have followed her as she walked right into the Oval Office of the White House on several occasions!

And, we were told she might never talk when she was born! She has now spoken where millions have heard her on television and thousands in other audiences! We couldn't have planned it all, and we couldn't have made it happen like it has if we *had* planned it. Miracles? We *know* them to be. We watch for God to work in mighty ways because we've seen him do the impossible. More than once! We've lost count on those, for sure!

On another invitation to visit the Oval Office she had asked if she could bring her grandparents and brothers and sister-in-law with her. This was really stretching an invitation list. Another surprise from Windy. David and I believed it was a bit cheeky to even ask! After that call, her dad asked for the business card Blake had given to her and put it in his billfold so Windy wouldn't be phoning in anymore requests. He had it for safekeeping, he explained to her. I was more than a bit suspicious when she handed it over immediately. The White House Staff said they would have to check and see and would call her back with the answer. They called her back within an hour and told her yes, that President Bush would love to meet her family! We couldn't believe it.

What a trip *that* was. It was awesome! Her Poppie got to tell President Bush that he had not been to the White House since he was a boy of twelve, when President Herbert Hoover had been in office. President Bush told him "You really should come back sooner than every seventy-odd years!" They shared a laugh over that. When the President extended his hand to shake hers, her Gaymom Flo told him, "Put that hand away I'm going to hug you instead!" He laughed and said he'd be a fool if he didn't take her up on the offer. They hugged. Then Grandmother Juanita, looked him in the eyes, and instead of saying, Hello, she blurted out, "I love you!" He answered her by saying, "Well, thanks. You people from Tennessee are *real* friendly!" and we all laughed.

Windy told him her Poppie loved to play golf. The President walked right over to a cabinet, opened one of the lower doors, took out a golf ball with the Presidential seal on it and gave it to him. Poppie was so pleased. (He couldn't stop smiling at his granddaughter the rest of the day!)

Then President Bush showed us around the office, explaining the oil painting he brought with him from Texas entitled, *"A Charge We Have To Keep,"* and he explained the personal feelings the artwork evoked for him as a president and as a citizen. Then he told us he had a bust of President Lincoln to remind him of the former President and of all the other presidents who had gone before him—those who had worked to see this great nation through many other rough times. We stayed a good twenty minutes or so. A private tour is far more than we ever thought possible.

Windy was so thrilled that she got to lead her grandparents and family members into the famed home of the Presidents of these United States. The grandparents couldn't help but be astonished at the happenings. We were all astounded at the way things had turned out for this young woman of ours!

Another visit to the Oval Office with the President occurred when Windy took a leather Bible, engraved with his name on the front, for his sixtieth birthday gift. She also took him a CD of one of her favorite Christian singers, Jeremy Camp. She knew the President had an iPod, and she thought he would enjoy listening to it after he downloaded the music. Then, several months later, she heard Jeremy Camp was coming to Knoxville for a concert. She got Dave to go with her and she somehow (not even Dave knows how) got to go backstage and meet Jeremy, and got the chance to tell him about his CD, now in the President's hands (and ears when he went jogging)! Dave couldn't believe he got to go backstage with her. We are all still a little unsure how she got to go, but she's not telling all the details, and we don't know Mr. Camp personally, so I guess it will forever remain a secret. Dave and Mike really like to hang out with their sister. She's loads of fun, all by herself, and an added bonus is: you never know who she'll get to hang out with!

Windy finds joy in doing for others and *adores* giving gifts to people. She looks for ways to bless others by buying them something she has overheard them saying they wanted or needed. She takes notes when they don't suspect she's writing about them. She feels the giving of the gift so deeply that she is usually on the brink of tears as she hands a gift to someone. Sometimes she buys something she feels someone should have. One of those times was on President George W. Bush's sixtieth birthday. She knew it was going to be a big day for him. Sixtieth birthdays *do* tend to be big deals, and she wanted to give him something special. (She had a meeting in D.C. near his birthday date, and she had called to ask if she could come by to see him for a brief moment while she was in town. Permission was granted immediately.) She asked me to stop at the Christian bookstore.

On this particular day she walked in with purpose. First she went to the CD's and found just what she was looking for: a new CD by the singer and songwriter Jeremy Camp, and she quickly went up front to buy it. I hung back and watched her in action. (When she was a little girl, and had *just* learned to talk in an understandable dialect, I had insisted upon her walking up to the counter and placing her own order for a meal at McDonald's. She got over being shy, even if she had been initially fearful and had tried several times, and in several conniving ways, to get me to do it for her. I always refused for her own good. I knew she was capable of the task, and she had to learn to function in society. I realized I couldn't be there to interpret for her every wish and desire. Consequently, she learned to talk in a way that the person could easily understand her, and she was gratified by the positive reinforcement and results. Onlookers probably thought I was a horrible mom—I would not give a food order for the precious little girl who obviously needed help talking and being understood. I didn't care. I stood my ground, for her sake and now I was witnessing the positive results.)

Windy went directly to the section of new Bibles at the bookstore. She had written down the version of her dad's Bible, all on her own. She asked the woman who worked in that department for one like it. She showed her the words she had copied down. Soon the clerk held up a thick study Bible bound in beautiful green leather that Windy had selected. Very masculine looking. That was just what she was looking for. She asked if they could put (engrave) a name on it. "Oh," the salesclerk asked, "Is this a gift for your dad?"

"No. It's just a gift for a friend," she answered in a soft voice.

"Okay, do-you-know-the-person's-full-name? Or-do-you-have-it-written-down?" The woman was trying to be kind to her, and she was talking slowly and deliberately to Windy, so she could understand what she was asking. I guess she surmised Windy had Down syndrome, and she felt a need to speak a bit louder for more clarity.

"Yes,- I -do. It's- George-W.-Bush," she said back, slowly and deliberately, so the lady could understand *her*. I think she surmised the woman had a hearing problem because she spoke louder than was necessary for a normal conversation.

The lady looked up in surprise, "Really? You want *that* name put on *here*?" She pointed to the front of the Bible as she questioned the name to be printed in silver lettering.

"I sure do. Thank you. When will it be ready?"

"In about an hour," she replied and then went right to work on the transaction without asking any more questions. Windy paid for it from her savings she had hoarded away for a while. She put a dollar and some loose change back into her purse, all in the proper places. Then she slung her purse over one shoulder and directed her next words to the salesperson. "I'll be back. Thanks for your help." Then she looked at her pink plastic wrist watch, then at me and said, so matter of factually, "We have to come back in an hour, Mom. It's 2:00. We have to be back here at 3:00."

It was my turn to tell the woman we would be back. Her gift to "a friend" for his important sixtieth birthday was a done deal. Now all she had to do was wrap it and deliver it. Small details to her. The hard part was thinking of the *right* gift. The hard part was over. The rest would be fun! She was already officially invited and 'on the books' to visit President Bush in the Oval Office. Now she was all set to celebrate his big day.

Windy was invited to meet Air Force One on several other occasions at the McGhee-Tyson Airport in Knoxville. Lamar Alexander was on the plane with the President on one particular landing on January 8, 2004. Windy's friend, Smoky Mountain artist Robert A. Tino, had given her a large, original oil painting entitled "Anthem" he had done after 9-11 to give to the Bush family. (The painting was a beautiful work of art depicting a torn American flag blowing in the breeze, with a regal looking American eagle flying in front of the flag. It was sent to the National Archives to be photographed, numbered and then eventually, we heard, it probably went on to the Smithsonian.) When they debarked and got to the location where she had been directed to stand, Tennessee Senator Alexander came out first, and came over to shake her hand in a friendly greeting, and said, "Hi, Windy. It's so nice to see you again. I hear from President Bush that you and he are not just friends but that you two are buddies. That's really special. To be buddies is much better than being just friends!"

David and I already knew they were true buddies. We had given nothing to his campaign, and Windy had given him twenty-five dollars of her hard-earned money. (She worked at Goody's Corporate Office at the time. Jason Zachary, a friend of hers at Farragut, was also a coworker and would later run for 2nd District Seat in the U.S. House of Representatives.) These people were not just about those who gave thousands to support them politically, sure that was greatly needed and they were grateful for it, but they were interested in all people, and had real values that they lived out in their daily lives.

Windy was sent an engraved invitation to attend the Opening ceremonies for the George W. Bush Presidential Library and Center at SMU campus in Dallas, on April, 2013. Every living, sitting President of the U.S. (Including Carter, Bush One, Clinton, Bush Two, and President Obama) were also invited. She had to turn down the kind offer as it was a special man's birthday in her life. Her nephew Caleb's sixth birthday was the same week, almost to the day, in Colorado, and she already had her plane ticket to be there to help him celebrate. I guess you could say any one of her boys will always take precedent over the Presidents! Faith, family and friends, in that order.

The moment she heard that George and Laura Bush had become grandparents she said to me, "Well, Mom! *Now* they will understand why I just couldn't make it to the Library's opening!" I'll bet she's right about that!

Troy and Trey are twin brothers who also worked in the White House, in the Domestic Policy Affairs office, and they befriended Windy and us, and led us through the halls on several occasions. Both brothers are fast movers and shakers even though they are confined to wheelchairs. They both overcame a physical disability and succeed in their personal careers. Climbing the ladder of success doesn't take physical and intellectual perfection, but it does require determination, perseverance, a great lack of self-pity, also a strong faith in God, and personal moral integrity is *most* helpful. We have seen it work that way for many, many people in our own lifetime. Both Troy and Trey proved this once again to be true. These men were very impressive communicators.

On one personal visit in the Oval Office, on a January morning, Windy and President G.W. Bush were talking about the decorations in the room, the pictures hanging on the wall, the big speech he had to make that night. (He was scheduled to make his State of the Union Address that very evening!) She had been there for several minutes, probably fifteen, and then all of a sudden he said, "Now come and give me a hug goodbye because I've got to go practice my speech for tonight, and before that I am going to eat lunch with my friend, Tony Blair. He's the Prime Minister of Great Britain, you know."

Windy walked toward him to throw her arms around him in a farewell hug. "Sure, I know about Tony Blair. Please tell him I pray for him, too!" (She always prayed for him, it was true. It may be because one of her favorite Sunday School teacher's name was Tim Blair, their names sounded so much alike. Regardless she prayed for him and England, too. She didn't try to analyze it, she just did it.

England sounded like a neat country to her. One of her all time favorite entertainers was Davy Jones, an English singer with the group *The Monkees,* so she reasoned it had to be a great place, right?)

"I sure will!" the President enthusiastically said. "Now, get out of here!" he teasingly said to her. She loved his ever ready sense of humor. (She has always said he reminded her of her dad's cute sense of humor.) Andy Card, who was standing over in the right side of the spacious room was smiling big at this line as Windy giggled and obediently hugged her President goodbye.

Andy was always standing in the background watching out for the President during his watch. He was a great friend and a trusted advisor to George W. Bush. He was also very kind and respectful to our daughter every time we saw him. (Even to this day he tells us he will never forget Windy and the wonderful thing she did for all of them by speaking at the RNC in 2000.)

Windy also became good buddies with the President's two Personal Assistants, Blake Gottesman and later, Jared Weinstein. Blake had been introduced to her by the President, and he must have informed Jared about Windy. She met Jared at a Christmas party after he came over to introduce himself to her, not long after he began his new job as Blake's successor. Both young men were very sweet and respectful to her. They would respond back immediately to her every email for the entire eight years G.W. was in Office! How miraculous and kind is that? We advised Windy not to write the President too often. We told her she should not abuse the privilege of keeping in contact with him. She said, "I know, I know. I wouldn't do that. I'm not that type of person!" Boy, is that the truth, and she knows it! So anyway, she purposely stopped communicating for awhile.

When the month of November rolled around, a beautiful engraved invitation came addressed to 'The Honorable' inviting her and her parents to a Christmas Reception at the White House. She was utterly astonished, and excited beyond belief. "Oh, Mom," she exclaimed, "what are we going to wear?" Oh boy, I thought, another shop till we drop trip will be required just to find two outfits and shoes that look good and feel good for long hours on concrete sidewalks and marble floors! Now there's a problem I would have never have believed my daughter and I would have had to face when I looked into her tiny face on the day of her birth.

> Isaiah 55:8 says, *"My thoughts are nothing like your thoughts," says the Lord. "And my ways are far beyond anything you could imagine . . ."* (NLT) How true this is for me, Lord, how true! Who would believe we would follow our Windy into the White House so many times that we lost count, and that she would also invite her brothers, Dave and Mikey, sister-in-law, Kari, and her grandparents to go with her all the way into the Oval Office? Unbelievable!

We did go to the party, and we did wear new clothes bought for the very special occasion. It was freezing cold, and we wrapped up in coats, gloves and sparkly scarves to keep us warm as we stood outside the White House before we were cleared by the tight security. There was only one problem, well, in actuality there were two: her two shiny black dress heels. The buckles kept releasing spontaneously, and she could only take a few steps before her feet came out of them. We were in a long line that moved ever so slowly, and it wasn't possible to stand perfectly still for long. We didn't think we had better get out of line because it would only delay the wait in the cold weather. We didn't want her to get miserably cold. Her dad came to her rescue. He bent down on one knee, on the freezing sidewalk, in his best suit pants and proceeded to make a new hole in the straps, one tedious try at a time, with the tiny prong that was there to stick through the existing holes.

After several attempts, sans hole punch or sharp object such as a pocket knife to expedite the process. (He's always been our "*MacGyver*". He has a knack for figuring a solution out for a particular problem, especially when few resources are readily available.) He patted her foot, stood up to brush himself off and straighten his pant legs out. What a sweet dad! Finally he had been successful, and she could walk unencumbered by ill-fitting shoes (At least until we were leaving that evening, when Windy lost a shoe on the grand staircase as she was descending to the cloakroom to find her hot pink wool overcoat. I caught her arm to steady her, and I reached down a step to retrieve the shoe. Looking up I saw a man in the Secret Service rush toward us, to help out. "Thank You!" Windy told him as she acknowledged his gesture.

"Yes, thank you for helping Cinderella find her lost shoe!" I said laughingly. He and Windy laughed together at that. (See, moms can be really funny sometimes, too!) It had been surreal . . . Sarah Evans came and stood in front of Windy at one point during the evening but Windy was, for once, too shy to speak to her. Later she said she should have told her she knew Kenny Chesney's dad. (He lived in our neighborhood at the time, and she always spoke to him at a local restaurant when she saw him there.) It would have been a good lead-in to a conversation, but meeting her was not to happen. To repeat Windy's words about the missed opportunity—"Darn it!"

At that same party, we also saw Jared, and he purposely walked up to hug and speak with Windy. He then asked why Windy had not written to the President in a long time. She explained *very* frankly that we had told her not to. She was nice about it, but sounded a little put-out with "the parents" about it. She spoke to him as if we weren't present.

He looked right into her eyes and said, "Please e-mail him soon, Windy. He loves hearing from you anytime." Then he looked at us and said, "Please allow her to e-mail the President. He *needs* to hear from her. She encourages him." Wow! How could we refuse this profound request? Well, we couldn't, and we didn't.

Our daughter was a friend and an encourager to the President of the United States. He respected this young lady, saw past her disabilities, and saw her true heart and her tremendous abilities to encourage and help others. He could have been too busy to hear from her or to respond back through his Personal Assistants. After all, he had an entire country to run and had a leading role among the leaders of the world! If he had been too busy to remember her, we would have understood. This . . . well, all *this* was beyond our wildest imaginations. Maybe this friendship—a surprise in her life and in ours—was to encourage us all. It sure has done that! And, do you know what? Now God has used it to encourage *thousands* of people. That's really awesome! And really surprising!

We walked out into the quiet night (especially quiet for D.C.), and we will never forget the image we saw that crisp, cold night on the driveway of the White House. Snow blanketed the grounds, reflecting the large lights at the doors and the post lights of the White House, making radiant pools of warm yellows on the white background. Outside of those perimeters, the landscape looked dark. The large, snow-dusted trees stood sentinel in the frozen silence. Walking with a decided limp was a soldier, whom we had met earlier at the reception, leaning heavily on a cane, to maintain his balance. He had been severely injured in Iraq during a raid and had lost an arm and a leg. He and his beautiful wife were leaving the party, just a little ahead of the three of us.

David grabbed my arm and whispered, "I will never forget this moment here in the moonlight, watching a true hero walk out of the White House he fought to protect. He fought for you, for me, for Windy. For our boys and their families. For all of the families in this great country we call America. God bless him, please bless him!" Then, in respect (we didn't want them to feel they needed to pick up their pace because we were so close behind them), we three held hands and waited back until he had haltingly walked out of the large, black iron gate, his bride pacing her steps to his, as they walked out into the night. Only then did we pass through the gate ourselves. This one time we had *his* back.

God, thank You for this and so many other moments that cause us to reflect on our lives and on those lives around us. Thank you for this solider, and for all those who put their lives in harm's way to keep America and Liberty and Freedom safe. In the powerful name of Jesus we pray. Amen.

In another line, this time standing outside of the White House to hear the President's Farewell Address in 2008, Windy seemed so solemn. She turned to look at the others who stood quietly in line behind, and in front of her.

Gathered there that night were people that the President and Miss Laura had personally asked to come to say goodbye to. They invited those who had meant so much to them during their eight years in office. Some were the firemen, and the policemen who had been active in 9-11. The two men who stood with President Bush as he addressed New York and the entire nation standing on the remaining rubble on Ground Zero were there with their wives. (Windy got to speak with them and have her picture made with them.)

Windy even got her turn to say goodbye. When his speech was done and everyone had filled the room with applause, several times, for many minutes, President Bush and Miss Laura began their walk to the back of the room to exit. The final walk took a long time to complete. Everyone had well-wishing words to speak to them. Shaking hands and saying farewell to as many people as they could, they made their way slowly down the aisle. When they got close enough that Windy felt they could see her, she said a quick "Bye" as they passed by. They both tenderly looked at her, and said, "Goodbye, Windy!"

Her eyes began to mist over. She wasn't going to make them sad by letting them see her tears, but when we walked out of the Gold Room, she cried silently all the way down the hall as we walked under the overhead, be-dazzlingly-lit, crystal chandeliers. Her tears sparkled like the crystals on the lights above her.

It was the end of an era for the Bushes. What an amazing eight years it had been for Windy! What miracles we had been allowed to see, and to be a part of. Yes, real miracles! Our daughter now called a President of the United States, a friend. She had spoken to millions on television. She had made friends with people all over Washington, D.C., around the country, and around the *world*. She had been asked to serve on a Presidential Committee and had helped to change the name of the very Committee. She had been part of a brave group who helped initiate a change from the horrible word "mental retardation" to a more acceptable term "intellectual disabilities". No wonder she was sad. She must have wondered how she would ever be able to help so many people like that again. She must have felt she had lost a big job. It was a huge letdown of sorts, but she was a strong woman . . . she will always find an avenue to help others, and to make her life count for something good. Of that we had no doubt!

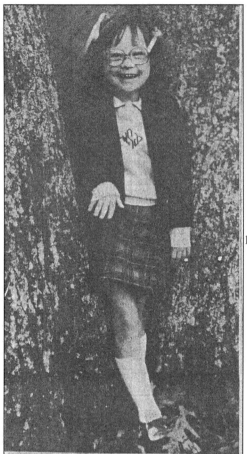

1981 ARC Poster Child

POSTER CHILD — Windy Jeanne Smith of Clinton has been chosen the 1981 Poster Child for the Association of Retarded Citizens for the state of Tennessee. The 7-year-old will be a guest at the TARC convention in June in Nashville, where she will meet Gov. Lamar Alexander and appear on television with Honey Alexander, honorary chairman of the association. Windy is the daughter of Dr. and Mrs. David L. Smith and attends Daniel Arthur Rehabilitation Center.

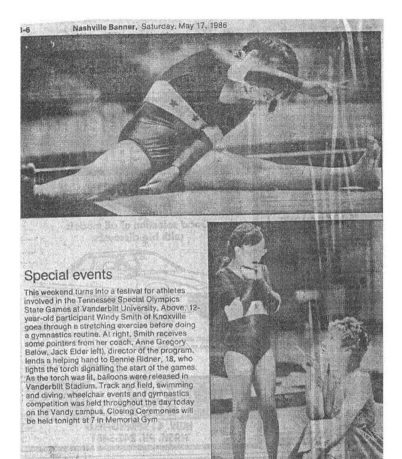

Nashville Banner, Saturday, May 17, 1986

Special events

This weekend turns into a festival for athletes involved in the Tennessee Special Olympics State Games at Vanderbilt University. Above, 12-year-old participant Windy Smith of Knoxville goes through a stretching exercise before doing a gymnastics routine. At right, Smith receives some pointers from her coach, Anne Gregory. Below, Jack Elder left), director of the program, lends a helping hand to Bennie Ridner, 18, who lights the torch signalling the start of the games. As the torch was lit, balloons were released in Vanderbilt Stadium. Track and field, swimming and diving, wheelchair events and gymnastics competition was held throughout the day today on the Vandy campus. Closing Ceremonies will be held tonight at 7 in Memorial Gym

Banner photos by Anthony Lathrop and Dave Findley

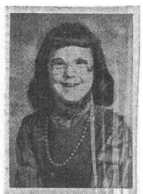

Windy Smith

Athlete to attend international games

Windy Jeanne Smith, 13, was one of 76 children chosen to represent Tennessee at the 1987 International Special Olympics Summer Games at Notre Dame University in South Bend, Ind., July 31 to Aug. 8.

She is the daughter of Dr. and Mrs. David Smith of Knoxville, formerly of Clinton, and the granddaughter of Dr. and Mrs. Charles Stansberry and Mr. and Mrs. Bill Smith. Windy has two brothers, Davey and Michael.

The Cessna Corporation with 400 Citation Business jets will transport the Olympians and their coaches to the games. There will be 4,600 athletes representing 73 countries participating at the international event.

ABC-TV will televise a two-hour special on the games Monday, Aug. 3, from 9 to 11 p.m. There will be additional coverage on the Wide World of Sports Saturday, Aug. 15, from 4:30 to 6 p.m.

Guest stars in attendance at the games will be Arnold Schwarzenegger, Patrick Ewing, Frank Gifford, Oprah Winfrey and Mary Lou Retton. Eunice Kennedy Shriver, founder and chairman of the Special Olympics International, said, "Special Olympics has opened a window to the world through which heads of nations, community leaders have come to appreciate the strengths and achievements of human beings who have met more challenges than most of us will ever face."

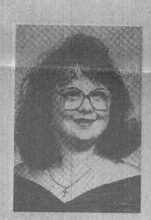

**Windy Smith
Farragut High
Senior**

Windy is in the school's Least Restricted Environment program. In her five years there she has served as an aide in several departments. She pays careful attention, working hard and cheerfully to establish the routine for her tasks. She recently tried out to be a speaker for graduation telling how important it is to the handicapped to be accepted by other students. Windy's acceptance and positive attitude have helped other students to be aware of their blessings and to develop compassion for those less fortunate.
**Nominator: Jean Hill
Farragut High**

Graduation was extra special for Farragut High's Windy Smith

By Cherie Kimmons
Staff Writer

Windy Smith came home from school a few weeks ago and told her mother, Vicki, that she would like some help writing a speech describing her experiences at Farragut High School. The words came easily when the two sat down late that evening and put together a 5-minute speech.

Vicki said she didn't give the speech another thought, assuming it was a homework assignment for one of Windy's classes. She was shocked when she learned that Windy had been selected to give the speech they had quickly composed during Farragut's graduation ceremonies. Once again, Windy would be leaving her own unique mark on the school.

In her speech, Windy, 22, spoke of how her dream came true at Farragut. Lonely and a little bit scared, she entered the high school as a student in Farragut's first Least Restricted Environment (LRE) class for disabled children five years ago.

The lovely young woman with shining dark hair and an infectious smile quickly made friends as she attended art and home economics classes. She trained as a teacher's aide, working for a while at Farragut Intermediate School and later at the high school, helping teachers with their bulletin boards and bringing them coffee.

An avid sports fan, she became a member of the Pep Club. This year she attended Homecoming, but not as a mere spectator. She was a Homecoming Queen candidate and enjoyed every minute in the limelight as her father, Dave, escorted her onto the football field at halftime.

She became a runner for the basketball coach, cheering on her brother, Michael, who also attends Farragut and plays on the varsity basketball and football teams. She attended the prom this year with one of her many male admirers, and Vicki has good-naturedly resigned herself to Windy's busy social schedule. Windy has another brother, David, who attends ETSU.

Although Windy transferred to Farragut from a small, private Christian school, she was no stranger to being the center of attention. The list of her activities is long and impressive.

She has been a poster child for the Association of Retarded Citizens and was pictured with

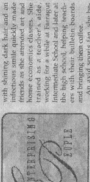

See GRADUATION, page 3A

THE WHITE HOUSE

July 27, 2001

Miss Windy J. Smith

1

Dear Windy,

Your note made my day!

Your cheerfulness and friendly manner make everyone around you feel happier, and reading the kind words of your note feels like being hugged.

President Bush and I were so pleased you could be with us when he made his speech to Congress. Here is a photo of that night for you to enjoy.

We are praying for you, too.

With best wishes,

Laura Bush

THE ARC OF TENNESSEE
A state organization on mental retardation and other disabilities

November 5, 2002

Windy Smith

Dear Windy:

It was so nice talking with you, your mother and your father last evening. As I state we are very proud to have a self-advocate such as yourself on the President's Committee. I am including some information that we have in our office that may provide some assistance in your roll on the committee.

I would like to strongly urge you to read the brochure on "Partners in Policymaking" This is a really a dynamic program that can provide you and your parents even more information plus give you a chance to visit with more self-advocates.

As I stated I will write a letter in support of the name change of the Presidents Committee but I would like to get the endorsement from our Board of Directors of the Arc of Tennessee. We have a full board meeting on December 7th and will send you the letter the week after.

Once again, thank you for talking with us and please feel free to use our telephone numbers any time you feel we can help.

Sincerely,

Walter F. Rogers
Executive Director

Enclosures

44 Vantage Way, Suite 550, Nashville, TN 37228
(615) 248-5878 Fax: (615) 248-5879 Toll free: (800) 835-7077
Web: http://www.thearctn.org

THE WHITE HOUSE

WASHINGTON

February 13, 2004

Ms. Windy J. Smith

Dear Windy:

It was a pleasure to see you and your family in Knoxville. Thank you for your kind note and for presenting the Robert Tino painting. I appreciate your thoughtful gesture, and I am grateful for your prayers.

Mrs. Bush joins me in sending our best wishes.

Sincerely,

George W. Bush

COLORADO SPRINGS, CO 80995 • (719) 531-5181

May 13, 2005

Miss Windy Smith

Dear Windy:

Greetings from your friends at Focus on the Family! Brady Tarr passed along your April 20 letter, and I wanted to respond personally. Your testimony touches my heart, Windy. It's clear that the Lord's love has taken deep root in your life, and you've done what so few seem to be able to do: trust Him with everything you are and have. Reading your story lifts my spirits, and I'm reminded of what God can do through a life that's surrendered to Him.

You have an impressive list of achievements – not many can say they have sat with presidents, spoken to thousands, and helped change government policies. And yet it's evident that all this is simply the result of your desire to honor the Lord by using your gifts as He directs. In doing so, you've also brought hope to others and inspired them to find their own unique area of contribution. What a great message!

Well done, Windy! Thanks so much for writing to me and for letting me know you've been praying for me and for Focus. That means more than I can say. It's been a tremendous encouragement to get to know you. I would love to meet you in person! God bless you as you continue to follow Him in the days ahead.

Sincerely,

James C. Dobson, Ph.D.
Founder and Chairman

> Jan. 2004
>
> Dear President Bush,
> I wanted to give you and miss Laura this painting because it reminded me of our country and of you.
>
> Maybe you can take it to Texas some day — but not for 4 more years!
>
> I'm still praying,
> I love you.
> Windy Smith
> IS. 40:31

THE WHITE HOUSE
WASHINGTON

March 4, 2005

Ms. Windy J. Smith

Dear Windy:

Thank you for your nice letter. I appreciate your support and especially your prayers. Like many Americans, I find strength and comfort in my faith.

I was glad to see you at the White House during the Detroit Pistons event. Please give my best to your family.

Sincerely,

George W. Bush

DEPARTMENT OF HEALTH & HUMAN SERVICES

ADMINISTRATION FOR CHILDREN AND FAMILIES
Office of the Assistant Secretary, Suite 600
370 L'Enfant Promenade, S.W.
Washington, D.C. 20447

NOV 1 6 2005

Windy J. Smith

Dear Ms. Smith:

It is my honor to congratulate you on your service with the President's Committee for People with Intellectual Disabilities.

The publication of the Committee's 2004 Report to the President: *A CHARGE WE HAVE TO KEEP... A Road Map to Personal and Economic Freedom for People with Intellectual Disabilities* has been lauded as a groundbreaking effort in support of President George W. Bush's New Freedom Initiative. Your service on the Committee has reflected the compassion of the President and the United States Department of Health and Human Services in improving the lives of people with intellectual disabilities.

It is my hope that your experience while a member on the Committee will serve you well through your continued leadership and advocacy for issues affecting those with intellectual disabilities.

Sincerely,

Wade F. Horn, Ph.D.
Assistant Secretary
for Children and Families

PRESIDENT'S COMMITTEE FOR PEOPLE WITH INTELLECTUAL DISABILITIES
Suite 701 Aerospace Building
901 D Street, SW
Washington, DC 20447

PRESIDENT'S COMMITTEE FOR PEOPLE WITH INTELLECTUAL DISABILITIES

November 29, 2005

Dear Windy,

What a pleasant surprise it was to recieve your wonderful letter, and to know that you enjoyed working with the President's Committee to make America a better place for all Americans. We will forever remember your role in the President's decision to change the name of the Committee from The President's Committee on Mental Retardation (PCMR) to The President's Committee for People with Intellectual Disabilities (PCPID). Thank you for this very sensitive and courageous act! We will always love you, Windy.

Madeleine C. Will

PRESIDENT'S COMMITTEE FOR PEOPLE WITH INTELLECTUAL DISABILITIES
Suite 701 Aerospace Building
901 D Street, SW
Washington, DC 20447

PRESIDENT'S COMMITTEE FOR PEOPLE WITH INTELLECTUAL DISABILITIES

11/30/2005

Windy,

Madeleine and I want to thank you for serving on the President's Committee for People with Intellectual Disabilities. Your courage in changing the Committee's name was greatly appreciated. Sally

STATE OF TENNESSEE
DEPARTMENT OF EDUCATION
6th FLOOR, ANDREW JOHNSON TOWER
710 JAMES ROBERTSON PARKWAY
NASHVILLE, TN 37243-0375

PHIL BREDESEN
GOVERNOR

LANA C. SEIVERS, Ed.D.
COMMISSIONER

June 01, 2006

The President's Committee for People with Intellectual Disabilities
Washington, D.C.

Dear Committee Members:

We are delighted to provide this information to you at the request of one of your committee members, Ms. Windy Smith. Recently Ms. Smith assisted the Tennessee Department of Education in our efforts to recruit special education teachers by joining us in a commercial aired in the Knoxville, Tennessee market area. The commercial she was in is included in these materials, and the television campaign is described below.

Since the 1980s when an increasing number of states began to heighten efforts to address the teacher shortage in certain subject areas, including special education, the Tennessee Department of Education devised ways to attract special educators to the classrooms. From Special Education Institutes and other models that provided financial support in the form of tuition remission and payment of associated fees for teachers working on employment standard waivers and probationary permits, through its Division of Special Education, the Tennessee Department of Education sought to address the current and anticipated mounting shortages in special education.

The success of these models was recognized; however, the shortage remained and even intensified, placing more special educators who were not properly licensed in the classrooms serving children with disabilities. Retirements, leaves of absence, sabbaticals, inadequate number of college graduates in special education, and attrition were contributing factors. With this recognition, the Tennessee Department of Education, Division of Special Education, recently launched the **B**ecome **A** **S**pecial **E**ducator in **Tennessee** (BASE-TN) Initiative.

BASE-TN uses a multi-dimensional approach that recognizes the complexities in addressing teacher shortages, including recruitment to the profession, recruitment to the classroom, teacher preparation, teacher recognition, and teacher retention. Several components are simultaneously implemented on a statewide basis as described in the following section.

·**Television-Based Multimedia Campaign with Branding**

- √ 30-second commercials were produced to attract high school graduates, mid-career professionals changing jobs, and college graduates to the field of special education. The commercials are broadcast in all Tennessee counties and into several contiguous states as well as the Caribbean Islands. (See the enclosed DVD that contains 6 of the commercials produced by the Department of Education.)

President's Committee for People with Intellectual Disabilities
Washington, D.C. 20447

June 27, 2006

Joseph E. Fisher, Assistant Commissioner
Division of Special Education
Lana C. Seivers
Tennessee Commissioner of Education
State of Tennessee
Department of Education
6th Floor, Andrew Johnson Tower
710 James Robertson Parkway
Nashville, Tennessee 37243-0375

Dear Mr. Fisher and Ms. Seivers:

I am delighted that Windy Smith, a former member of the President's Committee for People with Intellectual Disabilities (PCPID), assisted the Tennessee Department of Education in its efforts to recruit special education teachers by joining you in a commercial aired in the Knoxville, Tennessee market area, and that she asked you to share information regarding the Become A Special Educator in Tennessee (BASE-TN) Initiative with us.

Staff of the President's Committee for People with Intellectual Disabilities reviewed the informational materials and viewed the DVD that contains 6 of the commercials produced by the Tennessee Department of Education. Seldom has it been our good fortune to witness a more comprehensive initiative recruitment/public awareness initiative. Congratulations on a job well-done.

You may be interested to know that the PCPID is comprised of both citizen and ex officio members. The Secretary of the U.S. Department of Education, one of our ex officio members, has designated Donna Wiesner as his official representative on the Committee. Ms. Wiesner is Special Assistant to the Assistant Secretary of the Office of Special Education and Rehabilitative Services. We are taking the liberty of sharing the informational materials related to the Tennessee Department of Education efforts to recruit special education teachers to Ms. Weisner, with confidence that she, too, will find the materials most impressive.

Please accept our best wishes for continued success in your recruitment efforts.

Sincerely,

Sally Atwater
Executive Director

cc: ✓ Windy Smith
    Cleo J. Harris, Ed.D.
    Donna Wiesner

DEPARTMENT OF HEALTH & HUMAN SERVICES

ADMINISTRATION FOR CHILDREN AND FAMILIE
Office of the Assistant Secretary, Suite 600
370 L'Enfant Promenade, S.W.
Washington, D.C. 20447

NOV 1 6 2005

Windy J. Smith

Dear Ms. Smith:

It is my honor to congratulate you on your service with the President's Committee for People with Intellectual Disabilities.

The publication of the Committee's 2004 Report to the President: *A CHARGE WE HAVE TO KEEP... A Road Map to Personal and Economic Freedom for People with Intellectual Disabilities* has been lauded as a groundbreaking effort in support of President George W. Bush's New Freedom Initiative. Your service on the Committee has reflected the compassion of the President and the United States Department of Health and Human Services in improving the lives of people with intellectual disabilities.

It is my hope that your experience while a member on the Committee will serve you well through your continued leadership and advocacy for issues affecting those with intellectual disabilities.

Sincerely,

Wade F. Horn, Ph.D.
Assistant Secretary
  for Children and Families

THE WHITE HOUSE

WASHINGTON

November 30, 2005

The Honorable Windy J. Smith

Dear Windy:

Thank you for your service to the United States as a member of the President's Committee for People with Intellectual Disabilities.

Public service is a high calling and an expression of responsible citizenship. I appreciate your hard work and contributions to ensuring that individuals with intellectual disabilities have the opportunity to build a better future for themselves and their families.

Laura and I send our best wishes.

Sincerely,

George W. Bush

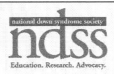

COPY

Ms. Windy Smith

Dear Windy:

Since you spoke at the Republican Convention, we have gotten a lot of positive feedback here! You are an inspiration to many people with Down syndrome and their families. I would like to invite you to write an article about your experience for the National Down Syndrome Society's magazine *News & Views*. The magazine is written for and by people with Down syndrome and is edited by Chris Burke. I spoke with your mom a few days ago and, as discussed, I have enclosed samples of the last two issues of *News & Views*.

The deadline for our next issue is soon – August 22. I would love it if you could get something to me by then, but if not, our next issue deadline is October 16. Your article should be 100-200 words. Please include 2-3 photos from your time in Philadelphia as well.

You may want to consider these questions when writing your article:

How did you end up speaking at the convention?
What did you talk about and how did you decide what was important to say?
What was it like speaking to all those people and being on TV?
Is there a message you want to send about politics to the people who read *News & Views*?

Please give me a call if you have any questions about your article.

Sincerely,

Jennifer Schell Podoll
Public Relations Manager

666 Broadway • New York, NY 10012-2317 • 212-460-9330 or 800-221-4602 • Fax: 212-979-2873 • www.ndss.org

E-newsletter from The Arc of the United States

From: The Arc <communications@thearc.org>
To: David Smith
Subject: E-newsletter from The Arc of the United States
Date: Mon, Oct 11, 2010 7:41 pm

Trouble viewing this message, click here.
To ensure delivery of this e-newsletter, please add communications@thearc.org to your address book and safe-sender list.

Oct. 2010

The President Signs Rosa's Law

On Friday afternoon, President Barack Obama presided over a celebration of Rosa's Law which was enacted on Tuesday; the law substitutes the term "intellectual disabilities" for "mental retardation" in many federal laws.

Self-advocates William Washington (The Arc's national office receptionist), Jill Egle (Co-Executive Director of The Arc of Northern Virginia) and Jeremy Jacobson (son of The Arc's Chief Development and Marketing Officer Trudy Jacobson) joined Paul Marchand, Director of the Disability Policy Collaboration, to represent the intellectual and developmental disability community whose advocacy resulted in this bill.

Read on:

This Just In

- The rock band Flame, a group of musicians with developmental and physical disabilities, is featured in the current issue of *People* Magazine. Their debut CD will be released in December and available for sale at www.flametheband.com.
- Welcome! The Arc has a new chapter – The Arc of Southeast Missouri in Cape Girardeau, MO.

U.S. Department of Labor   Office of Disability Employment Policy
200 Constitution Avenue, N.W., S-1303
Washington, DC 20210

MAY 28 2003

Ms. Windy Smith

Dear Windy,

Thank you, Windy, for your letter concerning your request for changing the name of the President's Committee on Mental Retardation (PCMR) to the President's Committee for People with Intellectual Disabilities. We all agreed this is a positive change as reflected in the votes at our last Board Meeting. The Office of Disability Employment Policy (ODEP) recognizes the importance of your request. We fully support any language that provides opportunities for increased respect and emphasizes the abilities of people.

Thank you for your faithful attendance and interest given to the PCMR Meetings. Nancy Skaggs and I look forward to seeing you again at future meetings. Please do not hesitate to contact us if we can be of further assistance.

Sincerely,

W. Roy W. Grizzard Jr., Ed.D.
Assistant Secretary

Windy, as you know now, I voted for the name change and it did pass. Best wishes for a nice summer.

Roy G

www.dol.gov/odep

Lana C. Seivers, Commissioner
Tennessee Department of Education

5/17/06

Dear Windy,
    I hope you've seen our commercial on television by now. You did a wonderful job, and I really enjoyed spending time with you. It was great to see you, your mother, your grandmother,

---

Office of the Chairman:

Stein Mart

March 13, 2009

Miss Windy Smith

Dear Windy,

It was a wonderful picture of you that I saw at the White House. On behalf of everyone who works here thank you for choosing your special outfit at Stein Mart. You are a great model for our clothing.

Sincerely,

Jay Stein

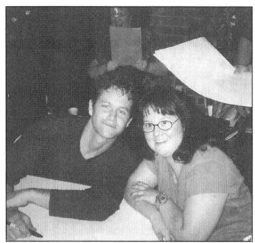

Kirk Cameron and Windy "hanging out"

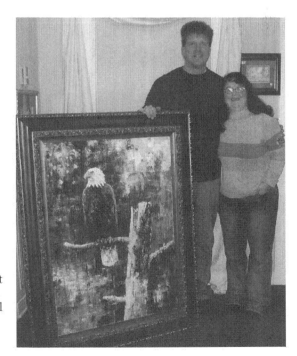

Artist Robert Tino giving Windy an oil painting

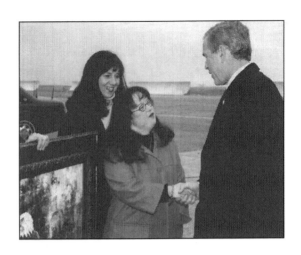

Meeting
Air Force One
with painting

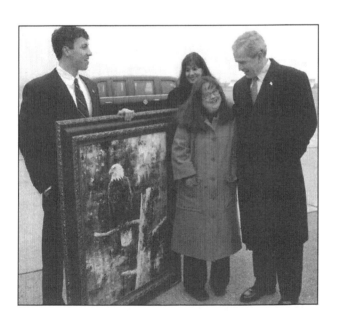

Chapter Twenty-Five
Tidbits and Giggles

Once, Windy was out behind our house helping me and her Nannie Juanita to plant a flowerbed. (She and her Nannie have a close relationship and love spending time together.) We were all digging away at the stubborn, hard soil to prepare the holes for our tender young plants. Windy stopped to watch us for a moment and focused on our hands as we worked away at turning the dirt with our hand shovels. She than looked down at her own hands, and said, "I wonder why my hands are so small?" as a flicker of a frown clouded her face as she pondered her smaller work gloves. Then she lowered her hands and started back to digging, saying to herself, ever so quietly, and completely content, "I guess God just made me that way!" She then smiled at the sun-warmed earth before her, shrugged her shoulders and fell to work. She had questioned something she found different about herself that set her apart from her mother and grandmother, and then she instantly accepted that difference as a choice made by her Creator, and she was content with the knowledge that He must have had good reasons for her to have been created as she was, and she trusted Him completely with it.

Windy is not a gossip. She doesn't talk about other people. She'll *hear* a comment made about someone, but she won't comment *on* it. She gets it, she knows the insinuation, but she refuses to lower her standards to talk behind someone's back. A quote by William Penn says it much better than I, "Never report what may hurt another, unless it be a greater hurt to some other to conceal it." Windy doesn't know who Mr. Penn was, but she lives out his observation and conviction on life. He would have liked her spunk and would have delighted in their shared belief of his statement, I think.

Ephesians 4:29, *Let no corrupting talk come out of your mouths, but only such as is good for building up, as fits the occasion, that it may give grace to those who hear.*

Windy prays *every* day for all who call her "Aunt Windy". She calls her nephews *her* boys. She has been able to exercise her excellent mothering skills: caring, protective, always teaching (especially in the manners department), and she loves the boys more than her own life. She and I have helped with Caleb and Jake since they were babies. She has fed them, dressed them, buckled them into car seats. She has been a lifesaver, a teacher, and a wonderful influence in the boy's lives. When her two nephews were adopted, she accepted Lookens and Kensley as her own flesh and blood. She loves all four boys and is crazy about them! She also loves going to their ballgames like she enjoyed going to their dad's games! Like all good aunts, she's still working on helping them polish their manners!

May our grandchildren come to know that their Aunt Windy is a person of strong faith, so they may be encouraged to live their own lives full of hopes and dreams and have strong faith in God, so that they may be able to carry all these things out to fruition. May she inspire them to answer God's call for excellence in each of their lives. We hope they realize they can become anything they want to be . . . a great research scientist, President of the United States, a doctor, a fireman, an educator, an attorney, an Evangelist preaching God's truth or a Christian singer, only a few vocations she has described to them. God can use you to glorify Him in *any* vocation.

After the death of our mother, my sister and I divided up her and our Daddy's possessions—probably another one of the hardest things I ever had to do in my lifetime. We had to ready the house to sell. Everything had to be sorted through. (Those of you who have gone through this have our compassion and sympathy. You just have to "face reality" like my dad once told me, and see it through.) When all was said and done, Windy had not asked for, or received, anything of much monetary value. Frankly, I was feeling sorry for her. She was so sweet and gentle over the entire process of cleaning out and redistributing my parents "worldly goods". She asked for very little, really all three of our grown kids were so unselfish and so "strong in the Lord" through the months after their grandparents' passing.

Their strong attitudes and words of encouragement were real help to me. It is in those dark, rough "stormy seas and seasons of our lives" that we prove, to ourselves and to others, how deep and real our faith really is. As we heard it put, years ago, "It is the rough times of life that show what we're really made of." When everything is going smoothly, it's easier to be kind, considerate, unselfish, and helpful. But in the rougher times—when we hit bumps along the road of life, when we are bumped—what spills out is what we are truly filled with. If we are filled with the Holy Spirit, His love and truth will flow out of us. If our faith is all just a show, a facade or shallow faith, then that too will be revealed.

I was grateful for what I saw in our kids in this difficult time in all our lives. I asked Windy if she would like to wear Gaymom's wedding band—the band she had worn for almost seventy years—

"So you can have a little piece of your Gaymom and Poppie with you every day." Windy declined, saying in her sweet voice, "Mom, I already have them with me in my heart. I don't need a ring to have that. Besides, I got a pair of her favorite socks, didn't I? I wear them every night like she did." As far as she was concerned the subject was closed. Don't get me wrong, she likes beautiful things (especially if they are bubblegum pink), but she knew Gaymom loved those little socks, and she felt close to her by wearing them nightly on her own feet.

She had gone into their bedroom, opened one of the drawers of a tall, narrow chest of drawers that sat back against the wall between their closet doors, and she searched for a pair that looked familiar to her and asked me if she might "have them for keeps." Mom would have loved that . . . her granddaughter had a heart of gold and had really, really loved her grandparents. No doubt about it. When she was "bumped"—out flowed 100% unselfish, pure love.

Another huge **WINDY LIFE LESSON** for everybody . . . don't get all caught up in making material possessions our main goal in life . . . don't let anything take precedent over the *true* meaningful things in life. And don't be greedy for Heaven's sake! (Literally for Heaven's sake and your own sake here!) Share from your blessings, and be a blessing to others! No matter how little or how much you have. We can all do something nice for someone else, give someone a break, the benefit of doubt, a smile, an encouraging word, a Bible verse, say a prayer for someone (a friend, an acquaintance, a stranger, *maybe* even a perceived enemy!), buy some food for someone that has very little, clean out your closet and give some of your clothes and coats away, give money and/or time volunteering at a local church, give to a ministry that helps children in orphanages, or helps out during times of disaster relief in America, and around the world.

Learn to love—100% pure love! You will be a blessing *and* be blessed. It's God's mathematical equation: you can't out-give God, and it's *amazing* how it works *every* time! But don't take our word for it, try it out yourself! Get going!

Birthday and Party Girl Stories

Windy's birthday is the one day a year she becomes a "little" self-centered . . . she used to talk about it so much, and plan so much in advance, that we had to make a pact . . . and she honors it totally. She is not allowed to mention her September birthday until August 1st. It is the only way we could have any peace over what she considers to be just this side of a national holiday! Each August 1st she releases her new plans (silently she has been planning all year long for this!), and we *always* have to downsize the plans considerable . . . no one we know could afford her large-scale gala plans. She would have been a fabulous professional party planner, no joke. Those of us that know her best, know this for a fact.

Every other day of the year she is one of the most thoughtful people in the world. On her birthday, *her* day, you had better come up with something, not material gifts necessarily (I said she liked pink things!) but *something*: a card, a phone call, a text is great to her . . . just don't forget, or her feelings are really hurt. She has been notorious for sending letters to people reminding them of the approaching day and then casually mentioning that she had a few suggestions in mind for their gift: a detailed list of what she has picked out, where they can find the item, and how much it costs. The list can be very extensive. I tried to be vigilant in confiscating her letters and explaining to her why this isn't very polite, but somehow each year some letters *do* go out in the mail without her dad's or my knowledge. She is very creative (and has now mastered how to send a detailed list—with websites—to friends) and thinks her mom is not completely right about this matter. (So, sorry to those of you who have received one of these lists, but I am not a super hero. It would take one to stay ahead of her sometimes.)

Birthday breakfast in bed is another thing that thrills her . . . and it can be as simple as a breakfast bar and orange juice. She just loves the planning you had to do to bring it to her, meaning you have REMEMBERED her day! Selfish or not, she celebrates her birth day in happiness and joy! Maybe this is just God's way of being sure I celebrate to the fullest on the anniversary date of one of the darkest days of my life . . . her day of birth. "No more crying, no more tears, only fun and celebration for us on *her* day—all through the years!" (My own quote. Well, give me a break, I think it's kinda cute! Plus, it sums up what the day has become for all of us.)

She always enjoyed going to the parties my first cousin, Sandie Bishop, and her husband, Archer, threw in Knoxville, before they moved to another state. She loved seeing her cousins and their kids there. Family, even extended family, is important to her. (I think their daughter, Kristen MacDermott is still on Windy's cell phone contact list because: number one, she has always liked Kristen, and number two, she and her husband, Michael live near L.A. You gotta keep that networking going, I guess!) Once, after we had just left their home, Windy turned to me, and said, "Now *that*'s how you host a party!" Well, well. Nice to know my daughter was trying to educate me on the way to give a fantastic party. Nice to know I couldn't possibly host one to please her! (She hopes her forty-fifth is going to be something really fun and special. Help!)

Windy and her friends get together every year with great pomp and circumstance, believing there's much reason for celebration. Windy has kept us laughing about birthday parties. So have some of her friends. A favorite story of ours is about Lisle, a friend of Windy's, who was so excited about his upcoming thirtieth birthday party, that he thought he would help his mother with the invitations, to help expedite the big day. On discovering the party invitations already written and addressed by his mother, and stacked neatly on the kitchen island, Lisle noted they were lacking the stamps. He logically found stamps, after a brief search of his home. Brief, because he remembered where his parents kept a large number of stamps. Brief, because his mother was due back from the beauty salon at any moment! He wanted to surprise her!

Methodically he chose, licked, and applied a lovely stamp on each envelope. Evidently he took some time in choosing each stamp with consideration for the recipient's personal taste or personality. Success came at last. They were finished and ready for the mail just in time to hand them over to the mailman as he walked down the sidewalk toward his house's mailbox. He couldn't wait for his mom to come home and be surprised with his efficiency.

Come to find out, she was *very* surprised. Lisle had found and licked forty invitations with stamps from her treasured stamp collection. (She called to suggest we might want to watch for the mail and save our stamps!) By the way, everyone invited came to the party, and Lisle had a ball! Windy and her friends couldn't wait to receive the invitations to his much anticipated yearly gala! He celebrates each year in high style!

Windy loves a party! She loves planning a party, and it doesn't necessarily have to be in her honor. She likes planning one for anyone, especially for someone she loves. One year I was really dragging my feet about making any plans for my own birthday. I was turning forty-five, and I really wanted to keep a low profile, and let the day slip on by without much of a "to do". I thought if I didn't make a big production over it, I could forget I was getting older, and no one would know any different, except for the family, of course. Windy felt completely opposite about the approaching date. When she saw I was doing nothing, she sneaked the call lists from church and school out of the kitchen drawer, set a time and date, called a whole bunch of people over, and even told them the nearby street names of where to park their cars. She did warn me to dress up some that afternoon, and suggested I might want to wash my hair. I did both, thinking her dad was taking us out to dinner.

When the guests started arriving, before I had dressed completely, I realized what she had done. God love her, she threw me a wonderful party! Even if I did have to go pick up my own cake that she had ordered at the grocery store nearest to our house. I was so happy they had respected her enough to make a cake at her request, nothing could have stopped me from going and picking it up and thanking them for my birthday cake. She would make a great Party/Event Planner. She comes highly recommended, with lots of experience! We nicknamed her "The Party Girl," and now you know why.

Windy and her friends are always excited for each other as they plan a year in advance for anticipated birthdays. Here is another **WINDY LIFE LESSON** the rest of us could imitate, and probably improve our own lives by doing so. Instead of the obsession with youthfulness our society seems to have, or pushes us into having, we should learn to be grateful for the years we have been given and not try to hide them. Rejoice and celebrate to the max with each passing year! It's an invaluable life lesson she has taught us.

I have said she loves parties and celebrations. And, as we all know, *sometimes* girls can get into some trouble over partying . . .

In Blount County we bought a farm with a small lake on it, and we built a white farmhouse connecting it to a rustic 1790s log cabin that stood on the property. A week after we moved in, one of the Ledbetter brothers came out to hook up cable for the televisions and the computer. A month later our first bill arrived in the mailbox that stood at the end if our gravel drive. I went down on the four wheeler to retrieve the mail, and I slit open the envelop to look inside. There, in print, was a charge of about eight dollars for one movie. A movie called something like "A Party Girl Always Has Fun, something, something, something". Don't remember the real title, but those two main words, "Party Girl", were in the title. They caught my attention and so did the inappropriate rating. Well, I was more than curious.

Who had rented this movie? There were our kids, now young adults, and their friends, who were in and out of our house at all hours. We always made room for any one of our kids' friends to spend the night with us. We had already hosted a whole group of kids for a week on a mission trip in our area. Surely not one of them? Had it been one of our boys? It had never happened before. Really, it hadn't. I didn't even know we had access to movies like this on our cable system. We enjoyed watching movies together as a family, but the key word here is *family* entertainment. We had been sure to ask for all the sports and kids channels. We must have accidentally gotten some kind of special programming package along with them!

I dialed up our cable installer, and he came by that afternoon. I told him about the charge on our bill and that we wanted all those choices off of our "options lists". He informed me that he could easily screen out all the channels we didn't want on our cable choices. He went around to each television cable box in our family room, kitchen, and den and got ready to leave. I reminded him that he had not done the one in our daughter's room yet. He promptly went upstairs to fix it. In a few minutes he came down the wooden steps laughing to himself. "I think I've solved the movie mystery! Your daughter's TV is the one that the movie was rented on."

"You're kidding! You can tell which television it was shown on? Are you sure?" I asked him, shocked. (I hadn't asked him to identify the TV. I hadn't known it was possible to do so.)

"Yep, it's on there all right, but it *was* stopped at the beginning and never watched. That should make you feel better. And I locked out all the questionable channels on that unit as well." He waved bye, and headed for his truck.

Oh, it did make me feel better . . . but the big mystery was still unanswered, until I went up to ask Windy about it. I will never forget her bewildered expression when she told me how she had seen the title, clicked on it, and settled into her hot pink velvet club chair "to watch a good old movie". She said, "All of a sudden, a picture of big . . . well, big . . . you know, a woman without her blouse on, and I knew it was *not* a nice movie, so I turned it off. It was disgusting! I was afraid you would be mad at me so I didn't tell you. I didn't watch it, Mom, I *promise*! It was gross!"

"It's okay, honey. I know you didn't watch it. The man said it had been stopped almost as soon as it had begun. I'm sorry that happened to you. This is a good lesson for all of us. Sometimes things sound good, but they may not really be good *for* us. You did the right thing, the honorable thing. When you saw it wasn't what you thought it was going to be, you turned it off. Thank you for using good judgment. Good discernment. You're such a good person, and you are *not* in trouble." She was terribly relieved. Bless her heart!

I told all this to David that night when he came home for dinner. (He later called the cable guy to tell him what had happened. The man said, "I "figured as much. She made the right choice.") We were real proud of her for making the right decision, especially when no one knew but her. Party girls can get into trouble sometimes . . . just not *our* party girl, at *that* particular time!

One day, a few years back, Windy couldn't wait to tell us the great news . . . Kirk Cameron was coming to speak at Concord First Baptist, and she wanted to go "real bad!" She left me a hand-written sticky-note on my calendar in the kitchen and an extra one on my purse calendar, just in case I needed more reminders, wanting me to commit it to our list of "must attend" events. I wrote it in bright green ink: Windy to go hear Kirk!!! When the date arrived, I fixed her hair. She knew he was married and a dad, but she wanted to look nice when she got to meet him. After all, he was a Star! He knew other movie stars! She loves movies and television shows. This was going to be fun!

On the way to the church, she urged us to hurry because the church would fill up fast. She was right about that! The gigantic new lobby and sanctuary were filling to capacity, and it was already hard to find a seat.

She was really interested in what Kirk said as he shared his faith with the audience. She listened and shook her head in that little bob she does when she's in agreement with something someone says. After he spoke, and a prayer was given by Pastor Sager, Windy got in the long line to get a chance to shake his hand and to get his autograph. When it was finally her turn she smiled up at him and said, "I've seen you on TV!" He smiled back and shook her hand and then took his pen and then just before he began to write, he asked her what her name was and how to spell it. "Windy Smith . . . W-I-N-D-Y."

"What a neat way to spell your name," he said, and then he stopped to look into her face, and he said, "Hey! Haven't I seen *you* on TV, *Maybe* with President George W. Bush?"

"Yes! You have!" she said, shaking her head in a big 'Yes', with a dazzling smile, as she looked him squarely in the eyes.

"I thought so! Wow! I never thought I would get the opportunity to meet *you* in person! What a big blessing to *me*! Windy come back here and sit with me while I sign autographs. You are more famous than I am, and they may want *your* autograph! Come tell me what President Bush is like and what it was like to speak live before millions of people? I don't think I could have done that. Did God give you the courage?"

"Yes, He did! I prayed about it, and I wasn't scared at all. My Mom panicked, but I didn't!"

He chuckled at that statement and motioned for her to come take a seat in an empty folding chair. She gladly walked to sit beside him as he took a seat at a large table set up in the lobby. They talked as if they were old friends. They *were* old friends in Windy's mind. She had watched him on sitcoms and in movies for *years*. She felt as if she knew him because of that, but mostly she knew him because he was a brother in Christ. She had heard him speak from his heart, and she discerned that his faith was real.

We were so impressed with him, and with his willingness to talk with her about her experiences. We took a picture of the two of them sitting like buddies. Every time we see the photo we are again reminded of God's Divine appointments that Windy seems to have on a regular basis. (Her brothers love hanging out with her just for who she is, but they also love the fact that God has so many wonderful Providential surprises when they are in her presence, as they are fond of saying.)

It was a very blessed evening, and one none of us will ever forget. How many people have a movie star tell *them* that they saw them on TV? Not many! What a lovely surprise for all of us. We were blessed by the events of the evening, and we hope Kirk was too!

Newt Gingrich and his wife, Callista, on 11-11-11 in Manchester, New Hampshire, came into a diner where David and I were having lunch. We had just flown in for a weekend training session that David had signed up for with Blanchard Contact Lens Laboratory, and we had been told this particular diner had great food. The young man who rented us a car at the airport had highly recommended it. Oddly, he almost seemed persistent that we go there. It was already about 1:30 p.m., and we were hungry. You know how it is on a plane trip, nothing to eat but a snack. The fellow gave us the directions, and since we were really close, we decided to give it a try. When we pulled up to the front, we almost didn't go in. It stood by a well-known hotel chain, but honestly, it looked like a bit of a dive, at least on the exterior. We went in anyway.

We had envisioned a lovely little ancient inn, tucked away on several rambling acres of New England soil. But, we were more than ready to eat lunch. We still had dinner time to find the perfect New England dining spot. Inside it looked great, and it sure was a hopping place. There were people eating at every booth and table. We hadn't been there twenty minutes when Newt and Callista walked in to have *their* lunch. We were seated at the counter near the front door (all the while watching actual chefs prepare several cuts *above* a Blue Plate Special!), and we stood up so we could shake their hands, just like everyone else was doing around us. When they got to us, Newt shook my hand and then looked me in the eye, still holding onto my hand, and he said, "Wait a minute! I've met you before. I know you. How do I know you?"

"Well," I said, surprised that he could remember my face, or anyone else's in the crowd that day, "We met you at the RNC in 2000. Our daughter, Windy Smith, was a keynote speaker. We're from Knoxville, Tennessee. We met you in Philadelphia."

"That's it! I *knew* I knew you all!" he happily replied.

We were quite impressed he would remember us. It *had* been several years, and he was now in the middle of a harried campaign, running for the 2012 Republican ticket as the Presidential nominee.

"Please take this card and give me a call about a project I am involved in concerning people with disabilities. I have wanted to get in touch with Windy and her parents for some time now. I hope Windy is doing well. I will *never* forget hearing her speak that night! She was great!" With that he handed David a business card with a number to call.

Wow! Even when Windy *wasn't* with us, David and I were remembered by well-known people. We had no idea they knew us because of her! Some neat lunch that day. Really, the entire trip was neat. David and I have never meet nicer people: Bob Martin and Richard Dorer at the lab, and even strangers at the restaurants, at the mall, everywhere we went. (Bob took us to a great dinner at an old historic inn, just like we had dreamed of, and during our dinner conversation we told him about running into Newt. He wanted to hear the rest of Windy's story. Afterwards, he opened up and told us a beautiful story about his son, John, nine years old at the time, who had been born with a disability. The love for his son was so evident and touching. It turned out to be a very special evening for all of us. Once again, a group of people were united over their love for people with disabilities!

We look forward to visiting New Hampshire again sometime. The people of Manchester were used to politicians coming and going in their town, but it was an unusual treat for us. By the way, the food was scrumptious! The Diner at the Holiday Inn was delicious, and dinner at Mambo's in Portsmouth was fab, and one of the most delicious and romantic dinners we have *ever* had. (We celebrated our fortieth wedding anniversary while we were there. Thanks to a gracious manager on duty, who gave us a surprise gift—he arranged for us a very special place for a couple celebrating an important event, at a grand piano, seated on tall stools, where we were served our meal. He was kind enough to quickly make room for two more people on his long list of diners for the evening. Sadly, he told us he didn't often hear of people making it to the fortieth year of marriage.

From our vantage point, at the more private spot next to the wall, in the large barn-like room, David and I could see out of the high windows of the beautiful old building, trussed with huge ancient wooden beams, out to a full moon reflected in the sea beyond the shore. The moon and stars were sparkling brightly, but not as brightly as the steel-blue eyes belonging to the man who sat so near me, lovingly gazing back into mine. Flying off with your lover can be quite spectacular . . . and greatly blessed by God. This *has* to be a miracle, too! Yep, has to be!

We (Windy, her dad and I, and two of her nephews, Caleb and Jake) were eating lunch at the Museum of Appalachia, not too long ago. (They have great home-cooked meals, and we are friends with Ed and Elaine Myers who run it. Elaine is the daughter of John Rice and Elizabeth Irwin, who founded the museum.) Windy enjoys visiting with all the people who work there, from the kitchen to the front desk. We feel close to our roots there for several reasons. My mom was born in 1918, in her grandparents' home nearby, at the site of the town of Norris's entrance. She later taught school at Glen Alpine. David's great-grandparents had once lived on a farm near the Norris Commons area. (If you've never been to the Museum of Appalachia you're in for a treat when you get the chance to visit. It's several acres of log buildings and artifacts depicting an earlier way of life for the people of Tennessee, and a fun stop. Windy highly recommends it!)

On that day Mr. and Mrs. Bates, of the televised reality series on The Learning Channel, *The United Bates of America*, and *Bringing Up Bates,* came in to eat, and with them was one of their 19 birth children, a lovely teenage girl. Windy, never shy, began to talk to their daughter and complimented her on the cute dress she had on. They chatted in a friendly manner for a few minutes. David and I were really impressed with the young girl's manners and the way she conversed with Windy. Windy, of course, was handling the situation delightfully. After we left to go home, I asked Windy if she knew who the Bates family was. She said, "No," and I told her they had a TV show all about their family. She said, "Really? I didn't know. I've never seen it. Their daughter is really sweet though. I do know *that*!" She was more impressed with the kindness of the girl than she was about the fact that they were on television all the time. Now that's impressive to me. Thanks, Windy, for another **WINDY LIFE LESSON**.

At Special Olympics my mom, Flo, used to shout out in her exuberant encouragement to Windy (and say with gusto like only Flo could), "Way to go, Windy!" She was always so thrilled to watch her granddaughter run past that finish line in hot competition. She was so proud that Windy loved sports like she had. Mom played basketball on an all girls' team in high school and in college at Carson Newman. If her heart ever ached for Windy, because of the sports venue she was involved in, or for me as a mom of a child with a disability, she never let on. Mom was always positive and buoyant, with poised lady-like posture, bouffant hairdo, and her rather loud, fun-filled voice. She never failed to stand straight with her shoulders erect, dressed in classic matching outfits, bedecked with matching jewelry, and to belt out her favorite phrase to Windy at the games. Well, Mama, your words have been our mantra for our daughter's life. We have spent these many years encouraging Windy by saying to her, "Way to go!" All the while God was showing all of us the 'way' to go through life by following Him. *Thank you Lord for showing us all the Way To Go and for giving us encouraging words to help us cross the finish lines in our lives triumphantly.*

"Way to go, Windy! Way to go!"

E-mail from Michael Tennery entitled **Look What Windy Started**:

In the e-mail was a link for an article from an E-newsletter of The Arc of the United States telling of the October, 2010, signing of Rosa's Law by President Barack Obama containing the following:

"The law substitutes the term "intellectual disabilities" for "mental retardation" in many federal laws. Self-advocates William Washington (The Arc's national office receptionist), Jill Egle (Co-Executive Director of the Arc of Northern Virginia) and Jeremy Jacobson (son of The Arc's Chief Development and Marketing Officer, Trudy Jacobson) joined Paul Marchand, Director of the Disability Policy Collaboration, to represent the intellectual and developmental disability community whose advocacy resulted in this bill."

An e-mail was forwarded to Windy from her friend, Laverdia Taylor Roach, Special Assistant to the Executive Director of the PCPID:

Acting Executive Director of the President's Committee for People with Intellectual Disabilities,
October 8, 2010
"Members and staff of the President's Committee for People with Intellectual Disabilities (PCPID) have long recognized the adverse impact of the term "mental retardation" on individuals diagnosed with the disability and on their family members, advocates, service providers, and a broad spectrum of Americans who understand that considerable damage frequently results from negative labeling."

Laverdia went on to inform her of the signing of the Law, S. 2781, which is now known as Rosa's Law, on October 5, 2010.

Wow! Just look at what you started girl! It's happened just like they told you it might happen several months ago! The much hated "R" word was to be replaced in America's legal, medical, and educational arenas. Hopefully, the new terminology would even filter down into everyday speech. But, it wasn't just your courageous efforts. It has taken many people and many years, bipartisan efforts, heroic efforts, and now . . . it has been done! Thanks to you, Windy, and thanks to *everyone* who has hung in there and helped to make this name change a reality. Most of all . . . Thanks be to God!

CONCLUSION

A fitting end to our story.

One sunny day in Denver, during the first week of September, 2013, Mikey was sitting in a room filled with attorneys, there to obtain their continuing education hours for the year. He had come to the lectures with two senior attorneys.

They were listening to a fellow attorney lecturing on new laws for the state when all of a sudden Mikey heard him say that the state of Colorado was probably the last state in the Union to embrace and change the term "Mental Retardation" to the term "Intellectual Disabilities" in any, and all, legal documents and laws pertaining to this people group. All the other forty-nine states had already made these changes. He was informing all present to be aware of the change and to make the appropriate changes in their individual practices.

Here was the fruition of his sister's bravery and tenacity during the time she served as a member of a Presidential Appointed Committee on a Federal level in Washington, D.C. (Mikey remembered us telling him what they had told Windy 12 years earlier: "Windy, this change in the wording is a huge deal. Not only will the President's Committee on Mental Retardation be changed to The President's Committee for People with Intellectual Disabilities, but the new words and terminology will someday be changed in the laws of the land, in every state, in the educational system, and even in the medical terminology and the medical dictionaries.") Believe me, miracles DO still happen today!

As soon as Mikey heard this awesome statement, he leaned over to them and whispered that Windy was partly responsible for making that change happen! They looked back at him, grinned, and said they couldn't wait to hear the *whole* story. He had quite a tale to tell!

At lunch Mikey related the entire story to both attorneys. They were amazed. We know the feeling—we all are still amazed at our Windy and the life she has lead up to this point. But, why not? She follows after an AMAZING God!

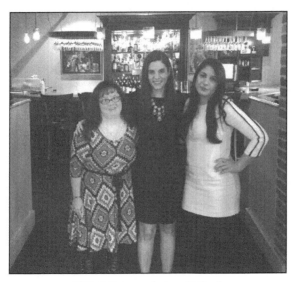

With Kristen and Amy Palumbo

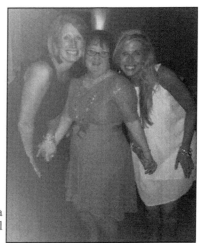

With the Moore girls, Beka Axon and Margaret Gill

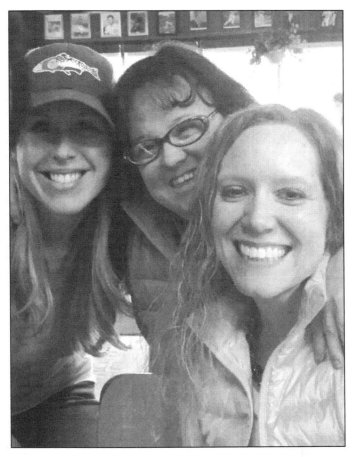

With sisters-in-law, Kari and Treva

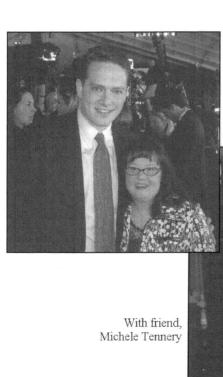

With Blake Gottesman

With friend, Michele Tennery

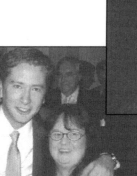

With Jared Weinstein

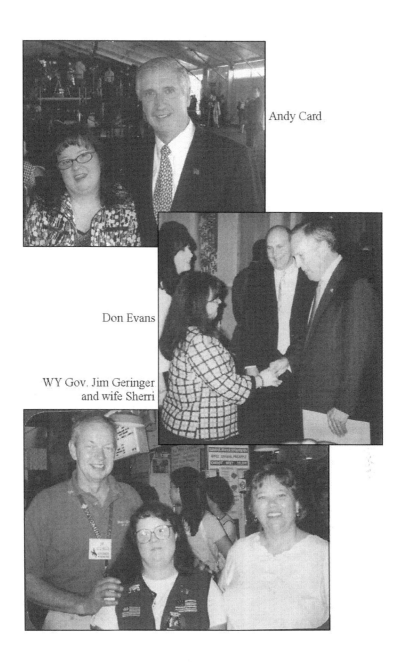

Andy Card

Don Evans

WY Gov. Jim Geringer and wife Sherri

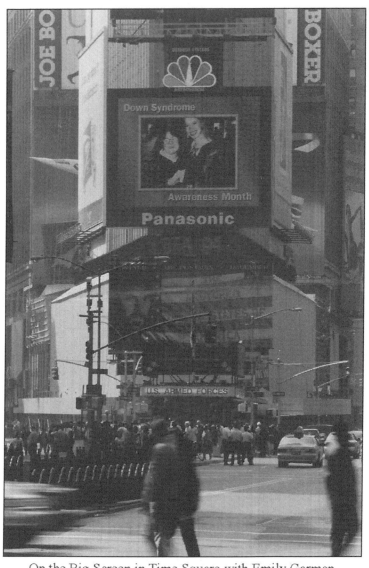

On the Big Screen in Time Square with Emily Garman
for Down Syndrome Buddy Walk

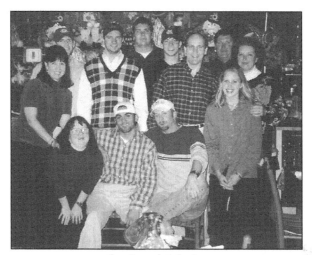

Family and Friends

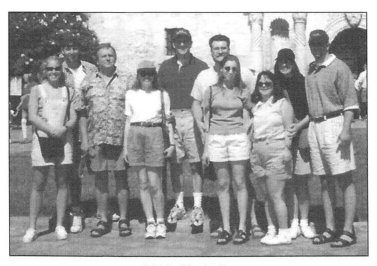

TX Smith Family

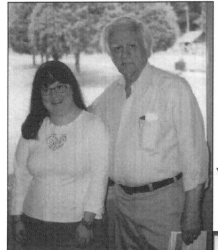
With John Rice Irwin

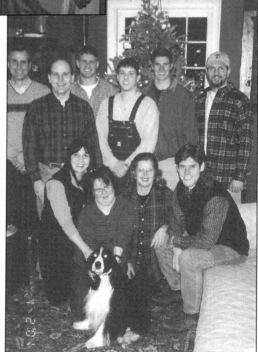
With Tarr Family

Afterword

When Windy was born, David and I faced our future head on—we had to face our inability to change our daughter's disability. We were a young couple feeling broken . . . and lost in despair. And yet, when we talked it all out, we realized that God was still there, even in our hurting . . . *especially* in our hurting. He was gently, but persistently, drawing our hearts *to* Him. He had a better plan for her life and for ours. We couldn't see it then, not even a small glimpse. We couldn't possibly have understood it all even if He had let us look into her future. We had to live each day, trusting in Jesus and allowing Him to grow and stretch us in His perfect timing.

Do we understand it all now? No way! We do understand that it is necessary for us to persistently keep reading His word, continue to pray to our heavenly Father on a daily basis. We continue to believe in miracles. Really, everyday is a miracle in itself!

I started writing this book about our life with Windy when she was only three days-old. I knew God wanted us to share her story to encourage other people. I just knew there was not much to tell that was of great interest to anyone at the time. About ten years after I had written my first words about her life, I wrote an article and sent it in to *Readers Digest*. It was soundly rejected. Unbeknownst to me, my dad gave a copy of my article to Alex Haley to read and to get his opinion. He was hoping he would like the article, or at least give me some advice. (Mr. Haley had bought a remodeled farmhouse as a get-away from the bright lights of fame, at the suggestion of his good friend, John Rice Irvin. The farm house and farm turned out to be the old home place of Windy's great, great-grandparents, Charlie and Ann Dail Weaver.)

Mr. Haley had kind words for me in a letter he wrote back to me. He said that it was a good story about Windy's life, but that it was no different from so many other stories of Down syndrome people. In other words, it was not very interesting, at least not interesting enough for the general audience of *The Digest*. It was really encouraging for me to hear that other kids, who had been born with DS, were out there doing great stuff. But I have to tell you, it was a let-down to hear that he thought the story wasn't appealing to the general audience.

Had I misinterpreted what I had believed to be God's calling on my own life? Was I not really supposed to share the story of Windy's life? Why did I still wake in the night with the urgency to put down on paper what I felt the Lord was leading me to do?

Now, I know. I had tried to write down something in my timing. It wasn't God's timing. God was communicating with me. He wanted me to write . . . just not 'right then'. Now, after all these years, there's so much to write about that I knew I was being disobedient if I didn't try to tell her story again. I had allowed rejection to feed my feelings of inadequacy. (How many of you can identify with that feeling?) The whole story had to be told to help and encourage others, and for the Glory of God to be shared. The only thing is, I have to confess, when I began to write her story again, I *really* resented it having such a political theme. It had not been my desire to be about politics.

David assured me, "It's not about politics. It's about a woman who has known many people, from both parties, who are in political office. It's about a woman who has been able to do amazing things in life by the empowerment of God Almighty." Politics wouldn't have been my personal choice for a strong storyline in her life's story, but I have had to accept and realize that it had been *exactly* how her life's story was supposed to unfold.

She enjoys her life to the fullest, looks beyond any disability, and loves with all her heart. This book is about her outlook on life, and the choices she has made to help other people. She has been blessed and has blessed others in many ways. Who could ask for more? Who could question the content? Her storyline? Not us. Not now.

Speaking of abilities, our daughter has the ability, as we had once heard a minister state, "to see the glory of her King in all people."

Lord, help us to see people as she does . . . the way You do! And to believe the way she does: that all things are possible. Oh, yeah Lord, and to expect miracles every day!

Windy has been the first to do many things in life. (Hey, someone has to be the first, right?) She is a courageous lady, and she has proved this time, and time again. There have been moments in her life when she volunteered to be first, others when she didn't hesitate to accept the challenge when she was asked to be "a first". Her quick response of, "Sure! Why not?" sums up and defines her true character and faith, as she unhesitatingly responds to callings that stretch her beyond herself, despite what someone else may think she is capable of achieving. Not much creates consternation for her. Windy has never allowed her disability to define her. That's her appeal, and her personal strength.

I found a church bulletin in my Bible the other day and read what she had written on it. I remembered the Sunday morning, a few years back, when I was seated between Windy and David. While the pastor was speaking, she had written the words, "I am free . . . I love Jesus Christ [with] all my heart," in her unmistakable child-like penmanship in pink ink. The script may be elementary, but make no mistake . . . the comprehension is exceptional. I kept the note. We all need that reminder in our own lives. I know I do.

Windy has done astonishing things in her life so far. But she never brags about her experiences. We have tried to talk to her about some of the memories we cherish, and usually she will listen for only a moment, and then she always says to us, "Let's don't talk about this anymore. Been there—done that!" It's her way of saying to us she did what she had showed up to do—jobs she felt God had given her to do. Now that was all in the past, and she is looking ahead to the future!

She's not the only person born with an intellectual disability to have done great and mighty things. She is one of *many*. (There are so many wonderful encouraging stories now. It's really awesome we can say that today!) She's just the only one we have had the pleasure and blessings of loving and living with for the past forty plus years.

Throughout the years, God has revealed *all the abilities* Windy has. Someone's abilities trump their disabilities! Surprisingly in the process of educating her, we have learned so much more than we have ever attempted to teach her. Because of our remarkable daughter, we now see the abilities in everyone's life. We have also learned how precious each life is. We are grateful for her, and what she has taught us about unconditional love—on a level we didn't know was possible. Our lives have been enriched beyond measure for having known her.

~ ~ ~

Thank you, Windy! Way to Go! We love you.

Love is patient, love is kind. It does not envy, it does not boast, it is not proud. It does not dishonor others, it is not self-seeking, it is not easily angered, it keeps no record of wrongs. Love does not delight in evil but rejoices with the truth. It always protects, always trusts, always hopes, always perseveres.

1 Corinthians 13: 4-7 (NIV)

APPENDIX

Times of Sadness

Our family has had its share, and then some, of adversity and heartaches. Windy has been through many difficult things in life that have brought her stress and caused her to pray for days. And I'm not kidding, for *days*. There have been other sad, hard times in Windy's life, times when it was hard for her to understand God's ways.

The day her Uncle Chip died in a car wreck when he was only thirty-five years-old was a dark, dark day. His little girls, Joey, age eight at the time, and Joni, age seven at the time, were with him. Their lives were spared thankfully. We all pulled close and walked through the shadow of death together. Her Poppie and Gaymom were devastated, but *knew* they would see their son again, someday. (Windy cried so hard and for so long, I really feared for her health. I had to take her home for a while before his funeral, so she could pull herself together.)

Another sad time in her life was when her Uncle Jack died of aplastic anemia. I thought her little heart would break then. We all loved Jack. We grieved with my sister, Dianne, and her three children, Jackie, Kristi, and Danny. (They had married when I was only nine years old, and Chip was only five—so he really was our big brother.)

Then her gentle, sweet, Uncle Richard, David's middle brother, died of cancer several years later. We all mourned along with his wife, Betty, and their children, Keisha and Roy.

Her heart was broken even more when her sweet great-grandmothers died. Then another big heartache was when she lost her grandfather, Bill, to cancer. (Her "eating buddy", as they had lovingly called each other, because they loved to go out and eat together.) She was unable to attend the invitation she got for the Inauguration for George W. Bush because of her Papaw's funeral. She never mentioned the invite to anyone in the family, except to show David and me the invitation. She didn't want anyone's thoughts to be on her, and not on her grandfather.

A Call from President Bush

Just five years ago Windy lost her Gaymom Flo and Poppie Charles, within just sixty-eight days of each other. Former President Bush called her on her phone to give her his condolences when he was told of her losses by a mutual friend. It reiterates his true compassion. She was very touched by his kindness. So were we. She has grieved deeply, and yet, still hangs on to a real hope in Jesus Christ, her Lord and Savior. She knows she will be with them all again someday. During these times she helped us all with our own faith and grief. That sweet hand slipped into ours, at just the right time, always bolstering our hope in life.

Family Update

Windy loves her brothers with all her heart. She gives them advice, and looks to them to give her advice. When they are happy, she is happy. When they are going through a rough time, she goes through it with them.

This book about Windy's life couldn't be written without her brothers being mentioned. Our sons' lives have been just as full of love and happiness and miracles as hers. Their lives have been so intricately entwined with her life. This is mainly her story, but they have their own life stories. We understand how someone would want to know how Windy's siblings grew up and "turned out." There are no family secrets. Our boys would tell you all of the following facts if you were standing here in person with them. (Maybe not all the *good* things they had done, they would consider it bragging.) They might ask you to pray for them. They might ask you what they could pray for in your life. I know our boys!

Windy's older brother Dave Smith, is a fine man, and she loves him with all her heart. They are *very* close, and born only sixteen-months apart.

Dave is tenderhearted and compassionate. He is a sincere prayer warrior for friends and family members. (There are people we know he has prayed for, for years, literally for years. He has been a witness to all of us because of his perseverance and faith in this area.) He is one *great* 'big' brother. He has always taken Windy to untold movies, ballgames, and chaperoned her at many church functions, dances and parties she has attended. He has been her special guest and escort to White House Christmas parties and functions. She always loves to "show him off" to people. He keeps in close touch with her. He'll often just call her up to hear her voice, and to check on her, to see how she is. She'll tell him without reservation. He knows he can be honest with his answer to her about how he is doing. He listens to her timely advice, and he knows she listens to him.

He played soccer in high school and was in the chorus where he sang solos in several productions. (Windy prays daily that he will continue to use his gift of singing for the Glory of God.) Many times he went to the downtown rescue mission to sing and minister to the people, who had no home and felt like they had no hope. He has spoken to countless people about the saving love of Jesus. He has helped to change other's predicament and lives in wonderful ways. He has made many friends through the years, and he remains life-long friends to many.

He graduated from a private Christian high school, Christian Academy of Knoxville, and from East Tennessee State University with a degree in Environmental Health and Safety. He works in the Safety and Health arena, and travels for different companies doing Occupational Health and Safety and Environmental Testing for various issues. He helps make workplaces safer places for people to work in, and he enjoys his field of work.

Dave's faith in God is deep, and real . . . but it took a tree. He was nearly killed in a tree cutting accident over six years ago. The tree, that someone else was cutting twisted as it was being felled, "seemed to turn in my direction, and hit only me, out of a crowd of people standing some distance away—as if it was meant to be." He now has some swelling and pain in his foot and back frequently from arthritis pain. He will always have that, but he is alive. (Those consequences are small compared to losing him forever!)

Our Dave healed from the inside out, completely and miraculously. He later prayed for a soul mate, a Christian woman, who he could spend his life with. We come from a *long* line of people who marry for life, on "both sides of the House", and it's what he has wanted for his own life.

One especially wonderful friend he brought home to meet us was named Treva. Treva is a southern girl. She is a fabulous, smart woman who loves the Lord and loves working with the students in a University setting. She is a daughter to us now, and a sweet sister to Windy. (Treva is an only child, so in a way, Windy *is* her sister!) We love her mom and dad, Ed and Betty, and her extended family. We always look forward to our visits with them and to eating Betty's wonderful meals and visiting with their many, lovely family members! She walked into his life, and into ours. We love her and know God sent her to him, and to us. She and her parents and their family have been a wonderful blessing to all of us. Just when you think there is not much hope left, God proves Himself, again and again, that He is powerful and mighty, as He restores our lives. We still pray for restoration in all things.

Dave had been married twice before he met, and married, Treva. He has a daughter from one of those marriages. He prays to be reunited with her someday.

He tells us he is the man he is today because of his little sis. She has inspired him to reach high and work hard to achieve goals. Her deep, abiding faith and unconditional love have sustained him. His love, prayers and protection for her have helped make her the woman she is today. There is no doubt in our minds. We are so proud of our oldest son.

Now for an update on Windy's younger brother, Mikey Smith. He is the typical younger brother (five years younger): he teases and jokes with her. Always has. They are *very* close. Somewhere on the timeline, he, being younger in age than his sister, became like an older brother.

He has had his own share of "fights" for his sister's honor in his growing up years. He has been her protector and friend, driving her to school and church functions, happily and openly sharing his friends and school days experiences. He and his wife, Kari have escorted her on several occasions to the White House. She always loves "showing him off" to everyone, too. In school he was a varsity athlete, who played basketball, football and track, and yet, had time to be in many extracurricular activities, especially church youth group, chorus, and acting in plays.

He has a gift of creativity and is a talented artist. He got a part in a movie, *October Sky,* filmed in TN, but turned it down because it required so much of his time. He would have had to quit college for a semester, so he chose school instead. (He really has enjoyed going to school!) He loves to paint pictures in oil, but he just doesn't have too much free time to do it these days. Kari says he will stay up once or twice a year to paint . . . and loses all track of time. In other words, he stays up all night and then has to go to work so . . . he has to contain his spontaneity! He also has an entrepreneurial spirit and enjoys law, business, sports and missions.

He graduated from Farragut High School and has a B.S. degree from Carson Newman University, and holds a Master's degree from University of Tennessee, and was in the *very* first graduating class of Liberty Law School at Liberty University in VA, where he served as the President of the class. He later interned at the White House in the Office of Presidential Personnel.

Mikey is an *amazing* Daddy to his four boys. They are crazy over their dad. His big sister, Windy, thinks he hung the moon! He and Kari took her with them to all the places and events they attended in high school. She was treated as a friend and a pal. She was a bridesmaid in their wedding. It's sweet to see her smiling so obviously happy in the photos we have of that special day. (She's convinced their marriage was the result of her successful matchmaking endeavors. She met Kari before Mikey did, in a Chorus class at Farragut, and Windy told her she needed to meet her brother. She thought they would make the perfect couple.) Wow, was she ever right!

Kari shares a history of our hometown with us. Her people have also lived in the area for several generations. We love her mom and dad, Jama and David. They are friends *and* family now. (We four attended the same high school where David and I were two years ahead of them.) We love Kari like a daughter. She is a caring R.N. She is most importantly, a godly woman and an awesome mom. They have been married for over thirteen years. Sometimes we have teased them that they "run in a pack"—there are so many of their school friends that they still see and speak with on a regular basis. They are all experiencing parenthood together. How cool is that?

For Windy's thirty-ninth birthday, Kari made her a special three-layer cake, after searching several recipes with her. Each layer was a shade of pink covered with a fluffy bubblegum pink icing. It was really beautiful and a labor of love for a sister-in-law she loves. She brought it to the big party Mikey threw her because he was uncertain if they would be able to see her on her fortieth birthday. They knew they were moving many miles away. Shared birthdays were going to be harder to celebrate in person. It was bittersweet for everyone.

Windy's younger brother is a man of integrity and has a strong faith. He had always been a warrior for God since he was a little fellow, and he has been a person his friends have wanted to emulate as he followed his Heavenly Father. He faces challenges head on, and has many friends whom he cares very much about. He believes in the power of prayer and lives his faith out every day. He and Kari have been on many mission trips to many places like: Spain, Mexico, Haiti and Alaska. (Once they were flown out of Alaska by Franklin Graham's own plane with the Christian organization, Samaritan's Purse.)

Mikey is now a Counselor at Law, who cares for his clients on a deeply felt personal level. He tells us that he would not be the man he is today if it wasn't for his sister and her great influence on his life. We know she would not be the woman she is today without his influence on her life. Parents could not wish for more than that. No one is more pleased and proud of her brothers than Windy!

One more interesting fact: both boys had some criteria for a lifetime soul-mate, decided before either of them married: it had to be understood that they came as a sort of package deal, meaning their sister. They asked the girls point-blank if they would allow Windy to come live with them if something ever happened to their mom and dad. When we heard this, we were astonished and humbled at the depth of love they both have for their sister. We even told them it wasn't totally fair to ask a spouse to take on a sister-in-law for life. Their answer: they both said it wasn't for life, it was for love. At last, our fears over how having a sister with a disability would affect our boys lives are laid to rest. It affected them all right—in such unexpected, blessed, wonderful ways! God had known that all along.

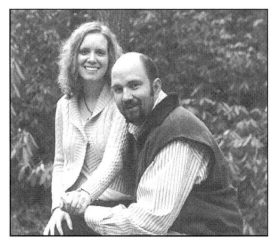

Dave and Treva

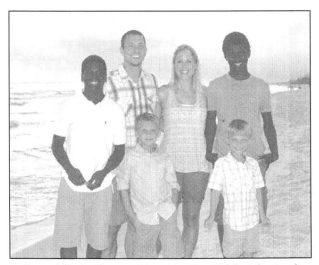

Mike and Kari with sons, l to r: Kensley, Caleb, Jake, Lookens

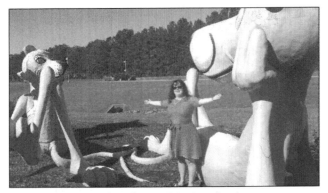

Loving all that pink! (panthers)

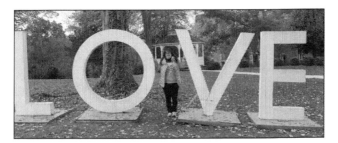

This says it all . . .

Words of Wisdom

God doesn't always do what we want Him to—but He knows what's best for us, and He can be trusted.
Billy Graham

Has it ever occurred to you that God may not want to deliver you from a situation, but to deliver you *through* it?
Chip Ingram

We are never closer to God than when trials come upon us.
Charles R. Swindoll

When we rest in the very situation where God has lovingly placed us, we find the fabulous freedom of following.
Jennifer Rothschild

Continuous effort—not strength or intelligence—is the key to unlocking our potential.
Winston Churchill

The best and most beautiful things in the world cannot be seen or even touched. They must be felt with the heart.
Helen Keller

Silently and imperceptibly, as we work or sleep, we grow strong or weak; and at last some crisis shows us what we have become.
B.F. Westcott

Life its self is the very best fairytale.
Hans Christian Andersen

God made you as you are in order to use you as He planned.
S.C. McAulay

With God, go over the sea; without Him, not over the threshold.
Russian Proverb

Our main business is not to see what lies dimly at a distance, but to do what lies clearly at hand.
Thomas Carlyle

This country will not be a good place for any of us to live in unless we make it a good place for all of us to live in.
Theodore Roosevelt

When one door closes another opens, but we often look so long and so regretfully upon the closed door that we do not see the one that has opened for us.
Alexander Graham Bell

More Information on Down Syndrome

www.ndss.org---National Down Syndrome Society

www.ndsccenter.org---National Down Syndrome Congress

www.globaldownsyndrome.org---Global Down Syndrome Foundation

www.ndsan.org---National Down Syndrome Adoption Network

www.TheArc.org---For people with intellectual and developmental disabilities

www.lejeuneusa.org---Jérôme Lejeune Foundation USA

For more information, please check out your local Down syndrome chapter or support group.

End Notes

[1] Stats from National Down Syndrome Society: The name of the syndrome came from the 19th century English physician, John Langdon Down, who published the first research on people with DS in 1866. He outlined a description of the characteristics shared by people with DS. In 1959, Jerome Lejeune, a French physician, identified the condition as a chromosomal anomaly. Instead of the usual 46 chromosomes present in each cell, he observed 47 in these individuals. Researchers later determined that it was an extra, partial, or complete 21st chromosome.

[2] Infant stimulation, just what was it? Years later The Down Syndrome Society would describe early intervention on their 07/07/11 dated website titled: Birth to 3: Early intervention is a systematic program of therapy, exercises and activities designed to address developmental delays that may be experienced by a child with Down syndrome or other disabilities. These services are mandated by a federal law called the Individuals with Disabilities Education Act (IDEA). The law requires that states provide early intervention services for all children who qualify, with the goal of enhancing the development of infants and toddlers and helping families understand and meet the needs of their children. The most common early intervention services for babies with DS are physical therapy, speech and language therapy, and occupational therapy.

[3] Editor: Tina Tossey. Printed by Caring, publisher of *Sharing Our Caring*, is a not-for-profit organization founded in 1972 by parents and professionals interested in the health and welfare of persons with Down's syndrome.

[4] "His Eye Is on The Sparrow", a Gospel hymn published in 1905, by Charles H. Gabriel and Civiilla D. Martin.

[5] Wikipedia explanation: "In the 1980's, the mainstreaming model began to be used more often as a result of the requirement to place children in the least restrictive environment (Clearinghouse, E.

2003). Students with minor disabilities remained in segregated, special classrooms, with the opportunity to be among normal students for up to a few hours each day. Many parents and educators favored allowing students with disabilities to be in classrooms along with their non-disabled peers."

About the Author

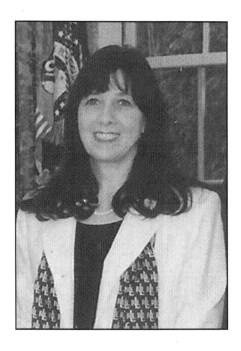

Vicki Stansberry Smith is a wife, a mom and a grandmother. She wrote *Born for This* from her home in the "Hills of East Tennessee". She and her husband, David, have three grown children. This is her first book.